AACVPR Cardiac Rehabilitation Resource Manual

Promoting Health and Preventing Disease

**American Association
of Cardiovascular
and
Pulmonary Rehabilitation**

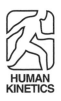

**HUMAN
KINETICS**

Library of Congress Cataloging-in-Publication Data

AACVPR cardiac rehabilitation resource manual / American Association of Cardiovascular and
   Pulmonary Rehabilitation.
      p. ; cm.
   Companion v. to: Guidelines for cardiac rehabilitation and secondary prevention programs.
c2004.
   Includes bibliographical references and index.
   ISBN 0-7360-4269-5 (soft cover : alk. paper)
   1. Heart--Diseases--Patients--Rehabilitation.   2. Heart--Diseases--Prevention.   I. American
Association of Cardiovascular & Pulmonary Rehabilitation.   II. Guidelines for cardiac reha-
bilitation and secondary prevention programs.   III. Title: Cardiac rehabilitation resource manual.
   [DNLM: 1. Heart Diseases--rehabilitation--Guideline.   2. Heart Diseases--prevention &
control--Guideline.   WG 210 A111 2006]
   RC682.A21 2006
   616.1'203--dc22   2005023142

ISBN: 0-7360-4269-5

Acquisitions Editor: Loarn D. Robertson, PhD; **Developmental Editor:** Judy Park; **Assistant Editor:** Lee Alexander; **Copyeditor:**
Julie Anderson; **Proofreader:** Kathy Bennett; **Indexer:** Nancy Ball; **Permission Manager:** Dalene Reeder; **Graphic Designer:** Nancy
Rasmus; **Graphic Artist:** Yvonne Griffith; **Photo Manager:** Sarah Ritz; **Cover Designer:** Keith Blomberg; **Photos:** © Washington
Hospital Center, except where otherwise noted; **Art Manager:** Kelly Hendren; **Illustrator:** Argosy; **Printer:** Versa Press

Printed in the United States of America   10 9 8 7 6 5 4 3 2 1

Human Kinetics
Web site: www.HumanKinetics.com

United States: Human Kinetics
P.O. Box 5076
Champaign, IL 61825-5076
800-747-4457
e-mail: humank@hkusa.com

Canada: Human Kinetics
475 Devonshire Road Unit 100
Windsor, ON N8Y 2L5
800-465-7301 (in Canada only)
e-mail: orders@hkcanada.com

Europe: Human Kinetics
107 Bradford Road
Stanningley
Leeds LS28 6AT, United Kingdom
+44 (0) 113 255 5665
e-mail: hk@hkeurope.com

Australia: Human Kinetics
57A Price Avenue
Lower Mitcham, South Australia 5062
08 8277 1555
e-mail: liaw@hkaustralia.com

New Zealand: Human Kinetics
Division of Sports Distributors NZ Ltd.
P.O. Box 300 226 Albany
North Shore City
Auckland
0064 9 448 1207
e-mail: info@humankinetics.co.nz

Contents

PART II   Role of Exercise in Heart Disease

PART III   Special Considerations

Foreword

As editor of the third and fourth editions of *AACVPR's Guidelines for Cardiac Rehabilitation and Secondary Prevention* and the upcoming fifth edition, I was extremely pleased to learn of the development of the *AACVPR Cardiac Rehabilitation Resource Manual,* which will serve as a companion text to the guidelines. Looking back, even to the beginning of the development process of the guidelines, the questions of what to cover and in how much detail have been troublesome issues. The purpose of the guidelines has been to give readers a basic structure of cardiac rehabilitation programs and recommendations for appropriate evaluations, interventions, and expected outcomes. Whether it was reasonable to provide an extensive review of the scientific literature has been debated at the onset of every new edition. The compromise was to provide some of the essential information as a basis for the more practical material, recognizing that the *Guidelines* itself could not be all encompassing. The development of the *AACVPR Cardiac Rehabilitation Resource Manual* solves, to a great degree, this ongoing dilemma by providing a wide-ranging review of topics critical to the understanding of the basis for cardiac rehabilitation and secondary prevention.

Although the *AACVPR Cardiac Rehabilitation Resource Manual* might be viewed as a logical extension of the guidelines, in reality the resource manual is the basis for the guidelines. I welcome this relationship as I see cardiac rehabilitation profession-als and students preparing for this field benefiting significantly from the opportunity to review the science behind the practice of cardiac rehabilitation and secondary prevention. The editorial board of the resource manual, including Kathy Berra, Dr. Terry Kavanagh, and Dr. Larry Hamm as editor in chief, has secured contributions from some of the world's foremost experts. These noted researchers and practitioners not only provide a relevant overview of the science but provide cutting-edge contributions in the field. The makeup of the editorial board represents the perspectives of physicians, cardiac rehabilitation nurses, and clinical exercise physiologists as members of the multidisciplinary cardiac rehabilitation team.

The editorial board is to be congratulated on this highly anticipated endeavor and for the extent to which the *AACVPR Cardiac Rehabilitation Resource Manual* will serve the cardiac rehabilitation practitioner. All professionals working in the area of cardiac rehabilitation and the secondary prevention of heart disease should find this book a valuable tool in understanding the scientific basis for program development as well as the modification of existing programs.

Mark A. Williams, PhD, FAACVPR
Editor in chief
AACVPR Guidelines for Cardiac Rehabilitation and Secondary Prevention, Fifth Edition

Contributors

Larry F. Hamm, PhD, FAACVPR,
Editor-in-Chief
  Department of Rehabilitation Medicine
  Georgetown University Medical Center
  Washington, District of Columbia

Kathy Berra, MSN, ANP, FAACVPR, Editor
  Stanford Prevention Research Center
  Stanford University
  Stanford, California

Terence Kavanagh, MD, FRCPC, DSc (Hon),
FAACVPR, Editor
  Faculty of Medicine
  Graduate Program in Exercise Science
  University of Toronto
  Toronto, Ontario, Canada

John C. Ashworth, MA
  FitnessNomad.com
  ExerciseCareers.com
  Madison, Wisconsin

Lauralyn B. Cannistra, MD
  Program for Cardiac Rehabilitation and Prevention
  The Memorial Hospital
  Blackstone Cardiology Associates
  Pawtucket, Rhode Island

Adam T. de Jong, MA
  Preventive Cardiology and Rehabilitation
  William Beaumont Hospital
  Royal Oak, Michigan

Barry A. Franklin, PhD, FAACVPR
  Preventive Cardiology and Rehabilitation
  William Beaumont Hospital
  Royal Oak, Michigan
  School of Medicine
  Wayne State University
  Detroit, Michigan

Neil F. Gordon, MD, PhD, MPH, FAACVPR
  Center for Heart Disease Prevention
  St. Joseph's/Candler Health System
  Savannah, Georgia

Matthew L. Herridge, PhD, FAACVPR
  Cardiac Rehabilitation Department
  Charleston Area Medical Center-Memorial Division
  Charleston, West Virginia

Suzanne Hughes, MSN, RN
  Center for Family Medicine
  Akron General Medical Center
  Akron, Ohio

Troy A. Klinger, MS
  Department of Cardiology
  Geisinger Medical Center
  Danville, Pennsylvania

Thomas P. LaFontaine, PhD
  PREVENT Consulting Services, LLC
  Columbia Missouri

Glenn N. Levine, MD
  Baylor School of Medicine
  Cardiology section
  Houston, Texas

John C. Linton, PhD
  Department of Behavioral Medicine
  West Virginia School of Medicine
  Charleston, West Virginia

Maureen E. Mays, MD
  Preventive Cardiology and Cardiac Rehabilitation
  Dean Medical Center/St. Mary's Hospital
  Department of Family Medicine
  University of Wisconsin Medical School
  Madison, Wisconsin

Patrick E. McBride, MD, MPH, FAACVPR
  Departments of Medicine and Family Medicine
  Preventive Cardiology Program
  University of Wisconsin Medical School
  Madison, Wisconsin

Timothy R. McConnell, PhD
  Graduate Studies in Exercise Science
  Exercise Science and Athletics
  Bloomsburg University
  Bloomsburg, Pennsylvania

Henry S. Miller, MD, FAACVPR
  Department of Internal Medicine/Cardiology
  Wake Forest University School of Medicine
  Winston-Salem, North Carolina

Jonathon N. Myers, PhD, FAACVPR
  VA Palo Alto Health Care System
  Stanford University
  Palo Alto, California

Jeffrey L. Roitman, EdD
  Cardiac Rehabilitation
  Research Medical Center
  Kansas City, Missouri

Ray W. Squires, PhD, FAACVPR
  Cardiovascular Rehabilitation Program/
  Cardiovascular Health Clinic
  Mayo Clinic
  Department of Medicine
  Rochester, Minnesota

Nanette K. Wenger, MD, FAACVPR
  Department of Medicine, Division of Cardiology
  Emory University School of Medicine
  Grady Memorial Hospital
  Atlanta, Georgia

Shu-Fen Wung, PhD, RN
  College of Nursing
  University of Arizona
  Tuscon, Arizona

Preface

This is the first edition of the *AACVPR Cardiac Rehabilitation Resource Manual,* which has been developed to be a companion text to the fourth edition of the *AACVPR Guidelines for Cardiac Rehabilitation and Secondary Prevention Programs* and a reference text for cardiac rehabilitation professionals as well as students in the field of cardiac rehabilitation.

It is a challenging task for any one book to cover the rapidly changing and expanding discipline of cardiac rehabilitation and our understanding of coronary heart disease. However, the publication of this book, in conjunction with the fourth edition of the *Guidelines,* provides pertinent, in-depth information on many important topics in contemporary cardiac rehabilitation and secondary prevention of coronary heart disease.

The focus of any cardiac rehabilitation and secondary prevention program guidelines publication is on the tools and information necessary for starting a new program or updating an existing program. It applies current position statements, recommendations, and scientific knowledge from the medical and scientific literature to the design and development of a safe, effective, and comprehensive cardiac rehabilitation program.

This *Resource Manual* complements the information in the *Guidelines* by expanding the discussion of selected topics related to cardiac rehabilitation, heart disease, risk factors, and secondary prevention. In addition, some of the chapters in this book provide information on topics not included in the *Guidelines,* such as the atherosclerotic disease process, cardiovascular and exercise physiology, exercise prescription, and the electrocardiogram. Other content in the *Resource Manual* is intended to complement, expand, or provide more background research data for some topics—risk factors for coronary heart disease, secondary prevention, psychosocial issues, and patients with special considerations.

The book begins with an overview of the many manifestations of heart disease by one of the early leaders in the field. The book is then divided into three sections. Information related to atherosclerosis, current revascularization techniques, secondary prevention, and psychosocial issues is included in the first section. Part II discusses exercise-related topics and use of the electrocardiogram in heart disease. The third section focuses on heart disease in women, elderly persons, persons with diabetes mellitus, chronic heart failure, and heart transplantation patients.

To help the reader coordinate the information in this book with that in the *Guidelines,* reference is made near the beginning of selected chapters to related information in the *Guidelines.* Also at the beginning of some chapters, current guidelines from national organizations that are pertinent to the chapter topic have been noted.

In the field, and in this book, specific terminology is used to describe the various types of cardiovascular diseases. The health care professional working in cardiac rehabilitation programs must understand these different terms and how they are used. Clinicians also need to be specific when relating statistics for diseases to patients or family members (e.g., prevalence, incidence, economic costs, and relative risk) because these statistics are different for cardiovascular disease and coronary heart disease. As illustrated in the figure, cardiovascular disease is the broadest category, including all diseases related to the circulatory system. Heart disease is the next broadest, dealing with all types of cardiac diseases but nothing outside of the heart. Coronary heart disease is the least broad, dealing only with that segment of heart disease that is atherosclerotic disease of the coronary arteries.

A chapter on exercise testing procedures was not included in this book. This decision was made because of the wide variation in clinical practice as to whether or not exercise testing is performed within cardiac rehabilitation programs, and whether or not patients entering cardiac rehabilitation programs have completed an exercise test. For information regarding exercise testing methodology, the reader is referred to resources from the American College of Sports Medicine, American Heart Association, American College of Cardiology, and various textbooks.

As is true with any book of this type, there are many people to thank. First and foremost, we extend our sincere appreciation to each of the health care professionals who wrote chapters for this book. Their combined expertise in so many areas of cardiac rehabilitation and heart disease is impressive, and their commitment to this new publication has been exemplary. In addition, the associate editors for this project, Kathy Berra and Terence Kavanagh, have been involved in the project since its inception, and their efforts were invaluable in bringing this book to publication. We also thank the professionals at Human Kinetics for their assistance on this project—especially Loarn Robertson, Judy Park, Lee Alexander, and Julie Anderson.

Cardiovascular Disease (CVD)

All of the diseases of the cardiovascular system; includes ICD/9 390 - 459, 745 -747.

- Stroke
- Hypertension
- Diseases of the arteries, arterioles, and capillaries
- Diseases of the veins, lymphatic, and other diseases of the circulatory system
- Heart disease, coronary heart disease, and heart diseases in those categories

Heart Disease (HD)

All diseases that affect the coronary circulation, electrical system or anatomical structures of the heart.

- Valvular heart diseases (ICD/9 424)
- Heart failure (ICD/9 428.0)
- Cardiomyopathies (ICD/9 425)
- Cardiac arrhythmias (ICD/9 426, 427)
- Congenital heart diseases and diseases in that category

Coronary Heart Disease (CHD)

Atherosclerotic disease affecting the arteries of the coronary circulation, synonymous terms used are coronary artery disease (CAD) or ischemic heart disease (IHD), includes ICD/9 410 - 414 and 429.2.

- Myocardial infarction
- Angina pectoris

Terminology used to describe various types of cardiovascular diseases. ICD/9 refers to the 2005 *International Classification of Diseases, Clinical Modification, 9th Revision*, Centers for Medicare and Medicaid Services.

Overview

Major Manifestations of Heart Disease

Henry S. Miller, MD

Editors' note: It is not often that we have the opportunity to read an overview of heart disease as seen through the eyes of a well-respected and experienced cardiologist. However, this chapter provides us with just such an experience. Henry S. Miller, Jr., MD, is Professor Emeritus at Wake Forest University School of Medicine, a founding Fellow of AACVPR, and a highly respected leader in the field of cardiac rehabilitation. In this overview, Dr. Miller walks us through several manifestations of heart disease and defines some related key concepts as he has observed them "at the bedside" during his illustrious career. This review provides personal insights, reflections, and perspectives that will enhance our understanding of heart disease from the clinical point of view. The chapter is not intended to be a detailed, referenced review of heart disease.

Coronary Heart Disease

Coronary heart disease (CHD) results from the development of atherosclerosis in one or more of the coronary arteries. CHD typically presents as either angina pectoris or acute myocardial infarction. Angina pectoris is caused by a temporary imbalance in the supply of oxygen to a portion of the myocardium (myocardial oxygen supply < myocardial oxygen demand) and it resolves when adequate myocardial oxygen supply is restored (myocardial oxygen supply ≥ myocardial oxygen demand). No permanent damage to myocardial cells results from an episode of angina. On the other hand, an acute myocardial infarction permanently damages the myocardial cells in the affected area. This occurs when myocardial oxygen supply to a specific area of the heart muscle is abruptly blocked or significantly reduced for several minutes or longer as a result of the atherosclerotic process.

Angina Pectoris

As so eloquently described by William Heberden in 1772,

There is a disorder of the breast marked with strong and peculiar symptoms, considerable for the kind of danger belonging to it, and not extremely rare, which deserves to be mentioned more at length. The seed of it and the sense of strangling and anxiety with which it is attended, may make it not improperly be called angina pectoris.

Those who are afflicted with it are seized while they are walking (more especially if it be up hill, and soon after eating) with a painful and most disagreeable sensation in the breast which seems as if it would extinguish life, if it were to increase or to continue; but the moment they stand still, all uneasiness vanishes.

Symptoms of angina pectoris have not been described any better in the ensuing 230 years. It is estimated that some 6,750,000 individuals have angina in the United States, with about 350,000 new cases each year. This disease occurs in 20% to 25% of men and 14% to 25% of women older than 65.

Angina pectoris is a discomfort (often described as dull pressure, uncomfortable ache, pain, tightness, or squeezing sensation) that typically occurs in the central chest near the sternum. However, in an individual patient, the symptoms may be experienced anywhere between the eyebrows and the umbilicus. Symptoms may radiate typically to the left neck, jaw, axilla, or arm. Symptoms termed *atypical angina* have different characteristics and anatomical locations. Angina pectoris occurs with exertion and is relieved partly or completely by rest. As noted by Heberden, the symptoms are much worse if exercise follows a meal and can be precipitated by anxiety and states of excitement.

Other symptoms may include progressive fatigue, shortness of breath, and diaphoresis (sweating) that are more significant than indicated by the level of exertion.

Palpitations or a rapid or slow heart rate may also accompany the angina symptoms.

Stable angina pectoris tends to be very predictable in its pattern and usually occurs at the same level of exercise under the same or similar circumstances. In a specific individual, the discomfort is usually in the same anatomical location and with the same associated signs and symptoms. It is described as new-onset angina if it has developed over the preceding 1 to 3 months. Nocturnal angina is characterized by symptoms that occur during sleep and are known to be triggered by emotional dreams or sleep apnea in some individuals. Unstable angina, which may recur at rest or while asleep, perhaps with periods of discomfort lasting 20 to 30 min, is now included in the acute coronary syndromes.

Patients may state that the angina occurs soon after they start to exercise, but if they decrease the pace, at times very slightly, the angina will gradually go away and they can continue to exercise at a normal level for long periods of time. This is known as *walk-through* angina.

Silent angina or *silent ischemia* is usually accompanied by other manifestations of coronary insufficiency such as breathlessness, rapid fatigue, and arrhythmias, in addition to ischemic electrocardiographic changes, but in the absence of any "angina-type" pain or discomfort. This is more common in diabetic persons and African Americans.

Asking questions about specific activities such as carrying laundry upstairs, carrying groceries in the house, walking up two to three flights of stairs, or pushing a lawnmower usually provides accurate information about the level of exertion that the person can tolerate with and without symptoms. Frequently, patients will discontinue activities that produce symptoms and therefore have no discomfort with their usual daily activities. Additionally, a family history of coronary disease and cardiovascular disease risk factors, as discussed in chapter 1, should be explored. All these facts are extremely important in determining the likelihood and probable severity of coronary artery disease, and they help determine the most appropriate diagnostic tests and medical and interventional therapy.

If the symptoms of crescendo, or unstable angina, are present, an exercise stress test is not needed to establish the diagnosis. Demonstrating the degree and location of the coronary obstructive disease and selecting the treatment are more appropriate. In silent ischemia and stable angina with or without classic symptoms, the exercise test, with and without myocardial perfusion assessment by echo or radioisotope, is very beneficial to determine the level at which the ischemia occurs, how it correlates with the patient's symptoms, and the occurrence of ischemic arrhythmias with physical activity.

Treatment of activity-limiting angina that is not controlled with medication should include demonstrating and treating the coronary obstruction causing the symptoms, if possible.

Medications are frequently successful in controlling anginal symptoms and allowing normal daily activities. The medications commonly used are nitrates, β-blockers, and calcium channel blockers.

Nitrates can be taken sublingually; by oral spray, transdermal patches, or paste; or orally. Angina is thought to be relieved by reduction of the preload and afterload of the left ventricle. The sublingual medication and mouth spray are more rapidly absorbed and may more quickly relieve symptoms.

β-blockers have a unique effect in that they decrease resting and exercise heart rate, decrease systolic blood pressure, and decrease myocardial contractility. The decrease in heart rate and myocardial tension increases the diastolic coronary perfusion time and improves distal coronary perfusion. This combination of decreased cardiac work and increased myocardial perfusion helps to control anginal symptoms. There are some unfavorable effects, but these are few and are outweighed by the benefits.

Calcium channel blockers are frequently beneficial for relief of angina when given in combination with β-blockers in the sustained action form. These vasodilators are helpful in controlling angina, arrhythmias, and hypertension.

Although angiotensin-converting enzyme (ACE) inhibitors have proven to be very beneficial in postinfarction patients, they are less effective in the treatment of myocardial ischemia unless there is concomitant myocardial dysfunction as a result of ischemic cardiomyopathy.

Physical activity and carefully prescribed cardiac rehabilitation exercise training can be extremely beneficial in patients with angina and will significantly improve their effective cardiac work without symptoms of angina. This improvement is related to physiological adaptations in both peripheral circulation and central cardiac function.

Myocardial Infarction

Myocardial infarction may be the first manifestation of coronary artery disease that a patient experiences, or it may be the result of the progression of unstable angina. Myocardial infarction can be associated with total and rapid occlusion of a single coronary artery or partial occlusion of one or more arteries depriving the myocardium of adequate blood flow (i.e., oxygen and nutrients) necessary to survive. The occlusion is frequently produced by a thrombus associated with a ruptured endothelial plaque in a coronary artery that may be only 40% to 60% obstructed and causing no symptoms of coronary insufficiency before the event. It is now thought that an artery with an unstable plaque is likely a frequent cause of myocardial infarctions as well as sudden death.

The primary objective of emergent therapy is to reestablish circulation in the occluded coronary artery as soon as possible. Even up to 12 hr after the initial symptoms of infarction, thrombolytics may be given under the proper circumstances. But, by far, the most successful therapy is initiated within the first 2 hr after the onset of symptoms. Whether intravenous thrombolytics or primary angioplasty is the best method of reperfusion is somewhat debatable. If there is a delay in starting an angioplasty of more than 90 min after arrival in the emergency department, thrombolytics are generally the treatment of choice. Rescue angioplasty is used in patients who fail to reperfuse the occluded arteries with thrombolytic therapy. Our policy is to initiate thrombolytics (30 min after first seen) if appropriate and if angioplasty cannot be performed within 90 min. In some jurisdictions, EMT personnel are authorized to administer thrombolytics at the scene after electrocardiograms have been transmitted and reviewed by a physician at the hospital. If reperfusion is established by normalizing the ST-segment elevation, then coronary arteriography can be used later to determine future therapy.

The medications given within a few hours after the perfusion is reestablished, or after a completed myocardial infarction, include the following. The medications are the same for Q-wave or non-Q-wave infarction:

1. Aspirin or other medications that may affect the clotting cascade such as clopidogrel, heparin, or coumadin are used. Thrombolytics are usually followed by heparin infusions to reduce the risk of reclotting at the culprit atherosclerotic lesion.

2. β-blockers are used to reduce likelihood of arrhythmias or to stabilize the myocardium.

3. ACE inhibitors reduce "remodeling" of the damaged ventricle and help to prevent the development of ischemic cardiomyopathy.

The primary complications of myocardial infarction are these:

1. Arrhythmias

2. Postinfarction angina pectoris

3. Left ventricular dysfunction—congestive failure

Arrhythmias may occur with minimal myocardial damage and with prolonged ischemic episodes that may not result in myocardial infarction. Inferior myocardial infarctions may be associated with complete atrioventricular block resulting in an idioventricular rhythm with rates of 30 to 35 beats·min^{-1} accompanied by 4- to 6-s pauses resulting in syncope. The slow rate and pauses may produce increasing myocardial ischemia resulting in ventricular tachycardia or fibrillation (brady–tachy syndrome). Treatment of the bradycardia by pacing will usually control this problem with or without arrhythmic medications. An atrioventricular (AV) block occuring with acute infarction is usually of short duration but may last up to 2 to 3 weeks and require temporary pacing.

Supraventricular arrhythmias are not uncommon and occur more commonly with atrial enlargement associated with the ventricular dysfunction attributable to infarction. Treatment is with antiarrhythmic drugs with or without direct current (DC) transthoracic electroshock to control the atrial fibrillation or flutter. These arrhythmias are easier to control as the myocardium becomes more and more stable after myocardial infarction. As noted, β-blockers are quite helpful in decreasing the occurrence of arrhythmias.

The development of postinfarction left ventricular systolic dysfunction is frequently associated with both ventricular and supraventricular arrhythmias. A combination of uncontrolled arrhythmias and left ventricular dysfunction that is severe enough to cause congestive failure is potentially lethal. Because of this, the use of implantable cardiac defibrillators (ICD) with pacing capabilities has proven to be life saving in patients with this sequela. Antiarrhythmic medications (e.g., amiodarone, procainamide, sotalol) are given to the patient with an ICD to control tachyarrhythmias and prevent the ICD from firing.

Postinfarction myocardial angina or ST-segment changes with exercise should be addressed by further evaluation of myocardial perfusion such as coronary arteriography or nuclear exercise or pharmacologic testing.

Postinfarction ventricular dysfunction that results in congestive failure is best treated with the medications given immediately after the infarction (β-blockers, ACE inhibitors, nitrates). Additionally, these patients may require diuretics or more sophisticated heart failure medical regimes.

After the first 24 hr following MI, lipid-lowering drugs, medications to control glucose abnormalities, and additional medications to control blood pressure, if not normalized by the ACE inhibitors and β-blockers, are typically started. Patients start to increase their activity level by beginning activities for daily living and progress to walking as tolerated. They also receive information concerning their risk factors for CHD and how to modify their lifestyle to decrease their risk of future problems (see chapters 3-5). At hospital discharge or soon thereafter, the patient should be referred to an outpatient cardiac rehabilitation program for exercise training and secondary prevention.

Sudden Death

Sudden death is almost always attributable to ventricular flutter or fibrillation, frequently starting as ventricular tachycardia, which at times starts as severe bradyarrhythmias with idioventricular rates of 30 to 35 beats·min⁻¹ and is not necessarily related to the severity of the myocardial damage. The severe bradyarrhythmias may produce myocardial ischemia that results in ventricular tachycardia or fibrillation.

Ventricular rupture can also be a mechanism of sudden death. This usually is preceded by symptoms of ischemia associated with an infarction and, therefore, results in a death that is not as sudden as with ventricular fibrillation.

Observed sudden deaths with ventricular fibrillation should be treated immediately with transthoracic electroshock. If this is done in less than 1 min from the onset, there is a much greater chance of normalizing the rhythm. If this fails, cardiopulmonary resuscitation and advanced life support are begun with subsequent DC electroshock, as required.

Survival after a sudden death event, even with immediate care, has a 25% to 30% poorer outcome if it occurs out of the hospital. Sudden death episodes not related to an infarction require an ICD for survival of subsequent episodes. All of these patients should have an electrophysiological study to determine the mechanism of sudden death. Then the proper therapy (IDC and medication) should be established.

Patients with angina frequently have more severe coronary obstructive disease than patients with a myocardial infarction as their initial event. Patients who habitually exercise and develop angina may have diffuse plaque in multiple arteries but have maintained myocardial perfusion and highly developed collateral circulation in the coronary system. These and peripheral circulation adaptations allow them to continue their physical activity. As has been noted by many observers, physically active patients are significantly less likely to die with a myocardial infarction (25%) compared with sedentary patients (see chapter 5).

Valvular Heart Disease

Valvular heart disease is either congenital or acquired (e.g., secondary to rheumatic fever, infectious endocarditis) and is classified as either stenosis or regurgitation of the valve. Valvular stenosis impedes the forward flow of blood through the valve because the valve orifice has become constricted and narrowed. In valvular regurgitation (also referred to as insufficiency or incompetence), blood is allowed to flow retrograde (backward) through the valve because the valve leaflets or cusps fail to close completely when the valve should be closed.

Etiology of Valvular Heart Disease

Valvular heart disease is a common clinical problem that can result from rheumatic fever, subacute bacterial endocarditis (SBE), calcific dilated ascending aorta, congenital heart disease, atherosclerotic heart disease with infarction of valvular supportive muscles, cardiomyopathy, valvular calcification, and aortic root dilatation.

Mitral Stenosis

Mitral stenosis is often a sequela to rheumatic fever but can also be the result of congenital heart disease. Atrial fibrillation or peripheral embolus may be the first symptom that the patient experiences. With severe stenosis (valve size <1 cm²), shortness of breath with exertion, cardiac arrhythmias, hemoptysis, pulmonary hypertension, and right heart failure may be noted. Recent-onset mitral stenosis in young individuals is uncommon now that untreated rheumatic fever is very infrequent in developed countries. Surgical correction with valve replacement or repair is often required, with arrhythmias controlled by medication or pacemaker insertion following AV node ablation.

Mitral Regurgitation

This is most commonly associated with prolapsed mitral valve (congenital) but may also result from rheumatic fever caused by or complicated by bacterial endocarditis. If mitral regurgitation is rheumatic in origin, it is frequently associated with mitral stenosis and aortic valve disease. Mild to moderate mitral insufficiency is usually well tolerated if there are no other complications. If the rhythm can be controlled, mitral regurgitation can frequently go for a number of years without requiring corrective surgery of the valve. Surgically, the valve can be repaired in almost all cases with either open heart or minimal access surgery. Occasionally, the valve will be replaced because of extensive destruction of the valve leaflets by using a tissue valve or a prosthetic valve (e.g., St. Jude). During valve replacement surgery, it is frequently necessary to also reconstruct the mitral valve supportive structure (any ruptured chordae tendinae, papillary muscle). Following mitral valve repair surgery, there is usually a significant improvement in hemodynamics.

Aortic Stenosis

If not associated with other valvular disease, aortic stenosis is almost always congenital disease with a bicuspid aortic valve or other congenital valve deformities. It is usually accompanied by some degree of aortic regurgitation. The congenital abnormality can be associated with a ventricular septal defect or coarctation of the aorta. Symptoms are related to the severity of the stenosis, degree of left ventricular thickness and compliance, and the extent of coronary artery disease. Dyspnea, syncope, and chest discomfort with activity indicate the need for surgical correction. Death will usually occur in 60% to 80% of patients who have symptomatic left heart failure secondary to aortic stenosis within a period of 6 months. Subvalvular asymetrical septal hypertrophy and midventricular stenosis are congenital in origin and are best treated with medications. Allografts and nonstented tissue valves (freestyle pig valves) are the most commonly used tissue valves for replacement, particularly in the elderly patients. The St. Jude valve is the most commonly used prosthetic valve, and outcomes are quite good with all these procedures. Replacing the aortic valve with the patient's pulmonary valve and the pulmonary valve with a tissue valve (Ross procedure) is more commonly performed in younger patients.

Aortic Regurgitation

Aortic regurgitation may be associated with congenital aortic stenosis, attributable to rheumatic fever or bacterial endocarditis, and is occasionally associated with aortic dissecting aneurysm involving the ascending aorta. Symptoms are related to the severity and duration of the aortic regurgitation. Mild to moderate aortic regurgitation can be well tolerated for years and does not always require therapy. However, it should be repaired surgically if the patient develops increased left ventricular size and significant symptoms. Sudden onset of aortic regurgitation with a dissecting aortic aneurysm that causes lack of support of the aortic leaflets or SBE destruction of the valve leaflets requires more immediate correction. Wide pulse pressure, accentuated pulses, femoral pulses, increased heart size, and a diastolic decrescendo murmur are signs that left ventricular function is worsening and the patient will require surgery.

Repair is difficult and replacement is almost always necessary and frequently involves reconstruction of the ascending aorta. Tissue valves (i.e., human allografts) and freestyle and nonstented freestyle pig valves have been very effective at our institution, and the size can usually be matched or the aortic root size changed to achieve the appropriate valvular fit. Under certain circumstances in young individuals, the Ross procedure will be used (i.e., pulmonary valve placement

in the aortic position and allografts in the pulmonary valve position) to allow a normal valve to be exposed to increased pressure load, as was previously noted with aortic stenosis.

Tricuspid Insufficiency

Tricuspid insufficiency can be associated with previous rheumatic fever or a dilated right ventricle and right atrium, as well as with the congenital downward displacement of the valve noted in Ebstein's anomaly. Tricuspid insufficiency is frequently repaired at the time of other valvular surgery, but it is very uncommon to repair this as an isolated valvular problem. Signs of worsening tricuspid valve insufficiency include prominent jugular A waves and a loud systolic murmur along the lower left sternal border; possibly a hyperdynamic right heart may occur as the insufficiency worsens and right ventricular failure develops. Tricuspid valve stenosis and insufficiency are almost always congenital in origin, except for a rare involvement with rheumatic fever or bacterial endocarditis. Bacterial endocarditis involving the tricuspid and pulmonary valve is more commonly found in intravenous drug users.

Pulmonary Stenosis

Pulmonary stenosis usually requires repair. Patients with pulmonary stenosis are primarily found to be short of breath, particularly with exertion, and have very loud systolic ejection murmurs over the left base of the heart radiating to the clavicle with associated bruits. These findings may be present even when surgical correction is not indicated. However, increased right ventricular hypertrophy and any symptoms of right heart failure would require correction of the stenosis.

For further information, the reader is directed to the following reference texts regarding heart disease.

Crawford MH, DiMarci JP, Paulus WJ (eds). *Cardiology*. Second Edition. New York: Mosby, 2004.

Fuster V, Hurst JW (eds). *Hurst's the Heart*. 11th Edition. New York: McGraw-Hill, 2004.

Topol EJ (ed). *Textbook of Cardiovascular Medicine*. Second Edition. Philadelphia: Lippincott Williams & Wilkins, 2002.

Zipes DP, Braunwald E (eds). *Brauwald's Heart Disease: A Textbook of Cardiovascular Medicine*. Seventh Edition. Philadelphia: Saunders, 2005.

PART I

Development, Intervention, and Prevention of Coronary Artery Disease

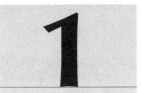

Atherosclerosis

Timothy R. McConnell, PhD, and Troy A. Klinger, MS

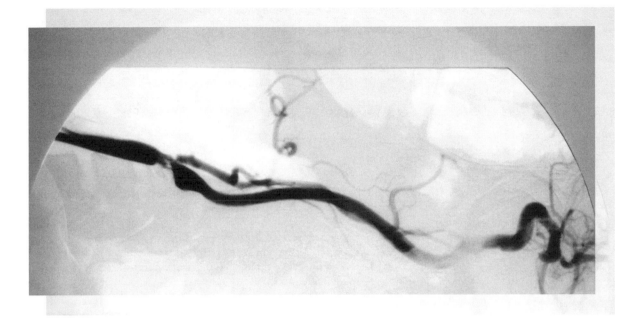

Atherosclerosis is, for all intents, coronary heart disease, which is the most common cause of death in the industrialized world. As a form of arteriosclerosis (thickening of the walls of arteries), atherosclerosis is initially characterized by changes in the intimal lining of arteries with eventual partial or full occlusion of the arterial lumen. Depending on lesion severity, coronary artery atherosclerosis manifests itself in an array of symptoms suggestive of such acute coronary syndromes as angina, myocardial infarction, and sudden death.

Traditionally, atherosclerosis was conceptualized as a simplistic model of a chronic progressive disease manifested once a threshold level of disease was obtained—total or near-total occlusion of the arterial lumen. The aim of acute treatment is to ameliorate symptoms and minimize myocardial damage, whereas chronic management depends on the degree of ventricular dysfunction and the recurrence of symptoms. Although atherosclerosis is still recognized as containing a chronic progressive component, newer biological, histochemical, clinical, and molecular assays have demonstrated that atherosclerosis is a dynamic, volatile, reactive process, particularly in the latter thrombotic stages.

Process of Plaque Formation

Although atherosclerosis has a complex pathogenesis, autopsies performed on U.S. wartime casualties as well as on children and adolescents have consistently demonstrated a high prevalence of early-stage atherosclerosis in American youth.[1,2] The

GUIDELINES, 4TH EDITION

- Appendix B, pages 207-208

Table 1.1   Lesion Classification

Early lesions	Type I (figure 1*a*)	• Usually found only in children • Characterized by an increase in the number of intimal macrophages and the accumulation of lipid droplets to form foam cells

	Type II (figure 1*b*)	• Include fatty streaks
		• First lesions that can be visualized
		• Layers of foam cells and vascular smooth muscle cells
		  • Type IIa—progression prone
		  • Type IIb—progression resistant

Intermediary lesions	Type III (figure 1*c*)	• Between type II lesions and mature atheroma • Pools of extracellular lipid droplets among the layers of vascular smooth muscle cells
Advanced lesions	Type IV (figure 1*d*)	• Atheromas • Well-defined collection of extracellular lipid within the intima (lipid core) • Frequently eccentric in location, causing a thickening of the arterial wall • Usually do not result in a significant narrowing of the arterial lumen and do not produce symptoms

	Type V (figure 1*e*)	• Formation of prominent new fibrous connective tissue (fibrous cap)
		• Generally present in the fourth decade of life
		• Can cause significant narrowing of the arterial lumen causing symptoms
		  • Type Va—lipid core covered with a thick fibrous layer composed of extracellular connective tissue matrix
		  • Type Vb—lipid core is calcified
		  • Type Vc—no lipid core and little if any lipid

	Type VI (figure 1*f*)	• Complicated lesion • Cause of most morbidity and mortality from atherosclerosis • Occur when type IV or V lesions undergo disruption of intimal surface, such as plaque ulceration or hemorrhage • Source of emboli or may cause arterial thrombosis • Acute coronary syndrome

Adapted, by permission, from H.C. Stary et al., 1995, "A definition of advanced lesions and classification of arteriosclerosis," *Circulation* 92:1355-1374.

primary assumption of the progression theory is that, over a period of years, these early lesions progress to more severe lesions at the same anatomical site.[3] These lesions progress at varying rates in different people.

Contemporary research has struggled with the complexity of events and constituents that comprise the atherosclerotic process. Although variations in disease development have been described, the American Heart Association (AHA) recently published lesion categories based on general agreement about the histological composition and structure of atherogenic plaque (table 1.1 and figure 1.1).[4,5]

Acute Coronary Syndromes

The manifestation of atherosclerosis is the gradual or sudden onset of signs or symptoms associated with what now is commonly referred to as *acute coronary syndromes*—and includes unstable angina, non-Q-wave myocardial infarction, Q-wave myocardial infarction, or sudden death. Although atherosclerosis is a long-term progressive process before clinical manifestation, the symptom-defining event or thrombus formation is now viewed as a dynamic, more rapidly evolving process that may occur unpredictably, regardless of the extent of plaque progression.

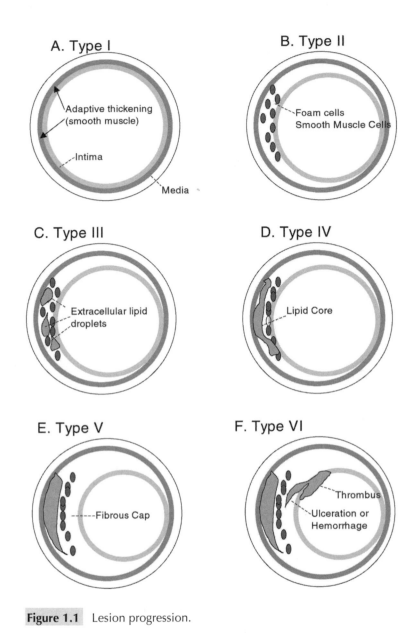

Figure 1.1 Lesion progression.

Lesion Progression

In summary, lesions progress from

- early benign deposition of fat droplets and the formation of fat cells,
  ↓
- formation of a lipid core within the vascular smooth muscle,
  ↓
- embolically and thrombotically dangerous disruption of the intimal surface, to
  ↓
- acute coronary syndromes.

Acute Coronary Syndromes

Unstable plaque

Rupture of a lipid-laden plaque with a thin cap is the most common cause of an acute coronary syndrome (ACS). The majority of these plaques are not hemodynamically significant before rupture. An inflammatory component is present in the subendothelial area and further weakens and predisposes the plaque to rupture. Blood flow velocity, turbulence, and vessel anatomy may be important contributing factors. Superficial erosion of a plaque occurs in a small percentage of patients.

Plaque Rupture

After rupture, a monolayer of platelets covers the surface of the ruptured plaque (platelet adhesion). Additional platelets are recruited (platelet aggregation) and activated. Fibrinogen cross-links platelets, and the coagulation system is activated with thrombin generation.

Unstable angina

A partially occluding thrombus produces symptoms of ischemia, which are prolonged and may occur at rest. At this stage the thrombus is platelet-rich. Therapy with antiplatelet agents such as aspirin and glycoprotein (GP) IIb/IIIa receptor inhibitors is most effective. Fibrinolytic therapy is not effective and may paradoxically accelerate occlusion by the release of clot-bound thrombin, which further activates platelets. An intermittently occlusive thrombus may cause myocardial necrosis, producing a non-Q-wave myocardial infarction (MI).

Microemboli

As the clot enlarges, microemboli may originate from the distal thrombus and lodge in the coronary microvasculature, causing small elevations of cardiac troponins, new sensitive cardiac markers. Patients in whom this occurs are at highest risk for progression to MI. This process is known as minimal myocardial damage.

Occlusive thrombus

If the thrombus occludes the coronary vessel for a prolonged period, a 0-wave MI occurs. This clot is rich in thrombin; fibrinolysis or direct percutaneous coronary interventions may limit infarct size if performed sufficiently early.

Pathophysiology

Atherogenesis (the formation of an atherosclerotic plaque) is a complex multifactorial process with chronic progression related to a variety of risks. The final stages of the process, or acute coronary syndrome, may be precipitated by the following:

- Injury
- Rupture
- Structural anomaly
- Inflammatory or infectious response
- Genetic predisposition
- Reactive endothelium

Response to Injury

The injury hypothesis conceptualizes the vascular wall as a reactive entity responsive to a variety of pathogenic factors including genetic constitution, chemical constituents of the blood, environmental influences, and hemodynamics.[7] Certain areas of the vasculature are more prone to atherosclerotic lesions, such as areas where there is turbulent flow and shear stresses are low (branches). As a result of the increased residence time for circulating particles, exposure of the endothelium to blood-borne atherogenic agents, such as lipoproteins,[7] is prolonged.

Consequently, the prolonged exposure of the endothelium makes it a focal activation point for plaque formation (figure 1.2).[8,9]

Role of Inflammation

Atheromatous plaques prone to rupture contain inflammatory mononuclear cells which have the potential to destabilize atheroma and lead to acute coronary thrombosis.[10(p. 59)]

Inflammation can cause a plaque to become vulnerable to disruption, leading to acute coronary

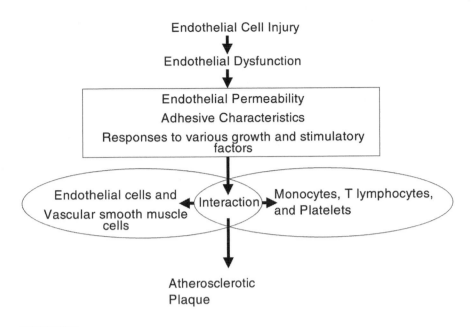

Figure 1.2   Atherosclerosis is, at least partially, attributable to the cellular response to endothelial injury.

syndromes.[11] Each stage of lesion progression is a manifestation of an evolving inflammatory process. Subsequently, if the inflammation continues, the eventual outcome is a mature atherosclerotic lesion and continued inflammation. So, "atherogenesis induces and promotes inflammation and inflammation induces and promotes atherogenesis."[11(p. 14)] Several processes support the theory that acute coronary syndromes is an inflammatory process: first, evidence of inflammation can be detected many years in advance of acute coronary syndrome; second, early or even later stage inflammatory processes appear to follow a common pathway to the ensuing acute coronary event; and third, there appear to be

effective, preventive anti-inflammatory measures.[10] Consequently, atherosclerosis appears to be a chronic inflammatory process that possibly can be prevented by early intervention.

Scientific American provided an excellent description and illustration of the many potential roles of inflammation in the atherosclerotic process (table 1.2 and figure 1.3).[12]

Role of Infection

The sclerosis of old age may simply be a summation of lesions arising from infectious or metabolic toxins.[13(p. 160)]

Table 1.2	Inflammation and the Atherosclerotic Process
1. Birth of a plaque	• Accumulation of LDL particles • Adherence to monocytes and T cells • Secretion of chemokines • Production of inflammatory mediators • Cell division • Development of fatty streak
2. Plaque progression	• Inflammation—growth of the plaque (lipid core) and formation of fibrous cap
3. Plaque rupture	• Inflammation contributes to plaque instability—weakens fibrous cap • Cap rupture—acute coronary syndrome

Note. LDL = low-density lipoprotein.

From Scientific American.

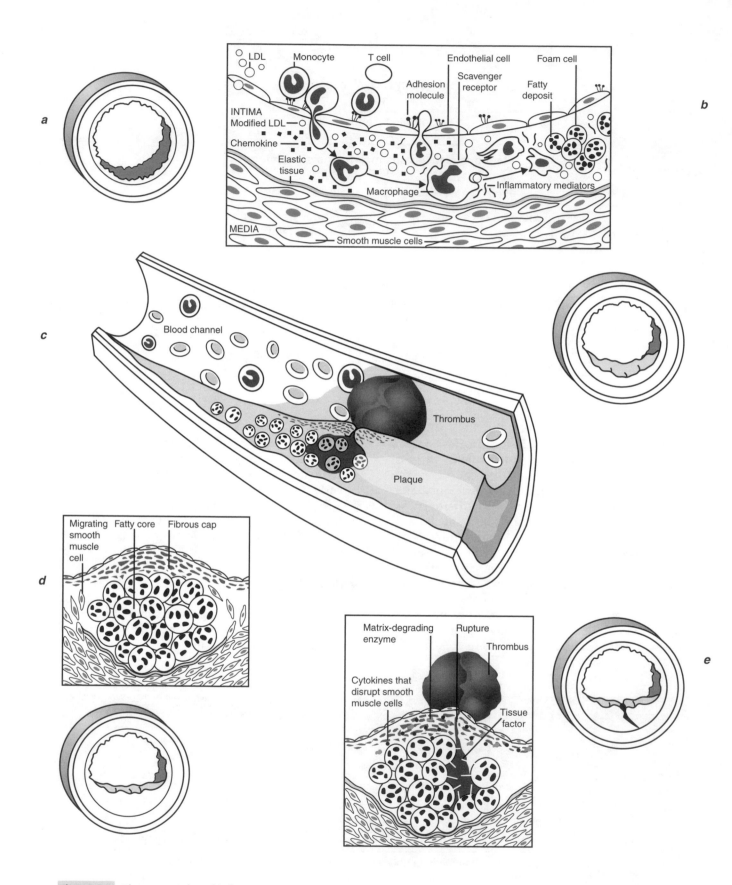

Figure 1.3 The many roles of inflammation.

Considering that more than one third of those dying of coronary vascular disease and one half of those with coronary heart disease do not have classic risk factors for coronary heart disease (CHD), additional factors such as infectious agents may facilitate the development, rapid progression, and instability of atherosclerotic plaques[14,15] as well as play a role in restenosis after atherectomy or angioplasty[16] and the progression of arteriosclerosis after heart transplantation.[17-19] Increasing the risk of acute coronary syndrome, infectious colonization in the atherosclerotic plaque can promote plaque instability by inducing endothelial injury, cell proliferation, and inflammation.[20] Suspected infectious agents include Coxsackievirus type B, herpesvirus, cytomegalovirus, *Chlamydia pneumoniae* (the most likely candidate), and *Helicobacter pylori*. Although not proved causal, these infectious agents evoke cellular and molecular changes of the vessel wall that strongly suggest an atherogenic role (table 1.3).[14,20]

There are other mechanisms by which infectious agents may promote atherosclerosis and acute coronary syndromes:

- Interactions within the plaque altering endothelial function[21]

- Activation of inflammatory mechanisms associated with an increase in plasma fibrinogen[22]

- Increased blood viscosity and hypercoagulability

- Alterations of serum lipid profiles (oxidize low-density lipoproteins)

- Induction of heat shock proteins (stress proteins)

Molecular Genetics

Family history has traditionally been recognized as one of the primary, unalterable risk factors for premature development of atherosclerosis. Family history consists of a number of gene-based alterations that predispose individuals to the premature onset of atherosclerosis. One gene-based alteration produces altered lipid metabolism—familial hypercholesterolemia[7]— whereas another includes genetic alterations that affect coagulation factors and fibrinogen responsible for increased thrombogenicity.[23] In addition, genetic alterations of the renin–angiotensin pathway result in hypertension and resultant cardiovascular disease.[24] Other genetic alterations may result in cell accumulation at sites of inflammation, regulation of tone of the arterial wall, obesity, and other indirect effects on the development of cardiovascular disease.[25,26]

Molecular genetics and the predilection to diseases go beyond the intent and scope of this chapter. The next exciting phase of molecular genetic research is the treatment and management of diseases through genetic manipulation.

Although family history is most commonly referenced regarding genetic makeup, one also must consider environmental or lifestyle factors. Individuals tend to develop the lifestyle habits learned from parents, who learned from their parents. For example, if eating habits consisted of traditional "three square meals," including eggs and bacon in the morning and meat and potato dinners, then these lifestyle habits are most likely perpetuated. In addition, atherogenic lifestyle habits, such as inactivity and tobacco use, will most likely be adopted. Patients must be aware that changing these unhealthy habits is one way to decrease the risk of developing atherosclerosis.

Table 1.3   Atherogenic Role of Infectious Agents

Infectious agents	Vessel wall changes

Smooth muscle cell accumulation	Inhibited p53 (tumor suppressor gene)
	    Increased smooth muscle cell proliferation
	    Decreased apoptosis
	Increased growth factor expression
	    Increased smooth muscle cell proliferation
	    Increased smooth muscle cell migration

Lipid accumulation	Decreased cholesterol esterase hydrolytic activity Increased scavenger receptor activity

Endothelial dysfunction	Procoagulant effects
	    Decreased vasodilator function
	    Increased expression of chemokines, cytokines, and adhesion molecules

Inflammation	Targeted to pathogen Targeted to pathogen products

Contemporary Revascularization Procedures

Glenn N. Levine, MD

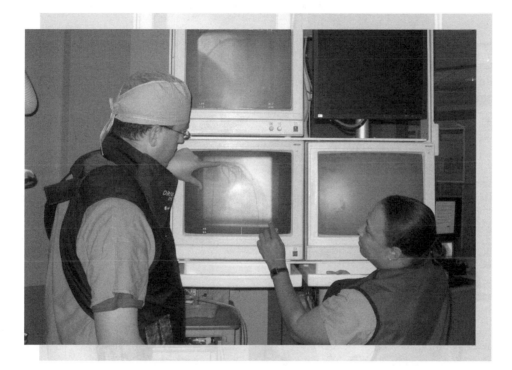

The last several decades have witnessed a new era in the treatment of coronary heart disease (CHD), with the development of coronary revascularization. The first coronary artery bypass graft (CABG) procedures were performed in the 1960s,[1] and the first angioplasty procedure was performed by Dr. Andreas Grunzig in 1977.[2] Since these hallmark procedures, dramatic advances in both CABG and percutaneous coronary interventions (PCIs) have increased the number of patients who can be treated with these procedures, reduced procedural complications, and improved long-term outcome. In this chapter, coronary heart disease is first briefly discussed. Then CABG and PCI are discussed, and the roles of these procedures in the treatment of various patient populations are reviewed. I also discuss complications and considerations relevant to cardiac rehabilitation and exercise training for each procedure and provide recommendations regarding cardiac rehabilitation in these patients.

Coronary Arteries and CHD

To understand coronary artery revascularization, it is useful to first briefly review the coronary arteries and CHD. The coronary arteries originate from the proximal ascending aorta and run along the outer surface of the heart. The *left main coronary artery* is a short segment of artery, usually 1 to 2 cm in length, that quickly bifurcates into the *left anterior descending artery* (LAD), which travels down the anterior aspect of the heart, and the *left circumflex artery*, which travels around the left side of the heart. Both arteries usually

GUIDELINES, 4TH EDITION

- Chapter 9, pages 146-149

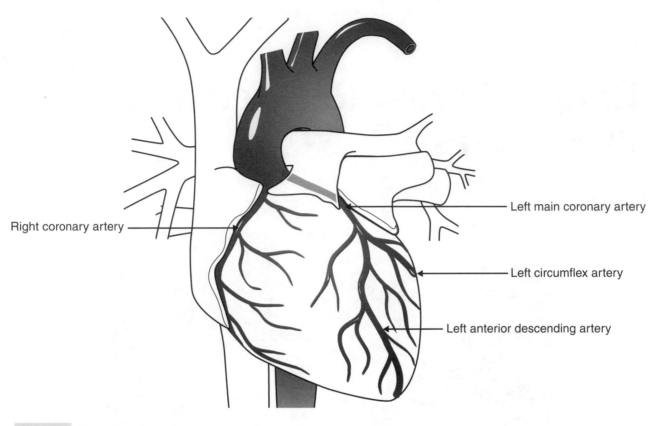

Right coronary artery

Left main coronary artery

Left circumflex artery

Left anterior descending artery

Figure 2.1 The coronary arteries.

give off several large branches. Branches of the LAD are called *diagonal arteries*, and branches of the left circumflex artery are called *obtuse marginal* (OM) arteries. The right coronary artery (RCA) travels around the right side of the heart and down to the inferior aspect of the heart. The RCA gives off branches called the *posterior descending artery* (PDA) and, usually, one or more *posterolateral branches*. The coronary arteries are shown in figure 2.1.

As discussed in more detail in chapter 1, over time, plaque made up of lipid and other materials can develop within the lumen of the coronary arteries. As this plaque grows, larger lesions develop within these arteries. This development of these lesions can have two adverse effects. If the lesion continues to encroach on a greater percentage of the arterial lumen, the lesion can begin to impede blood flow to the myocardium distal to the stenosis. Although blood flow through a significant stenosis may be adequate to supply the myocardium with oxygen-rich blood when the patient is at rest, during exercise and other periods of increased oxygen demand the lesion may limit the supply of oxygen-rich blood reaching the myocardium, resulting in myocardial ischemia and the sensation of angina. This phenomenon usually begins to occur when lesions are 70% or more of the arterial lumen diameter.

The second adverse process that can occur is that at some time, a lipid-filled plaque may rupture, leading to platelet aggregation, triggering the coagulation cascade, and resulting in thrombus formation at the site of the ruptured plaque. When this occurs, the thrombus may partially or completely occlude the coronary artery, leading to unstable angina (angina occurring at rest) or myocardial infarction. These two adverse processes are shown in figure 2.2.

Because the left main coronary artery subtends such a large proportion of left ventricular myocardium, lesser degrees of stenosis are considered clinically important. Studies (discussed subsequently) have shown that in patients with lesions that are 50% or more of the left main artery's diameter, treatment of these lesions with coronary artery bypass surgery increases life expectancy.

Coronary Artery Bypass Graft Surgery

Since the dawn of CABG in the 1960s, surgical bypass of coronary stenoses has undergone dramatic improvements in technique, accompanied by higher

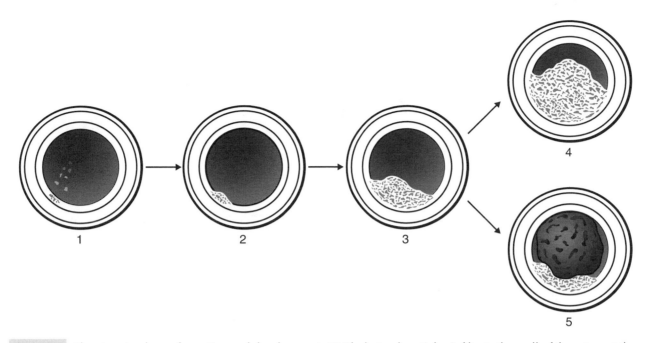

Figure 2.2   The steps in plaque formation and development. (1) Cholesterol particles infiltrate the wall of the artery at the site of the damaged inner lining of the artery; (2) a plaque develops in the artery; (3) as more cholesterol and other materials are incorporated into the plaque, the plaque grows; (4) the plaque may continue to grow, blocking blood flow through the artery, resulting in exertional angina, or (5) the plaque may rupture and a blood clot may form, resulting in unstable angina or myocardial infarction.

success and lower complication rates. In the United States, more than half a million CABG procedures are performed annually,[3] making it the most commonly performed surgery. Next I describe the CABG procedure and issues regarding the post-CABG care of patients.

CABG Procedure

During the CABG procedure, a median sternotomy is performed, in which the sternum is literally cut in two and spread apart, allowing access to the heart (figure 2.3). Special catheters are inserted into the heart and ascending aorta so that cardiopulmonary bypass (CPB) can be performed while the heart is stopped. CPB allows for the oxygenation of blood during the bypass procedure, and this complex machine also uses specialized devices to maintain a phasic forward flow of blood to the tissues of the body (particularly the brain) during the bypass procedure. As CPB is initiated, the heart is stopped, allowing the surgical team better access to the coronary arteries and a more stable surgical field in which to anastomose bypass grafts into the diseased coronary arteries.

The number of bypass grafts the patient receives depends on the number of diseased arteries that need to be bypassed as well as the suitability of these arteries for being bypassed. The saphenous vein is harvested from the leg and used to bypass diseased coronary arteries. One end of a saphenous vein segment is anastomosed to the ascending aorta, and the other end is attached to the coronary artery distal to the arterial stenosis. Such grafts are referred to as *saphenous vein grafts* (SVGs). In most current procedures, the left internal mammary artery (LIMA) is carefully dissected away from the chest wall, and then the distal end of the LIMA is anastomosed to the left anterior descending artery (LAD). The proximal end of the LIMA remains attached to the left subclavian artery (figure 2.4). Most procedures use the LIMA to bypass the LAD because, as discussed later, it has a greater long-term patency than an SVG, and its use is associated with a greater incidence of long-term survival. At the end of the procedure, the heart is restarted, and the sternum is closed and held together with wires (figure 2.3).

After the procedure, patients typically require 1 to several days of intensive care unit management and then up to a week more of further care. In current practice, a "fast-track" management is used, with the goal of achieving patient discharge around the fifth postoperative day. Full recovery requires approximately 4 weeks (and in some cases significantly longer).

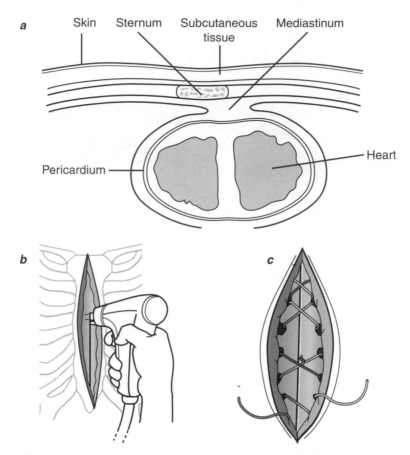

Figure 2.3 Sternotomy during CABG. *(a)* Incisions must be made first through the subcutaneous tissue and then in the sternum itself to expose the coronary arteries for treatment. *(b)* The sternum is cut using a specialized drill and then spread using specialized "spreaders." *(c)* After the procedure, the two halves of the split sternum are wired back together. It may take some time for the sternum to heal, an important consideration in rehabilitation after CABG.

Reprinted from *Ischemic heart disease surgical management,* B. Butson et al., 1999, Copyright 1999, with permission from Elsevier.

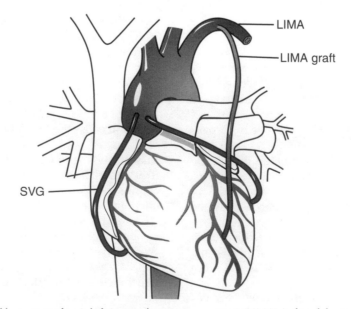

Figure 2.4 Illustration of bypass grafts. A left internal mammary artery (LIMA) is freed from the chest wall and anastomosed to the left anterior descending artery. Saphenous vein grafts (SVGs) are attached proximally to the ascending aorta and anastomosed distally into the right coronary artery and left circumflex coronary artery.

Specific Conditions

CABG may be performed both to improve symptoms and to extend life expectancy. These various conditions are discussed next.

- Multivessel CHD

  Compared with medical therapy, CABG resulted in a greater improvement in anginal status. In the Coronary Artery Surgery Study (CASS), at 5-year follow-up, surgically treated patients used less antianginal medications; 63% of surgically treated patients were completely angina free, compared with 38% of the medically treated patients. These differences, however, were no longer present at 10-year follow-up.[4] As discussed in the section on PCI, CABG has generally been shown to decrease anginal status to a greater degree than multivessel PCI, at least over the short to intermediate term.[5-12] Whether this advantage over PCI is sustained over the long term, as SVGs become diseased and occluded with increased frequency, remains to be seen. There is no advantage in survival with CABG compared with multivessel angioplasty, and neither clearly decreases the incidence of future myocardial infarction (MI).[5-12]

- Depressed Ejection Fraction

  Three major trials performed in the 1970s, comparing CABG with medical therapy, provided data on the benefits of CABG in patients with multivessel disease and depressed left ventricular ejection fraction. Data from these trials demonstrated that in patients with three-vessel disease (or two-vessel disease if one of the two stenoses was located in the proximal LAD), CABG improved life expectancy.[1,13]

- Left Main CHD

  Those same three studies from the 1970s comparing CABG with medical therapy demonstrated a clear survival advantage with CABG. In the CASS trial, median survival for surgically treated patients was 13.3 years, compared with a median survival in the medically treated patients of 6.6 years.[13] Four-year survival curves are shown in figure 2.5.

- Diabetic Patients

  In the largest of the trials comparing multivessel PCI with CABG, the Bypass Angioplasty Revascularization Investigation (BARI), diabetic patients fared better with CABG than with balloon angioplasty. At 5-year follow-up, both all-cause mortality rate (19.1% and 34.7%, respectively) and cardiac mortality rate (5.8% and 20.6%) were significantly lower in those patients randomized to CABG.[14]

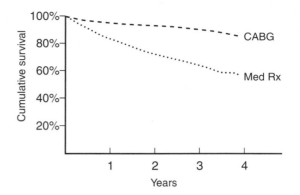

Figure 2.5   Kaplan-Meier survival curves for patients in the Coronary Artery Surgery Study (CASS) with left main coronary heart disease treated with either coronary artery bypass surgery (CABG) or medical therapy (Med Rx).

Adapted from *American Journal of Cardiology* Vol. 48, B.R. Chaitman et al., Effect of coronary bypass on survival patterns in subsets of patients with left main coronary artery disease. Report of the collaborative study in coronary artery surgery study (CASS) pgs. 765-777, Copyright 1981, with permission from Elsevier.

Complications and Considerations

Rehabilitation specialists should be aware of several important complications and considerations in post-CABG patients that can affect the care of these patients and their exercise prescription.

The most important risk factors associated with an increased incidence of complications and adverse outcome in patients undergoing CABG include age, left ventricular ejection fraction, and the urgency of the operation (e.g., whether it was emergent, urgent, or elective). Other important risk factors include the presence of diabetes, chronic obstructive pulmonary disease (COPD), renal disease, and peripheral artery disease (PAD).[7] Patients with poor exercise capacity pre-CABG usually can be expected to take longer to recover and regain good functional status. Specific complications and considerations are discussed next.

Central Nervous System Deficits

Both focal motor and sensory deficits and general cognitive deficits can occur after CABG. Stroke with resultant focal deficits is believed to be most frequently caused by atheroembolisms that become dislodged from the proximal aorta during the CABG procedure. Cognitive changes may be attributable to intraoperative hypotension, inadequate cerebral perfusion, and the use of CPB. The incidence of significant focal deficit (motor or sensory stroke) is approximately 3%.[7,15] The incidence of cognitive deficits post-CABG is controversial and depends on the definition of a cognitive deficit, how a deficit is diagnosed, and other study-related variables. Rates as low as 3% and as high as 50% have been reported,[7,15-17] and I believe that the incidence of clinically apparent and clinically relevant cognitive deficits is more toward the lower end of this range. Relevant to the rehabilitation of the post-CABG patient, one well-designed study demonstrated that cognitive function was the lowest at discharge, with incremental improvements in cognitive function at 6-week and 6-month follow-up.[15]

Mediastinitis and Sternal Healing

Deep sternal wound infections are referred to as *mediastinitis*. Patients who are more prone to mediastinitis and in whom a higher index of suspicion should be maintained include those who are obese, have diabetes, or have undergone a previous CABG operation.[7,18,19] Significant pain and tenderness in the sternal area, persistent oozing from the wound, or failure of the sternum to properly heal may suggest the presence of mediastinitis and warrant further evaluation.

As shown in figure 2.3, the sternum is literally cut in half and then sewn together with wires at the end of the procedure. Healing of the sternum may take 1 to several months, and in some cases the sternum may never completely heal properly (a condition referred to as *sternal nonunion*). Exercise and rehabilitation specialists must pay particular heed to this issue, particularly in patients in whom resistance training is planned. Unfortunately, musculoskeletal pains associated with sternotomy and sternal healing, as well as other musculoskeletal issues (e.g., ribs, cartilage), may be a cause of chest pain, particularly during physical activity, and may be difficult both for the patient and health care professional to differentiate from angina.

Atrial Fibrillation

Atrial fibrillation is an arrhythmia in which there is unorganized, chaotic depolarization of the tissue of the atria (see chapter 8). Atrial fibrillation occurs in up to one third of post-CABG patients. This arrhythmia presents two related problems to the cardiac rehabilitation specialist. First, baseline heart rates in these patients are often rapid, even at rest before beginning exercise. Second, the heart rate response to exercise may be exaggerated, confounding and complicating decisions about exercising patients at specific target heart rates.

Graft Closure

Bypass graft closure is not a complication but an accepted limitation of CABG. Studies have shown that by 10 years post-CABG, approximately half of all SVGs will be either severely diseased or occluded.[20] In contrast, the left internal mammary artery (LIMA) has been found to be resistant to the development of atherosclerosis and has excellent long-term patency. Because most patients undergoing CABG are treated with a LIMA anastomosed to the LAD and one or several SVGs anastomosed to other diseased coronary arteries, it can be expected that even in patients who have received a LIMA as part of their CABG, many

will be susceptible to the phenomenon of long-term SVG degeneration. Thus, cardiac rehabilitation specialists should approach patients who have had CABG many years ago with more caution than those who have undergone recent revascularization.

Less-Invasive Surgery

Significant progress and research have been achieved over the last half-decade on less-invasive methods for performing CABG. For the purposes of clarity, it has been proposed that these invasive methods be divided into three categories: off-bypass (or "off-pump") CABG, minimally invasive direct CAB (MIDCAB), and port-access CABG.[7] During off-bypass CABG, the bypass operation is performed through a standard median sternotomy (splitting of the sternum), generally with a smaller skin incision. The bypass anastomoses are performed while the heart is still beating, without the use of CPB. A MIDCAB is performed though a small incision in the left anterior chest wall, with or without thorascopic techniques, while the heart is still beating. This procedure can be used to anastomose the LIMA to the LAD (figure 2.6). Port-access CABG is performed using CPB on an arrested heart but with the cannulae inserted into the femoral artery and vein instead of the aorta and right atrium.[7]

In the United States, 10% to 20% of CABG operations are performed with one of these less-invasive strategies, and that percentage is expected to increase significantly over the coming decade. Compared with conventional CABG, less-invasive CABG decreases hospital stay and results in a lower incidence of chest infection, atrial fibrillation, and need for blood transfusion.[17,21,22] However, the rates of periprocedural Q-wave

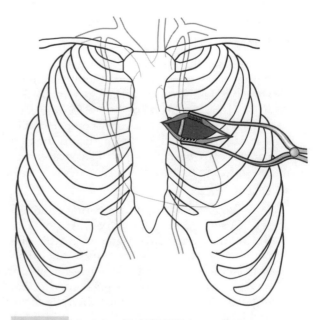

Figure 2.6   Incision for MIDCAB procedure.

myocardial infarction and short-term mortality are similar whether or not less-invasive surgery is used.[17,21] Although there are theoretical reasons to believe that patients who undergo off-pump surgery (e.g., without cardiac arrest and CBP) would suffer less impairment in cognitive function, current data on this are limited and contradictory and do not establish any clear benefit with off-pump surgical procedures.[17,23,24] Several concerns remain about less-invasive CABG, including the ability to achieve complete coronary revascularization (e.g., bypass all the stenosed arteries), the quality of graft anastomoses (particularly the LIMA), and long-term graft patency, issues that will only be resolved with further research and follow-up.

Exercise and Cardiac Rehabilitation

The American Association of Cardiovascular and Pulmonary Rehabilitation recommends that some post-CABG patients can initiate secondary prevention as soon as 1 week post-surgery. Recommended initial assessment of the post-CABG patient includes inspection of incision sites (chest and leg) for signs of infection, assessment of mood and social support, and evaluation of physical functioning.[25]

In theory, patients who have undergone recent CABG should be fully revascularized. Nevertheless, exercise stress testing before exercise training seems prudent both as a screen for unexpected inducible ischemia (which may be caused by incomplete revascularization or early graft closure) and an assessment of exercise capacity.

An American Heart Association (AHA) Science Advisory noted that stretching or flexibility activities can begin as early as 24 hr post-CABG. Upper and lower extremity range of motion exercises are initially recommended in the rehabilitation process. These range of motion exercises may be beneficial in preventing the tissues in the sternal area from developing adhesions and in preventing the upper-body musculature from becoming weak and foreshortened. Resistance training that may cause pulling on the healing sternum should be avoided for the first 3 months, and the sternum should be checked for stability by an experienced health care professional before resistance training is initiated.[26] Further and more specific recommendations for both aerobic and resistance training are provided in chapter 7.

Percutaneous Coronary Interventions

As percutaneous revascularization has evolved, so has the terminology describing the procedure. For the first decade that percutaneous revascularization existed, the only procedure available was balloon angioplasty (described later). During this time, the procedure was described as either *percutaneous transluminal coronary angioplasty*, better known by the acronym PTCA, or simply as *angioplasty*.

Over the last decade and a half, additional devices (discussed subsequently) have been used during percutaneous revascularization procedures, including directional coronary atherectomy (DCA), rotational atherectomy (Rotablator), laser procedures, and, most important, coronary stenting. To better encompass all these different procedures, the term *percutaneous coronary intervention* (PCI) is now used in the literature to refer to any of these percutaneous revascularization procedures. Health care practitioners should note, however, that many patients and family members, understandably naive to the nuances of the many different percutaneous procedures, will simply inform health care professionals that they have undergone an "angioplasty" or "balloon procedure."

PCI Procedure

During an angioplasty procedure, a strawlike tube (called a *sheath*) is first inserted into the femoral artery (or occasionally into the brachial or radial artery). A specially designed catheter, called a *guiding catheter*, is then threaded through the sheath, in a retrograde direction up the aorta and into the left or right coronary ostium. A very thin *guide wire* (usually only 0.014 in. [0.036 cm] in diameter) is carefully manipulated into the target coronary artery and across the arterial stenosis. Over this guide wire, a thin balloon is passed to the area of stenosis, and the balloon is then inflated to several atmospheres of pressure. Inflation of this balloon enlarges the arterial lumen both by displacement of the plaque and by "stretching" the artery.[27,28] This is shown schematically in figure 2.7.

In most patients a thin metallic *stent*, mounted on another angioplasty balloon, is then passed to the area of stenosis. When the angioplasty balloon onto which the coronary stent is mounted is subsequently inflated, the coronary stent is expanded and embedded into the wall of the coronary artery. By keeping the coronary artery scaffolded or "stretched" open to a greater degree than can be achieved with balloon angioplasty alone, stent implantation leads to a larger luminal area at the site of stenosis.

Most coronary lesions are treated with a combination of balloon angioplasty followed by coronary stent implantation. However, other devices are occasionally used, and it is useful for the health care professional to be familiar with these other devices.

- Directional Coronary Atherectomy

  During DCA, a small cylindrical cutting device, rotating at a rapid rate, is used to cut away small pieces of atheroma from the coronary lesion. Although the introduction of this novel device

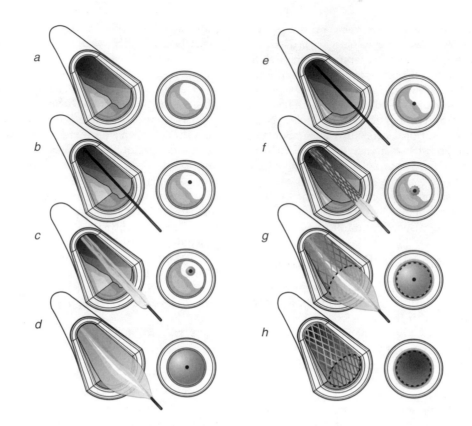

Figure 2.7   Percutaneous coronary intervention procedure. *(a)* Plaque partially obstructing the coronary artery; *(b)* the angioplasty guide wire is maneuvered across the obstruction; *(c)* a thin angioplasty balloon is passed over the guide wire to the site of the obstruction; *(d)* the angioplasty balloon is inflated, compressing and displacing the plaque and "stretching" the artery open; *(e)* increase in the arterial lumen after balloon angioplasty; *(f)* a metal coronary stent, mounted on an angioplasty balloon, is then passed over the guide wire to the area of obstruction; *(g)* the angioplasty balloon in then inflated, expanding the stent and embedding it into the arterial wall; *(h)* the expanded stent serves as a scaffold to keep the artery maximally expanded.

Reprinted, by permission, from the American Heart Association.

was initially greeted with great enthusiasm, after the disappointing results of several large trials conducted in the 1990s comparing DCA with plain balloon angioplasty,[29-31] use of this device decreased dramatically, and DCA is now only occasionally performed at a small number of hospitals.

- Rotational Atherectomy

In rotational atherectomy, a diamond-studded burr (figure 2.8), rotating at 140,000 to 160,000 rpm, is advanced within the coronary artery to the area of stenosis and is used to ablate the atheromatous material, somewhat analogous to how a drill bit turns wood into sawdust. Rotational atherectomy may be used in very long or calcified lesions, often to facilitate subsequent implantation of a coronary stent. The procedure is commonly referred to by the brand name of the device, the Rotablator. Patients will often report that they underwent a "Roto-Rooter" procedure.

- Laser Atherectomy

Although the concept of using a laser to ablate plaque had much appeal, clinical results were generally disappointing, as only a modest amount of plaque was actually ablated and complications such as vessel artery perforation plagued the procedure.[32-35] Laser atherectomy procedures are currently performed only rarely and only at a small number of institutions.

- Cutting Balloon

The cutting balloon is the latest novel interventional device. The cutting balloon is basically an angioplasty balloon fitted with three to four very fine razors distributed circumferentially on the balloon. When the balloon is inflated, these razors are pressed against the arterial wall. This process is purported to help dilate the coronary artery. The cutting balloon may be used in patients with lesions in the ostium of a coronary artery or branch, at an arterial bifurcation, or in a stent in which restenosis has occurred. Although

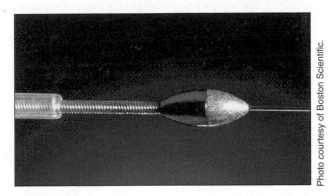

Photo courtesy of Boston Scientific.

Figure 2.8 The diamond-tipped Rotablator. In contrast to balloon angioplasty, which leads to small tears in the artery, the Rotablator may lead to a more uniform enlargement in lumen area.

the cutting balloon is a popular new treatment, actual data supporting its preferential use over other percutaneous revascularization modalities are modest at best.

Specific Conditions

Numerous well-designed and well-conducted studies have evaluated the efficacy of PCI in several important anatomical and clinical conditions. Information that is relevant to health care providers is discussed next. Each of the following PCI procedures uses the sheath, guiding catheter, and guide wire process previously described.

Single-Vessel, Stable CHD

The long-term prognosis of patients with single-vessel stable coronary heart disease is excellent.[36] In a retrospective review of survival rates in patients with single-vessel coronary heart disease treated in the 1970s with medical therapy who would have been amenable to treatment with coronary angioplasty (had it been in existence at the time), the 10-year survival rate was 91%.[37] Data from the Duke Database demonstrate that adjusted 5-year survival rates in patients with single-vessel coronary heart disease were 93% in those treated with medical therapy and 95% in those treated with PCI.[38] Thus, it is extremely unlikely that PCI will ever be demonstrated to decrease the incidence of future MI or death in patients with stable single-vessel coronary heart disease. Instead, its main role may be in improving anginal status and exercise capacity.

The Angioplasty Compared to Medical Therapy (ACME) study, published in 1992, remains the only true randomized trial comparing PCI (angioplasty alone without stenting) with medical therapy in the treatment of patients with stable angina and single-vessel coronary heart disease, regardless of the location of the stenosis.[39] The mean decreases in episodes of angina each month in the angioplasty and medical groups were 15 and 7, respectively ($p = .06$), and the mean decreases in number of nitroglycerin tablets taken each month were 15 and 7, respectively (p = not significant). Patients undergoing angioplasty had greater improvements in quality of life scores, in terms of both psychological well-being and physical functioning.[40] A price was paid, however, for this benefit, because a small number of patients in the angioplasty group suffered myocardial infarction or required emergency CABG or later repeat angioplasty. Thus, treatment with angioplasty led to a modest increase in exercise test duration and a modest improvement in anginal status, as well as quality of life scores, although some risk was associated with undergoing the procedure.

In the only other randomized study comparing balloon angioplasty with medical therapy, 214 patients with stenosis in the proximal LAD were enrolled in the Medicine, Angioplasty, or Surgery Study (MASS) study and followed for 3 years. The primary study end point was cardiac death, MI, or refractory angina requiring revascularization. In the angioplasty group, repeat angioplasty was not considered an end point because this was considered to be an accepted part of an angioplasty revascularization strategy. The primary end point occurred in 24% of angioplasty patients, 17% of medical therapy patients, and 3% of CABG patients. These differences were primarily attributable to the need for revascularization in patients who had undergone angioplasty or medical therapy; no significant differences were reported in mortality or infarction rates among the three groups. At 3-year follow-up, the percentages of patients in the angioplasty, medical therapy, and CABG groups who were angina free were 82%, 32%, and 98%, respectively.[9] The results of this study reinforce the ACME study finding that angioplasty of a stable coronary artery stenosis does not prevent future myocardial infarction or cardiac mortality but can improve anginal status.

No randomized trials have compared coronary stenting with medical therapy in patients with significant angina and stable coronary heart disease, nor are any likely to be conducted in the future.

Multivessel CHD

Only very limited data are available comparing PCI with medical therapy in patients with stable multivessel coronary heart disease. In a report based on prospectively collected data in nonrandomized patients, Mark and coworkers[38] compared 5-year survival probability in patients with multivessel coronary heart disease treated with PTCA, CABG, or medical therapy. Adjusted 5-year survival probabilities for patients with two-vessel disease were 91%, 90%, and 84%, respectively. Adjusted survival rates in patients with three-vessel disease were 81%, 87%, and 69%, respectively.

The investigators in the ACME study reported on 101 patients with two-vessel coronary heart disease who were randomized to angioplasty or medical therapy. At 6-month follow-up, there were no statistically significant differences in improvements in the balloon angioplasty or medically treated patients in exercise capacity as measured by treadmill testing (1.2 and 1.3 min, respectively), time to onset of angina during exercise testing (0.7 and 1.1 min, respectively), or freedom from angina (53% and 36%, respectively). There was also no significant difference between treatment with angioplasty or medical therapy in the decrease in monthly angina episodes achieved with these therapies or in quality of life scores.[41,42] No studies have compared coronary stenting with medical therapy in patients with stable multivessel coronary heart disease.

Seven major randomized trials have compared PCI with CABG in the treatment of patients with multives-

Table 2.1   Results of the Seven Major Randomized Trials Comparing PCI With CABG in Multivessel Coronary Artery Disease[a]

Trial	Follow-up (years)	Primary end point	PCI (%)	CABG (%)	Comments
ARTS[138]	1	Death, MI, CVA, TIA, need for repeat revascularization	26.2	12.2	Only trial to use routine stenting in PCI patients. The increased event rate in PCI patients was driven almost completely by a greater need for repeat revascularization; death, MI, and stroke rates were similar in the two groups.
BARI[5]	5	Death	13.7	10.7	(1) Largest of the randomized trials with longest follow-up period; (2) 5-year survival notably worse in diabetic patients treated with PTCA (65.5%) vs. those treated with CABG (80.6%); (3) repeat revascularization required in 54% of PTCA group vs. 8% of CABG group.
CABRI[6]	5	(1) Mortality	(1) 3.9	(1) 2.7	(1) Only 1 coronary lesion had to be suitable for PTCA in order to qualify for the study.
		(2) Symptom status (>CCS class I angina)	(2) 13.9	(2) 10.1	
EAST[10]	3	Death, Q-wave MI, or large ischemic defect on thallium	28.8	27.3	(1) Repeat revascularization procedures required in 54% of PTCA group vs. 13% of CABG group; (2) angina and need for antianginal medications more common in PTCA group; (3) activity level and employment status similar at 3-year follow-up.
ERACI[12]	1, 3[b]	Death, angina, or MI	47.0	77	(1) Recurrence of angina more frequent in PTCA group; (2) cumulative costs at 3-year follow-up notably higher in CABG group.
GABI[8]	1	Freedom from angina (<CCS class II)	71.0	74	(1) Study terminated prematurely when interim analysis showed the two treatment groups did not differ in regard to the primary end point; (2) internal mammary artery used in only 37% of CABG patients; (3) cumulative risk of death or MI at 1-year follow-up higher in CABG group (13.6%) than PTCA group (6.0%).
RITA[11]	2.5	Death or MI	9.8	8.6	(1) Trial included 45% of patients with 1VD; (2) in patients with 3VD, >63% of PTCA patients were completely revascularized (vs. 87% with CABG); (3) angina and use of antianginal drugs more common in PTCA group; (4) physical activity and employment status were similar at 2-year follow-up.

Note. ARTS = Arterial Revascularization Therapy Study; BARI = Bypass Angioplasty Revascularization Investigation; CABRI = Coronary Angioplasty vs Bypass Revascularization Investigation; EAST = Emory Angioplasty vs Surgery Trial; ERACI = Argentine Randomized Trial of Percutaneous Transluminal Coronary Angioplasty vs Coronary Artery Bypass Surgery in Multivessel Disease; GABI = German Angioplasty Bypass Surgery Investigation; RITA = Randomized Intervention Trial of Unstable Angina; PCI = percutaneous coronary intervention; CABG = coronary artery bypass graft surgery; MI = myocardial infarction; CVA = cerebrovascular accident; TIA = transient ischemic attack; PTCA = percutaneous transluminal coronary angioplasty; CCS = Canadian Cardiovascular Society; 1VD = one-vessel coronary artery disease; 3VD = three-vessel coronary artery disease.

[a]Only one trial, the ARTS trial, routinely used stent implantation in PCI patients; [b]interim analyses published at 1 and 3 years.

sel coronary heart disease (table 2.1). Only one of these studies was conducted in the modern era of coronary stent implantation and potent antiplatelet pharmacotherapy. In general, these studies found no significant differences in hard end points such as stroke, myocardial infarction, or cardiac mortality. Not surprisingly, the need for repeat revascularization was significantly higher in those undergoing angioplasty. As discussed later, only the BARI study suggested that CABG may lead to better outcomes in patients with diabetes.

Unstable Angina and Non-Q-Wave MI

Unstable angina is the clinical condition in which patients develop rest angina, usually caused by the rupture of a coronary plaque with subsequent thrombus formation that partially or temporarily occludes the involved coronary artery (refer to chapter 1). Non-Q-wave myocardial infarction (NQMI) similarly involves the development of rest angina, also believed attributable to plaque rupture and intracoronary thrombus formation. In NQMI, patients present without ST-seg-

ment elevation, do not develop pathological Q waves on the electrocardiogram (depending on how NQMI is defined), or both, but these patients do show enzymatic evidence of myocardial infarction (e.g., elevated levels of troponin or isoenzyme of creatine kinase with muscle and brain subunits). Unstable angina and NQMI are now considered part of a spectrum of disease states called acute coronary syndromes (ACS). Patients who develop rest angina and are without ST-segment elevation on the electrocardiogram are now said to have non-ST-segment-elevation acute coronary syndrome (NSTE-ACS). This terminology nuance is important because recent studies of PCI in unstable patients have included patients who were previously referred to as having either unstable angina or NQMI.

Four randomized trials have compared a treatment strategy of early cardiac catheterization and PCI (if indicated by findings on angiography) with a treatment strategy of initial medical therapy, with cardiac catheterization and revascularization only for recurrent angina symptoms (table 2.2). The first two of these

Table 2.2 Results of the Four Trials Randomizing Patients With Non-ST-Elevation Acute Coronary Syndromes to Either Early Invasive Strategy or Initial Medical Therapy

Study	Study design	Primary end point	Early invasive strategy	Initial medical therapy	p value	Comments
TIMI IIIB[43]	Unstable angina and NQMI patients	Death, MI, or positive ETT at 6 weeks	16.2%	18.1%	NS	Secondary end points, including hospital length of stay, need for rehospitalization, and number of antianginal medications were all lower in the early invasive group.
VANQWISH[137]	NQMI patients	Death or MI at 12 months	24.0%	18.6%	.05	The higher event rate in the early invasive group was driven by a high incidence of death in those who underwent CABG. There were no deaths in those who underwent PCI and were no differences in the composite end point at 3-year follow-up.
FRISC II[44]	Non-ST-elevation ACS	Death or MI at 6 months	9.4%	12.1%	.031	Secondary end points such as presence of angina and need for readmission were halved by an early invasive strategy. At 12-month follow-up, total mortality rate was lower in the early invasive group (2.2% vs. 3.9%, $p = .016$).
TACTICS-TIMI18[45]	Non-ST-elevation ACS	Death, MI, or rehospitalization for ACS at 6 months	16.5%	19.4%	.025	

Note. TIMI = Thrombosis in Myocardial Ischemia; VANQWISH = Veterans Affairs Non-Q-Wave Infarction Strategies in Hospital; FRISC = Fragmin and Fast Revascularization During Instability in Coronary Artery Disease; TACTICS-TIMI 18 = Treat Angina with Aggrastat and Determine Cost of Therapy with an Invasive or Conservative Strategy-Thrombolysis in Myocardial Infarction-18; NQMI = non-Q-wave myocardial infarction; MI = myocardial infarction; ETT = exercise tolerance test; NS = not significant; CABG = coronary artery bypass surgery; PCI = percutaneous coronary intervention; ACS = acute coronary syndrome.

studies, the Thrombosis in Myocardial Ischemia (TIMI) IIIB study[43] and the Veterans Affairs Non-Q-Wave Infarction Strategies in Hospital (VANQWISH) trial,[42] did not detect any significant difference in outcome between the two treatment strategies. The two more recent studies, the Fragmin and Fast Revascularization During Instability in Coronary Artery Disease (FRISC) II[44] and Treat Angina with Aggrastat and Determine Cost of Therapy with Invasive or Conservative Strategy-Thrombolysis in Myocardial Infarction-18 (TACTICS-TIMI 18) studies,[45] both enrolled patients with NSTE-ACS and randomized them to early or relatively early cardiac catheterization and revascularization or to initial medical therapy. Patients undergoing PCI were treated with more recent pharmacological and device advances, including potent platelet inhibitors and coronary stents in most cases.

At 1-year follow-up in FRISC II, patients treated with an early invasive strategy (catheterization and angioplasty), when compared with those treated with initial medical therapy, had a statistically significantly lower incidence of myocardial infarctions (8.6% vs. 11.6%), death (2.2% vs. 3.9%), and need for readmission (37% vs. 57%).[46] In TACTICS-TIMI 18, the combined 6-month end point of death, MI, or need for rehospitalization occurred in 15.9% of early invasive strategy patients and 19.4% of initial medical therapy patients, a statistically significant reduction in adverse events of 22%. The difference in outcome was particularly striking in patients who presented with enzymatic evidence of myocardial damage (elevated cardiac troponin levels), with event rates of 14.3% versus 24.2%, respectively, representing a reduction of 48%.[45]

These latter two more recent studies provide compelling data that patients who present with NSTE-ACS should preferentially be treated with a strategy of early catheterization and revascularization (assuming patients are reasonable candidates for revascularization), particularly if they have evidence of myocardial damage as evidenced by elevated cardiac troponin levels. This strategy was recently officially endorsed by a committee of experts from the American College of Cardiology (ACC) and American Heart Association (AHA).[47]

Primary Angioplasty

In the late 1980s and early 1990s, patients who presented with acute MI with ST-segment elevation on the electrocardiogram were usually treated with thrombolytic therapy, the administration of a potent "clot buster" that could restore normal blood flow in the occluded coronary artery in approximately 50% of cases. As experience with angioplasty grew, practitioners began to triage patients with ST-segment-elevation MI directly from the emergency room to the cardiac catheterization laboratory and mechanically open the occluded artery. This procedure became known as *primary angioplasty*. In the United States, approximately 20% of patients who present with ST-segment-elevation MI (or in current terms ST-segment-elevation acute coronary syndromes) are treated with primary angioplasty.

Seven randomized trials have been conducted comparing primary angioplasty with thrombolytic therapy in ST-segment-elevation MI patients. These studies were generally performed during the early 1990s, during which period the potent antiplatelet agents available today were not present, and equipment used in the procedure was less advanced than that currently available. Nevertheless, in the majority of these trials, patients treated with primary angioplasty tended to have lower mortality rates than those treated with thrombolytic therapy (figure 2.9).[36] When the results of these trials were combined, major end points were consistently statistically significantly lower in the primary angioplasty group compared with the thrombolytic group (figure 2.10).[48] In the United States, primary angioplasty is often used preferentially if patients present to a hospital that is equipped to perform angioplasty and if the patient can be quickly brought from the emergency room to a ready catheterization laboratory.

Complications and Considerations

Most PCI are performed without significant peri- or postprocedural complications. However, there are several complications and safety issues for health care professionals, particularly those involved in cardiac rehabilitation or exercise training.

Vascular Complications

Some degree of bleeding in the groin area may occur during and shortly after the PCI procedure. Although the presence of ecchymosis (a purplish discoloration of the skin resulting from bleeding in the superficial layers of tissue) in the days to weeks after PCI is not uncommon and does not warrant further evaluation, the finding of a very tender or tense groin or thigh area may reflect significant bleeding into the deeper tissues of the body and should be assessed before an exercise program is begun.

A femoral pseudoaneurysm can form postprocedure after the sheath used during the PCI procedure is removed from the femoral artery. Instead of the artery sealing at the site of sheath insertion, a communication forms between the artery and the overlying fibromuscular tissue, resulting in a blood-filled cavity (figure 2.11). The reported incidence of pseudoaneurysm ranges from 0.5% to 6.3%.[49] A painful or tender groin, a palpable pulsatile mass, or a bruit in the groin area may suggest the presence of a pseudoaneurysm. Because there is a small but real risk that a pseudoaneurysm may rupture and lead to significant bleeding, patients in whom a pseudoaneurysm is suspected should undergo an ultrasound examination before engaging in an exercise program.

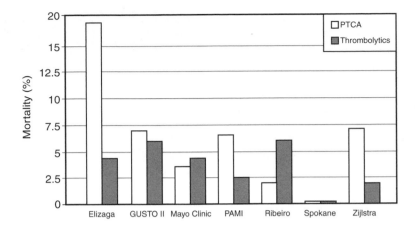

Figure 2.9 In-house (all trials except GUSTO IIb) or 30-day (GUSTO-IIb) mortality rates in the seven randomized trials of primary angioplasty (percutaneous transluminal coronary angioplasty, PTCA) versus thrombolytic therapy in patients with acute ST-segment elevation myocardial infarction (ST-segment-elevation acute coronary syndrome). GUSTO = Global Utilization of Strategies to Open Occluded Coronary Arteries; PAMI = Primary Angioplasty in Acute Myocardial Infarction.

Reprinted, by permission, from G.H. Levine et al., 1997, "The role of percutaneous revascularization in the treatment of ischemic heart diseases," *Chest* 112: 805-821.

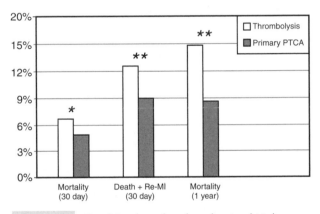

Figure 2.10 Combined results of randomized trials comparing primary angioplasty (percutaneous transluminal coronary angioplasty, PTCA) with thrombolytic therapy. There are statistically significant lower rates in primary angioplasty-treated patients for 30-day mortality, 1-year mortality, and 30-day mortality or reinfarction. MI = myocardial infarction; * = P=0.02; ** = P=0.01.

Adapted, by permission, from K.B. Michels et al., 1995, "Does PTCA in acute myocardial infarction affect mortality and reinfarction rates?" *Circulation* 91: 476-485.

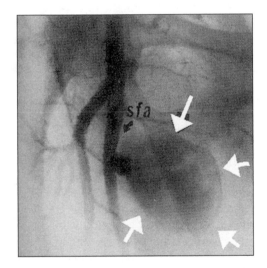

Figure 2.11 Angiogram revealing a large pseudoaneurysm (white arrows) arising off of the superficial femoral artery (sfa).

Adapted, by permission, from J.J. Skillman, D. Kim, and D.S. Braim 1988, "Vascular complications of percutaneous femoral cardiac interventions. Incidence and operative repair," *Archives of Surgery* 123: 1207-1212.

An arteriovenous fistula can result from sheath-mediated communication between the femoral artery and femoral vein. The presence of an arteriovenous fistula may be suggested by the presence of a bruit and confirmed by Doppler ultrasound examination. The reported range of arteriovenous fistula is 0.2% to 2.1%.[49,50] A large arteriovenous fistulae can result in decreased arterial blood flow to the affected leg through a "steal phenomenon" and can, at least in theory, lead to claudication in that leg.

Stent Subacute Thrombosis and Thienopyridine Therapy

Because many patients referred for cardiac rehabilitation and exercise training will have undergone a recent PCI with coronary stent implantation, health care professionals must understand the phenomenon of stent thrombosis and thienopyridine therapy in the period after stent implantation. Stent thrombosis is the process in which the implanted coronary stent "clots off," occluding the coronary artery. Stent thrombosis is a catastrophic complication, associated with 30-day mortality rates in recent series of up to 26%.[51-53] Stent thrombosis most frequently occurs in the first days to weeks after stent implantation. *Acute thrombosis* is the occurrence of thrombosis of the implanted stent within the first 1 to 2 days after the PCI procedure; *subacute thrombosis* is the occurrence of thrombosis of the stent in the days to weeks after stent implantation.

Early attempts to prevent stent thrombosis through the use of intensive anticoagulation were associated with extremely high bleeding complication rates and unacceptable rates of stent thrombosis.[54-59] Improvements in stent deployment technique,[50-62] as well as the use of antiplatelet therapy, have decreased the incidence of stent thrombosis to approximately 1%.[51,63-69] Paramount in antiplatelet therapy is the use of a thienopyridine, an oral antiplatelet agent somewhat more potent than aspirin. In early studies, the thienopyridine used was ticlopidine (Ticlid).[67,68,70,71] More recently, the thienopyridine of choice is clopidogrel (Plavix).[65,66,72-77] Because subacute thrombosis occurs during the days to weeks (or months on rare occasions) after stent implantation, most patients are now treated with at least 3-6 months of clopidogrel therapy (in addition to indefinite aspirin therapy). The risk of subacute stent thrombosis is not a contraindication to exercise training, but patients who report abrupt onset of significant or severe angina should be immediately evaluated to ensure they are not suffering stent thrombosis. Although the risk of bleeding is probably slightly increased by both aspirin and clopidogrel therapy, such therapy must not be stopped under any circumstances in the first 2 to 4 weeks after stent implantation without consultation with the interventional cardiologist who performed the stent procedure.

Restenosis

Restenosis is the process in which a treated artery narrows over time. Restenosis is believed to occur because of negative arterial remodeling (arterial "constriction"), intimal hyperplasia, and other complex processes.[78-80] Although most patients who develop restenosis will manifest symptoms, a small percentage of patients who develop angiographic restenosis will remain asymptomatic. The restenotic process occurs over the first 1 to 8 months after PCI. Because of this, most patients with symptomatic restenosis manifest symptoms during a similar time frame.[81-83] The presenting symptom for the majority of patients with restenosis is exertional angina, with much fewer patients presenting with unstable angina and only rarely with acute myocardial infarction (table 2.3).[81,84-91] Most patients who present between 1 and 8 months after PCI with recurrence of typical anginal chest pains will be found to have restenosis.[92]

Table 2.3	Clinical Presentations of Patients With Restenosis From Combined Data
Symptom	**Occurrence (%)**
Asymptomatic	1.4-20.0
Exertional angina	28.0-85.5
Unstable angina	11.3-41.0
Acute myocardial infarction	1.0-6.0

Adapted from reference 80. [80,84,85,88-91]

The incidence of clinical restenosis (i.e., restenosis causing clinical symptoms) in patients who were treated with balloon angioplasty alone is approximately 25% to 40%.[54,58,93-106] No systemically administered pharmacological agent has been convincingly demonstrated to decrease restenosis. Novel revascularization devices such as directional coronary atherectomy (DCA), rotational atherectomy (Rotablator), laser atherectomy, and cutting balloon have never been clearly demonstrated to decrease restenosis compared with plain balloon angioplasty.[29,78,107,108] The greatest advance in decreasing restenosis was the introduction of coronary stents. Early studies comparing coronary stenting with plain balloon angioplasty demonstrated that implantation of a coronary stent could reduce the incidence of restenosis by approximately one third.[54,58] Most recent trials that have enrolled patients treated with coronary stents report repeat revascularization rates of only approximately 10% to 20%.[106,109-122]

"Drug-eluting" stents are coated with a drug that decreases the restenosis process. The drug elutes from the implanted stent over a period of weeks to months, into the walls of the coronary artery, and inhibits the processes (such as intimal hyperplasia) that lead to restenosis.[123,124] Drugs that have been shown to be beneficial in clinical studies include rapamycin and paclitaxol. In clinical studies, implantation of a drug-eluting stent has been shown to decrease the incidence of restenosis to approximately 5% to 8%. Patients who are treated with drug-eluting stents require longer-term antiplatelet therapy, usually at least 3 to 6 months of clopidogrel (Plavix) plus aspirin, because of the possible risk of late stent thrombosis. Other than this, patients are treated in a manner similar to other patients who undergo percutaneous coronary revascularization.

Cost remains the main issue limiting the use of drug-eluting stents. The cost of a drug-eluting stent is approximately $2,700 to $3,100 (although this may decrease a little over time as competition increases among companies), compared with the cost of a "bare metal" stent of between $800 and $1,500. In Canada and Europe, the percentage of patients that receive drug-eluting stents varies widely. The majority of patients who now receive coronary stents, receive drug-eluting stents.

The prognosis of patients with asymptomatic restenosis (i.e., restenosis that would be demonstrated by angiography but does not manifest itself clinically) is generally excellent.[81,125-128] Using routine exercise testing to detect restenosis in the months after PCI has not been shown to be of general benefit and is not recommended[77,129,130] (although exercise testing may be indicated before patients begin formal cardiac rehabilitation programs). Even many patients who develop restenosis with just mild exertional anginal symptoms can continue to be treated medically and do not necessarily need to be referred for repeat revascularization.[81]

Exercise and Cardiac Rehabilitation

There is a paucity of formal recommendations regarding when post-PCI patients can begin exercise programs. Balady and colleagues[131] demonstrated that in patients who had undergone uncomplicated balloon angioplasty, treadmill exercise testing (Bruce protocol) could be performed safely as early as 1 to 3 days (38 ± 14 hr) postprocedure. The study, performed during the relatively early days of coronary angioplasty, demonstrated that such exercise testing could allow physicians to recommend patients return to various activities at an earlier date.[131] With much more experience available in the post-PCI management of patients undergoing PCI, such testing is not usually required or performed in the immediate post-PCI period.

In patients in whom restenosis is a concern, simple electrocardiographic treadmill testing has proven to be an insensitive predictor of restenosis and has little clinical utility.[77,81,132] For this reason, patients undergoing stress testing in the evaluation of possible restenosis should be referred for an imaging study. Such studies include nuclear imaging studies,[77,81,130,133,134] for which there is the most experience, or a stress echocardiogram study.[81,135,136]

Patients who have undergone recent cardiac catheterization and PCI, were found to have no other significant stenoses other than the one treated by PCI, had an uncomplicated PCI, have no other significant cardiac disease (e.g., severely depressed ejection fraction, significant valvular disease), and do not have significant exertional angina (or any rest angina) may not require formal stress testing evaluation before beginning exercise programs. At my institution, most patients who undergo PCI, assuming they have not suffered a recent myocardial infarction, are instructed not to perform any heavy lifting for 2 days (so that their femoral arteries and groins can heal adequately) and then resume all normal activities (including work and sexual relations). In patients who have suffered a recent myocardial infarction, have complex or extensive coronary heart disease, or have significantly depressed left ventricular ejection fraction or valvular heart disease, I recommend stress testing before initiation of an exercise program.

Summary

Dramatic changes in technology, pharmacotherapy, and knowledge, as well as an accumulation of experience, have expanded the number of patients who can be treated with coronary revascularization procedures, who have decreased adverse outcomes, and who have improved long-term benefit. Both CABG and PCI can improve anginal status and exercise capacity. Important considerations in the post-PCI patient relevant to cardiac rehabilitation include groin status, the risk of subacute thrombosis, and the phenomenon of restenosis. In post-CABG subjects, important considerations include sternal healing and stability, deconditioning, postoperative atrial fibrillation, and graft occlusion. With proper evaluation and only modest special considerations, however, both groups of patients should be able to participate in cardiac rehabilitation and exercise training.

Efficacy of Secondary Prevention and Risk Factor Reduction

Jeffrey L. Roitman, EdD, and Thomas P. LaFontaine, PhD

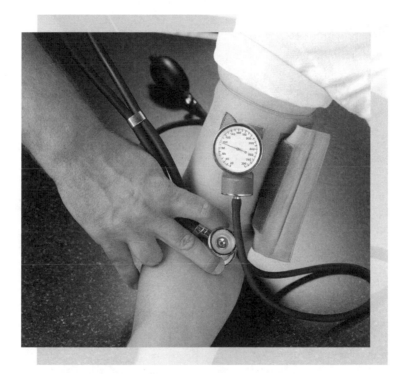

Secondary prevention is the process of reversing or stabilizing underlying disease to reduce the risk of subsequent events. Studies of secondary prevention of coronary heart disease (CHD), including meta-analyses of cardiac rehabilitation and exercise, consistently indicate that prevention of mortality and morbidity is achievable.[1-3] Both prescription drug (e.g., statins, β-blockers, angiotensin-converting enzyme [ACE] inhibitors, aspirin) and lifestyle therapies have been shown to reduce morbidity and mortality rates in populations with cardiovascular disease.[4,5] Lifestyle therapies include diet, exercise, stress management in the form of meditative or relaxation exercises, weight loss and control, smoking cessation, and limiting alcohol intake. Table 3.1 is a compilation of important secondary prevention studies.

Established risk factors (RFs) for CHD are shown in table 3.2 and appendix A. The Framingham Heart Study is a comprehensive, long-term epidemiological study of CHD risk that has elucidated RFs.[6,7] A recent

study reinforces the RF theory and its application to large populations. The study also supports the notion that RFs are important by showing that more than 90% of attributable risk can be accounted for in modifiable risk factors, which are discussed later. This is in direct contradiction to information previously published that attributed 50% or less of the risk to these factors. The important conclusion is that CHD is preventable and that established risk factors are the culprits to attack.[8]

RFs have been classified in various ways, but the American Heart Association (AHA) provides one of the most common classifications—"major" RFs for CHD (see table 3.2). A landmark publication from the 27th Annual Bethesda Conference of the American College of Cardiology (ACC) specifically addressed efficacy of intervention in RFs.[9] This conference categorized risk according to the availability and strength of the evidence "for which interventions have been proved to lower CVD risk." Recently, the ACC convened the

Table 3.1　Secondary Prevention Studies

Study	Study group	Intervention	Event reduction (%)
O'Connor GT[2]	Meta-analysis	Cardiac rehabilitation	–20%
Oldridge NB[1]	Meta-analysis	Cardiac rehabilitation	–20%
Hammalainen H[17]	MI patients	Exercise and physical activity	–37% (sudden death)
SCRIP[11]	Patients with CHD	Multiple risk factors with usual care vs. risk reduction	–36%
STARS[4]	Patients with CHD	Diet; diet + cholestyramine	–71% in diet-only group
DART[46]	Patients with CHD	Fish oils or 1,500 mg omega-3 supplement	–34%
Lifestyle Heart Trial[12]	Patients with CHD	Exercise, <10% fat diet, weight loss, stress management	–60%
Heidelberg[23]	Patients with CHD	Exercise, <20% fat diet	NS
Lyon Heart Study[45, 47]	Patients with CHD	Mediterranean-type diet	–72%
4S[31]	Patients with CHD	Lipid lowering—simvastatin	–35%
LIPID Trial[5]	Patients with CHD	Lipid lowering—pravastatin	–25%
GISSI[39]	Patients with CHD	Omega-3 supplement—1 g/day	–45%

Note. MI = myocardial infarction; CHD = coronary heart disease; NS = no significant difference; SCRIP = Stanford Coronary Risk Intervention Project; STARS = St. Thomas Atherosclerosis Trial; DART = Diet and Reinfraction Trial; 4S = Scandinavian Simvastatin Survival trial; LIPID = Long-term Intervention with Pravastatin in Ischemic Disease; GISSI = Gruppo Italiano per lo Studio della Sopravvivenza nell'Infarto Miocardico.

33rd Bethesda Conference on Preventive Cardiology.[10] The conference addressed the fact that primary and secondary prevention of CVD still has not established an appropriately strong position in the overall care of patients with CVD. The conference provided precise recommendations regarding how providers can better implement programs for the prevention of CHD. Cardiac rehabilitation (CR) professionals need to become intimately familiar with this report.

RFs are "associated" with CHD but do not necessarily cause the disease. RFs may be divided into those that are amenable to change and those that are not (see table 3.2). However, the major, traditional RFs identified by AHA and the ACC are all independently related to risk of CHD. Additionally, patients may exhibit any combination of risk factors; thus, prioritizing risk is important with respect not only to the efficacy of intervention but also to the behavioral aspects of changing long-standing, complex behaviors (see table 3.3).

There are complex and variable interactions among and between RFs; for example, obesity affects blood pressure, diabetes, blood lipids, ability to exercise, thrombogenic risk factors, and even endothelial function. Effective management of several risk factors simultaneously affects risk to a greater extent than single RF intervention. In addition, treating an emerging RF (e.g., high blood levels of homocysteine) may have less influence on overall risk than treating one or more of the major risk factors. The literature leads to the conclusion that aggressive intervention with as many RFs as possible is the most efficacious approach.[3,11-14] Indeed, aggressive lipid lowering may be more efficacious than even invasive treatments for CHD.[15,16] However, management of and intervention with multiple RFs are complex and difficult. Risk for CHD is almost always multifactorial and requires aggressive and persistent management for optimal secondary prevention.

GUIDELINES, 4TH EDITION

- Chapter 5, 7, and 8

Cardiac Rehabilitation

Meta-analyses of randomized, controlled trials of outpatient CR demonstrate a 25% reduction in long-term, all-cause, and cardiovascular mortality rates.[1,2] Hamalainen and colleagues,[17] in a 15-year follow-up of a randomized trial of CR, reported a 37% reduction in sudden death among post–myocardial infarction (post-MI) patients who participated in a comprehensive CR program. A recent prospective study of men with documented CHD reported that those who remained active over the follow-up period had a reduced risk of mortality of 30% to 79%. Men who became active during the follow-up period had a 44% lower risk of combined fatal and nonfatal

Table 3.2   Risk Factors for Coronary Heart Disease

Risk factor	Amenable to change	Evidence for association	Efficacy of intervention
Smoking[a]	Yes	+++	Proven to lower risk
Hypertension[a]	Yes	+++	Proven to lower risk
LDL cholesterol [a]	Yes	+++	Proven to lower risk
High-fat diet	Yes	+++	Proven to lower risk
Left ventricular hypertrophy	Yes	+++	Proven to lower risk
Thrombogenic risk factors	Yes	+++	Proven to lower risk
Diabetes mellitus[a]	Yes	+++	Likely to lower risk
Inactivity[a]	Yes	+++	Likely to lower risk
HDL cholesterol	Yes	+++	Likely to lower risk
Triglycerides, small dense LDL	Yes	++	Likely to lower risk
Obesity[a]	Yes	+++	Likely to lower risk
C-reactive protein (hs-CRP)	Yes	++	Unknown
Postmenopausal status	No	+++	HRT trial failed
Psychosocial factors	Yes	++	Might lower risk
Lipoprotein(a)	Yes	+	Might lower risk
Homocysteine	Yes	++	Might lower risk
Oxidative stress	Yes	+	Might lower risk
Lack of alcohol consumption	Yes	+++	Unknown
Age	No	+++	NA
Male gender	No	+++	NA
Low socioeconomic status	No	+++	NA
Family history	No	+++	NA

Note. LDL = low-density lipoprotein; HDL = high-density lipoprotein; CRP = C-reactive protein; HRT = hormone replacement therapy; NA = not applicable.

[a]Major risk factors according to American Heart Association classification ("high cholesterol" replaced by LDL).

CHD events.[18] Another recent study of Hispanic and non-Hispanic men and women participating in CR demonstrated a 60% to 78% lower risk for reinfarction among patients who entered CR and remained active throughout a 7-year follow-up period.[19] Other prospective studies have shown a strong relationship between directly measured maximal oxygen uptake and survival in patients with documented CHD.[20,21] Finally, a recent randomized trial of prognosis post-MI reported that exercise training favorably modified long-term survival provided that it was associated with a clear shift of the autonomic nervous system toward an increase in vagal activity.[22] Several comprehensive and randomized secondary prevention trials of lifestyle management of CHD also have shown significant reductions in clinical events in intervention compared with the control or usual care groups (see table 3.4).[11,12,23] In summary, recent interventional and epidemiological trials have established the efficacy of physical activity and comprehensive CR in reducing the risk of mortality and morbidity among patients with documented CHD (see table 3.5).

Smoking

Smoking has long been known to be a significant, major risk factor for CHD. Two Surgeon General's Reports have centered on the health risks associated with smoking.[24,25] Smoking interacts with other risk factors to affect plaque stability, endothelial function, and thrombogenesis, and thus smoking can amplify other risk factors.[26] Smoking cessation decreases both mortality and morbidity rates.[27] Smoking is closely

Table 3.3   Methods for RF Intervention

Major risk factor	Behavioral methods	Pharmacological agents	Efficacy
Smoking	Counseling	Buproprion, nicotine replacement	Lifestyle: + Medication: ++
Hypertension	Diet, exercise, weight loss, relaxation, omega-3 fatty acids	Many	Lifestyle: ++ Medication: ++
LDL cholesterol	Diet, exercise	Statins	Lifestyle: ++ Medication: ++
High-fat diet	Diet		Lifestyle: ++
Left ventricular hypertrophy	HTN control, diabetes, weight loss, exercise	ACE inhibitors, angiotensin receptor blockers	Lifestyle: + Medication: ++
Thrombogenic risk factors	Exercise, diet, weight loss	ASA, other antiplatelets	Lifestyle: ++ Medication: ++
Diabetes mellitus	Diet, exercise, weight loss	Insulin and many oral agents	Lifestyle: ++ Medication: ++
Inactivity	Exercise	NA	Lifestyle: +++
HDL cholesterol	Diet, smoking cessation, weight loss	Nicotinic acid, fibrates, statins	Lifestyle: ++ Medication: ++
Triglycerides, small dense LDL	Diet, exercise, weight loss, omega-3 fatty acids	Nicotinic acid, fibrates, statins	Lifestyle: ++ Medication: ++
Obesity	Diet, exercise, counseling	Orlistat, meridia	Lifestyle: +++ Medication: +
Postmenopausal status	NA	HRT (limited recommendations)	Medication: ++
Psychosocial factors	Stress management, counseling	Many	Lifestyle: ++ Medication: +
Lipoprotein(a)	None known	Nicotinic acid, fibrates	Lifestyle: NA Medication: +
Homocysteine	DASH diet	Folate, B_6, B_{12} vitamins	Lifestyle: ++ Medication: +
Oxidative stress	Diet, exercise	Numerous vitamins, supplements—vitamin E, C, selenium, CoQ10, lipoic acid, grape seed extract	Lifestyle:++ Medication: +

Note. LDL = low-density lipoprotein; HDL = high-density lipoprotein; HTN= hypertension; NA = not applicable; DASH = Dietary Approaches to Stop Hypertension; ACE = angiotensin-converting enzyme; ASA = acetylsalicylic acid (aspirin); HRT = hormone replacement therapy. The + signs indicate the strength of the effect.

Table 3.4   Reduction in Cardiac Events in Five Key Secondary Prevention Lifestyle Trials

Study	N	Control events	N	Intervention events	% Reduction	Risk ratio
LHT[1]	25	45	20	20	−60	0.36
Heidelberg[2]	53	19	43	20	NS	1.30
SCRIP[3]	155	34	145	20	−36	0.57
STARS[4]	28	10	27	3	−71	0.31
Lyon[5]	204	90	219	27	−72	0.28

Note. LHT = Lifestyle Heart Trial; SCRIP = Stanford Coronary Risk Intervention Project; STARS = St. Thomas Atherosclerosis Trial; Lyon = Lyon Diet Heart Study; NS = no significant difference. Risk ratio <1.0 indicated reduction in clinical events in the intervention group; >1.0 indicates an increase in intervention group.

Table 3.5	Diet, Exercise, and Weight Loss in Five Key Secondary Prevention Studies								
Study	Calories	% Fat	% SF	% MUFA	% PUFA	Fiber	Cholesterol	Exercise	Weight loss
LHT[1]	1,884	8.2	2.5	NA	NA	NA	18.6	3.6 hr·week^{-1}	5.8 kg
Heidelberg[2]	NA	<20	<7	NA	NA	NA	<200	~2.5-3.0	NA
SCRIP[3]	NA	23.8	6.8	NA	NA	NA	143.4	NA	3.0 kg
STARS[4]	NA	27.0	7.0	12.1	8.0	3-6 g per 1,000 kcal	~180	NA	NA
Lyon[5]	1,947	30.4	8.0	13.0	5.0	18.6 g·day^{-1}	203	NA	NA
Mean	1,916	21.9	6.3	12.6	6.5	NA	149	3.18 hr·week^{-1}	4.4 kg (9.7 lb)

Note. SF = saturated fats; MUFA = monounsaturated fats; PUFA = polyunsaturated fats; LHT = Lifestyle Heart Trial; SCRIP = Stanford Coronary Risk Intervention Project; STARS = St. Thomas Atherosclerosis Trial; Lyon = Lyon Diet Heart Study; NA = not applicable.

related to and interacts with blood pressure, sedentary lifestyle, diabetes (especially in women), dyslipidemia, and thrombogenic risk factors.

Methods for intervention include both lifestyle and pharmacological interventions. Counseling and formal cessation programs have been shown to be effective, but long-term recidivism is high. The Agency for Health Care Policy and Research (AHCPR) Report on Smoking Cessation states that more than 70% of the 50 million smokers in the United States made at least one prior quit attempt; 46% of smokers attempt to quit each year. The recidivism rate appears to be almost 93% at 1 year after the attempt to quit.[28] More recently, pharmacological intervention with nicotine patches or gum and buproprion (Zyban) has been shown to be effective.[29] Long-term compliance to smoking cessation remains a problem, probably because it is both chemically and behaviorally addictive at various levels.

Dyslipidemia

The National Cholesterol Education Program (NCEP), Adult Treatment Panel III (ATP III) recently issued new guidelines for lipids and lipid management.[13] Serum cholesterol, low-density lipoprotein (LDL), high-density lipoprotein (HDL), and other lipoproteins have been shown to be independently related to incidence of CHD. Both primary and secondary prevention clinical trials of lipid lowering therapy have proven to be efficacious in preventing morbidity and morality from cardiovascular disease.[4,13,30-32] See table 3.6 for NCEP ATP III goals for lipoproteins.

Intervention methods necessarily include both lifestyle modification (diet, exercise, tobacco use cessation, and weight loss) and drugs. Lifestyle modification can

Table 3.6	Adult Treatment Panel III Goals for Patients With CHD and CHD Equivalent
Lipid	Goal (mg·dl^{-1})
Cholesterol	<200
LDL	<70[a]
HDL	>40
Triglycerides	<150
Non-HDL cholesterol	<130

Note. LDL = low-density lipoprotein; HDL = high-density lipoprotein.

[a]Amended July 2004

be successful but may also be quite difficult for patients without assertive and aggressive long-term reinforcement of dietary changes. It appears that the content of the diet, outside total fat and saturated fat content, can be quite helpful in altering lipid profile. Table 3.7 summarizes dietary changes that can be efficacious in altering lipid profile. See table 3.3 for efficacy and methods for intervention in lipid RFs.

Diet

Dietary intervention (usually a step 1 AHA diet) has been part of virtually all prospective trials using lipid-lowering drugs. Major statements from AHA, ACC, and other organizations all recommend dietary intervention in secondary prevention of CHD.[33-38] Standard dietary intervention produces mild to moderate effects in lipid alteration but potentiates the effects of pharmacological therapy.[39] Exercise therapy also potentiates the effect of diet and lipid-modifying drugs.[40,41]

Table 3.7   Dietary Recommendations

Statement/study	Dietary fats	Other recommendations
AHA/ACC Secondary Prevention Guidelines	Fat: NR SAFA: <7% total calories TC: <200 mg·day^{-1}	Consume omega-3 fatty acids Increase physical activity Lose weight
AHA Dietary Guidelines	Fat: NR SAFA: <7% total calories TC: <200 mg·day^{-1}	Monitor patients on very low fat diets (<15% calories) for increased triglycerides and decreased HDL
NCEP ATP III	Fat: 25-35% total calories SAFA: <7% total calories TC: < 200 mg·day^{-1} MUFA: up to 20% total calories PUFA: up to 10% total calories	Recommendations about fiber (20-30 g/day), total calories (balanced with activity), and protein (15% total calories); additionally trans fatty acids and carbohydrates are included; moderate exercise (200 kcal·day^{-1})
Guide to Preventive Cardiology for Women	Fat: <30% total calories SAFA: <7% total calories TC: <200 mg·day^{-1}	Limit sodium intake (<6 g·day^{-1}) Dietary fiber 25-30 g·day^{-1} >5 servings fruits, vegetables/day
MUFA statement	MUFA: 15% total calories PUFA: 10% total calories SAFA: <8% total calories	NA
Dietary fatty acids statement	Increase: MUFA, PUFA, omega-3 fats Decrease: SAFA	NA
Stanol-sterol statement	Those with dyslipidemia and CHD may include for secondary prevention (2-4 g·day^{-1})	NA
Fish consumption/omega-3 statement	Increased intake of omega-3 fatty acids, especially EPA, DHA	Intake of ALA also recommended in prevention efforts (both secondary and primary)

Note. AHA/ACC = American Heart Association/American College of Cardiology; NCEP ATP III = National Cholesterol Education Program Adult Treatment Panel III; TC = total cholesterol; CHD = coronary heart disease; HDL = high-density lipoprotein; ALA = alanine aminotransferase; EPA = eicosapentaenoic acid; DHA = docosahexaenoic acid; NR = no recommendation; NA = not applicable; MUFA = monounsaturated fatty acids; PUFA = polyunsaturated fatty acids; SAFA = saturated fatty acids; Stanol-Sterol = incorporated into food (mainly margarine) from soybean and pine tree oil.

More aggressive dietary changes (similar to step II AHA or the diet described in NCEP ATP III) produce significantly greater improvements in lipids, although there is large variability in response.[41] Recently, recommendations for dietary intervention have broadened and include significantly more than limiting dietary fat and saturated fat. Recommendations for incorporation of selected types of fat, addition of fiber, and other nutrients have become standard for lowering and control of lipids (see table 3.7).[36,37,42]

The AHA has issued several statements regarding dietary macronutrients with respect to cardiovascular disease, blood lipids, and disease prevention.[33-37] The epidemiological literature shows that diets should contain monounsaturated (MUFA) and polyunsaturated fatty acids (PUFA) in place of saturated fatty acids (SAFA) and hydrogenated and partially hydrogenated fats; that refined carbohydrates should be limited and replaced by whole grains, fruits, vegetables, and nuts; and that omega-3 fats from fish oil or plant sources should be increased.[42-44] SAFA should be limited to <7% of total calories. The Lyon Diet Heart Study and the Diet and Reinfarction Trial (DART) are landmark trials of dietary intervention in secondary prevention of CHD.[45] The replacement of saturated and hydrogenated fats with monounsaturated, polyunsaturated, and particularly omega-3 fats has been shown to lower cholesterol, triglycerides, and LDL and to modestly raise HDL and is associated with lower all-cause and cardiovascular mortality rates in patients with CHD.[44,46] Intervention with a Mediterranean-style diet lowered risk of recurrent events by 50% to 70% in the intervention group of the Lyon trial, whereas the DART trial reported a 32% reduction in recurrent cardiac events with just two fatty fish meals per week.[44,46,47] It appears that this high MUFA, PUFA, omega-3, and soluble fiber diet using a variety of fresh fruits and vegetables, along with whole grains and increased omega-3 fatty acids from fish consumption, is an excellent tool for both lipid alteration and secondary prevention.

LDL Cholesterol

Total cholesterol remains an important risk factor for CHD in ATP III, although not a primary treatment goal. It may be used in the risk estimate tables for secondary prevention.[13] ATP III emphasizes that LDL is the "primary target" of lipid-lowering therapy for CHD. Oxidized LDL has potent negative effects on endothelial function and plaque stability. Modifying blood levels of LDL, both concentration and particle size, has been shown to be effective in lowering both mortality and morbidity rates.[13,48]

The target LDL for secondary prevention is <70 mg·dl^{-1} in high-risk persons and in those with diagnosed CHD.[49] Tables 3.8, 3.9, 3.10, and 3.11 summarize the effects of various pharmacological agents on LDL

and other lipids. Exercise, a low-fat diet, and modification of the type of dietary fat consumed have been shown to lower LDL as well as have positive effects on other lipids. Other therapeutic options for lowering LDL include the addition of soluble fiber, plant stanols-sterols, and monounsaturated fatty acids.[36,37,50] Aggressive lifestyle management for LDL should be a central part of all secondary prevention of CHD.[49]

HDL Cholesterol

Raising the proportion of HDL cholesterol is also a major objective of lipid management. The Veterans Affairs High-Density Lipoprotein Cholesterol Intervention Trial (VA-HIT) involving patients with known CHD recently showed a 22% reduction in mortality

Table 3.8   Summary of Statins

Available drugs	Lovastatin, pravastatin, simvastatin, fluvastatin, atorvastatin, rosuvastatin
Major use	To lower LDL cholesterol
Lipid/lipoprotein effects	LDL cholesterol: decreased 20-60%
	HDL cholesterol: increased 5-15%
	Triglycerides: decreased 10-40%
Contraindications	Active or chronic liver disease
Use with caution	Concomitant use of cyclosporine, fibrates, or nicotinic acid—increased risk of myopathy
	Known interaction with grapefruit and grapefruit juice
Reduce CHD risk	Yes
Long-term safety	Evidence from >15 years of extensive clinical use and in up to 6-year controlled trials
Major adverse side effects	Elevated hepatic transaminase, myopathy, and upper and lower gastrointestinal complaints
	Statin + anticoagulant may increase prothrombin time, may deplete coenzyme Q

Note. LDL = low-density lipoprotein; HDL = high-density lipoprotein; CHD = coronary heart disease.

Table 3.9   Summary of Bile Acid Sequestrants

Available drugs	Cholestyramine, colestipol
Major use	To lower LDL cholesterol
Lipid–lipoprotein effects	LDL cholesterol: decreased 10-20%
	HDL cholesterol: increased 3-5%
	Triglycerides: may increase
Contraindications	Familial dysbetalipoproteinemia
	Triglycerides >500 mg·dl^{-1}
Use with caution	Triglycerides >200 mg·dl^{-1}
Reduce CHD risk	Yes
Long-term safety	Yes
Major adverse side effects	Upper and lower gastrointestinal complaints Decreased absorption of other drugs Pancreatitis in patients with hypertriglyceridemia

Note. LDL = low-density lipoprotein; HDL = high-density lipoprotein; CHD = coronary heart disease.

Table 3.10   Summary of Nicotinic Acid

Available drugs	Crystalline nicotinic acid, niaspan Sustained-release (or slow-release) nicotinic acid (not FDA-approved); Niaspan is an intermediate-release, FDA-approved formulation
Major use	Useful in most lipid and lipoprotein abnormalities
Lipid/lipoprotein effects	LDL cholesterol: decreased 10-25% HDL cholesterol: increased 15-35% Triglycerides: decreased 20-50%
Contraindications	Chronic liver disease
Use with caution	Non-insulin-dependent diabetes mellitus, gout, or hyperuricemia
Reduce CHD risk	Yes
Long-term safety	Yes for nicotinic acid, Advicor, and Niaspan
Major adverse side effects	Flushing, hepatotoxicity (especially for sustained-release form), hyperglycemia, hyperuricemia or gout, and upper gastrointestinal complaints

Note. FDA = Food and Drug Administration; LDL = low-density lipoprotein; HDL = high-density lipoprotein; CHD = coronary heart disease.

Table 3.11   Drug Selection for Combination Therapy

Lipid levels	Single drug	Combination drugs
Elevated LDL cholesterol and triglycerides <200 mg·dl⁻¹	Statin Nicotinic acid BAS	Statin + BAS Statin + nicotinic acid[a] Nicotinic acid + BAS
Elevated LDL cholesterol and triglycerides 200-400 mg·dl⁻¹	Statin Nicotinic acid	Statin + NA[a] Statin + gemfibrozil[b] Nicotinic acid + BAS Nicotinic acid + gemfibrozil
Elevated LDL cholesterol and low HDL	Advicor[c] (lovastatin–niacin combination drug)	Nicotinic acid + mevacor

Note. LDL = low-density lipoprotein; HDL = high-density lipoprotein; BAS = bile acid sequestrant.

[a]Possible increased risk of myopathy and hepatitis; [b]increased risk of myopathy, must be used with caution; [c]Advicor is the first combination drug approved by the Food and Drug Administration for treatment of dyslipidemias.

rate for a 6% increase in HDL with Lopid therapy.[51] Low HDL cholesterol is related to the prevalence of CHD even when optimal levels of total cholesterol and LDL are present.[13] Raising apolipoprotein A-I (the primary protein in the HDL molecule) and overall HDL cholesterol and changing the ratio of HDL to total cholesterol (or to LDL) are effective secondary prevention tools.

Initial approaches to raising HDL cholesterol include exercise, weight loss, and smoking cessation. Drug therapy may also be appropriate depending on success with lifestyle intervention. Tables 3.8 and 3.9 show some pharmacological methods for raising the level of HDL cholesterol.

Non-HDL Cholesterol

ATP III also recommends using "non-HDL" cholesterol as a secondary goal, particularly in patients with triglycerides >200 mg·dl⁻¹ and those patients with the metabolic syndrome (three or more of the following: abdominal obesity, elevated triglycerides, low HDL cholesterol, elevated blood pressure, and insulin resistance).[13] Non-HDL has recently been suggested to be a better predictor of cardiovascular risk than LDL.[52] Non-HDL cholesterol consists of all atherogenic lipoproteins (LDL, very low density lipoprotein [VLDL], intermediate-density lipoprotein [IDL], and lipoprotein(a) [Lp(a)]) except HDL. Non-HDL cholesterol can be measured by subtracting HDL from total cholesterol, both of which can be determined reasonably accurately in a nonfasting blood sample. The targets for non-HDL cholesterol are then calculated by adding 30 to the standard LDL targets.

Triglycerides

ATP III has changed recommendations concerning triglycerides. Triglycerides should be assessed in all persons with CHD, particularly those with the metabolic syndrome and diabetes mellitus. Diabetes is a "CHD equivalent" in ATP III; that is, patients with diabetes have equivalent risk for a cardiac event as patients with known CHD. Elevated triglycerides are an independent RF for CHD, and both lifestyle and pharmacological therapies are recommended depending on the level. The presence of elevated triglycerides with elevated LDL (combined dyslipidemia) is an especially ominous combination, because much of the LDL is likely to be of the "small dense" variety that is quite atherogenic.[13]

Exercise, low-fat diet, weight loss, and avoidance of alcohol, caffeine, simple carbohydrates, and processed or refined carbohydrates are effective lifestyle interventions for lowering triglycerides. Tables 3.10 and 3.11 provide general guidelines for medical therapy.

Diabetes Mellitus

Diabetes mellitus (DM; both type 1 and type 2) is considered a "CHD equivalent" in the most recent statements and treatment guidelines issued by the AHA/ACC and American Diabetes Association as well as ATP III.[13,53,54] Management of RFs in people with DM but without CHD should be as aggressive as in those with documented CHD. All RFs should be addressed and intervention recommendations strongly advised. Patient follow-up in this population must be aggressive and frequent.[53,54]

DM can markedly accelerate atherogenesis through predisposition to inflammatory reactions, endothelial dysfunction, and oxidation reactions.[53,54] Hyperglycemia is associated with dyslipidemia, metabolic dysfunction, and insulin resistance and deficiency, all of which predispose individuals to atherogenesis. Treatment of both hyperglycemia and other RFs, including aggressive treatment of lipids with exercise, diet, and

medication, is indicated. See the following discussion of obesity and metabolic syndrome.

Obesity and Metabolic Syndrome

The association of obesity, defined by a body mass index (BMI) of >30, with increased risk for CHD is well established.[55] However, the association of obesity with many of the RFs for CHD (e.g., diabetes mellitus, blood pressure, and dyslipidemia) confounds the issue. Obesity is related to endothelial dysfunction in those with normal or mildly diseased coronary arteries.[56] Studies have shown that the risk ratio of individuals with obesity in the presence of any of the aforementioned RFs is increased approximately 1.5 to 5.5 times.[57] Central obesity (increased waist girth and waist-to-hip ratio) seems to be related to these risk factors (especially in women) as does increased insulin resistance, although some studies have suggested that the association is correlative and not causative.[58,59]

Both the ATP III and Joint National Committee on Prevention, Detection, Evaluation and Treatment of High Blood Pressure (JNC VII) statements recognize the significant, and perhaps central, role that the metabolic syndrome occupies in cardiovascular risk.[13,60,61] The ATP III defined the metabolic syndrome as the presence of three or more of the following conditions:

- Abdominal obesity: waist circumference greater than 102 cm (40 in.) in men and greater than 88 cm (35 in.) in women
- Glucose: fasting glucose greater than or equal to 110 $mg \cdot dl^{-1}$ or 6.1 $mmol \cdot L^{-1}$
- BP: 130/85 mm Hg or more
- High triglycerides: greater than or equal to150 $mg \cdot dl^{-1}$ or 1.70 $mmol \cdot L^{-1}$
- Low HDL cholesterol: less than 40 $mg \cdot dl^{-1}$ or 1.04 $mmol \cdot L^{-1}$ in men and less than 50 $mg \cdot dl^{-1}$ or 1.30 $mmol \cdot L^{-1}$ in women

Related to the fasting blood glucose value used in the definition of metabolic syndrome, the American Diabetes Association (ADA) recently established the clinical identification value of 110 $mg \cdot dl^{-1}$ or more.[62]

Intensive lifestyle changes should be strongly recommended and pursued in all persons with CHD who have metabolic syndrome. Drug therapy should be instituted as necessary to improve each of the components.

Although no prospective clinical trials have shown that weight loss changes mortality rates in patients with CHD, many studies have shown that weight loss positively affects RFs that are associated with obesity.[63] Additionally, it is well documented that "moderate" weight loss (5-10% of total body weight) is sufficient to positively affect these RFs.[10,63] Wing and others have demonstrated that weekly caloric expenditure of more than 2,000 kcal/week is necessary to sustain significant weight loss.[63,64] In the recently published Diabetes Prevention Study of more than 3,000 patients at risk for diabetes, there was a 58% reduction in new cases of type 2 diabetes over 3 years in the group that lost 7% of body weight, exercised 30 min, 5 days per week, and consumed a low-fat, high-fiber diet.[63] Remarkably, in the subgroup of those older than 55 years, there was a 70% reduction in new cases of type 2 diabetes. The lifestyle changes were nearly twice as effective as the diabetic drug, Metformin, in preventing the onset of diabetes. Secondary prevention programs are clearly obligated to include weight control and weight loss interventions as part of their services. Successful weight loss programs include both dietary intervention (both type and amount of food intake) and exercise and activity components.[63] Increased exercise and activity are strong, long-term predictors of maintenance of weight loss.[65,66]

Hypertension

National guidelines for blood pressure are published by the Joint National Committee on Prevention, Detection, Evaluation and Treatment of High Blood Pressure.[60] Table 3.12 provides JNC VII recommendations for blood pressure. The efficacy of lowering blood pressure for secondary prevention is well established.[60] JNC VII recommends using lifestyle measures for blood pressure treatment in those with "prehypertension" and oral antihypertension drugs in combination with lifestyle treatment in those with stage 1 hypertension or greater (table 3.12). JNC VII also advises this more aggressive step in those with "compelling indications" as defined in that report. Blood pressure is closely related to, and interacts with, cigarette smoking, dyslipidemia, and diabetes.[67] See table 3.3 for methods and efficacy for lowering elevated blood pressure.

Blood pressure is affected by diet, exercise, weight loss, and moderate alcohol consumption. Modification of lifestyle through improved diet, increased physical activity, and weight control is the cornerstone of effective management of hypertension.[60,67] The Dietary Approaches to Stop Hypertension (DASH) diet has been shown to be efficacious not only for controlling blood pressure but also for improving blood lipids and homocysteine levels and is a highly recommended tool.[60,67-69] The 1,600 mg·day^{-1} sodium restriction of this diet is lower than other recommendations but has been shown to be more effective in lowering blood pressure.[67] The diet includes increased fiber and complex carbohydrates, calcium, and potassium consumption, along with reduced fat and saturated fat compared with the AHA Step One diet or, especially, the average American diet. A recent meta-analysis showed that increased physical activity is effective in lowering both systolic and diastolic blood pressure in both genders of all ethnic groups and in older adults.[70]

Sedentary Lifestyle

Aside from the meta-analyses showing that exercise intervention (with cardiac rehabilitation—see preceding section) reduces mortality, many studies indicate that regular exercise is an effective measure in both primary and secondary prevention and that fitness level is a powerful predictor of mortality.[20,21,71-73] Epidemiological studies have demonstrated that more than 1,250 to 2,000 kcal of excess energy expenditure per week is necessary to raise $\dot{V}O_2$max in CHD patients as well as to provide a cardioprotective effect and to stabilize or reverse CHD.[23,74,75] (See chapter 5 for further discussion.)

Recent statements by the American College of Sports Medicine (ACSM), ACC, AHA, and others have called for daily (or "almost every day") exercise and activity.[76-79] It appears that the benefits of aerobic exercise training in secondary prevention of CHD events accrue from both the long-term (e.g., increased fitness level, improved lipid profile, and reduced inflammation) and short-term (e.g., acute improvement in endothelial function, blood pressure, blood glucose, and insulin sensitivity) benefits. Thus, a combination of regular structured exercise aimed at increasing fitness level and increased daily lifestyle physical activity appears necessary to obtain the greatest efficacy. Although 3 days per week is sufficient to raise fitness level, it may be inadequate to provide benefits for secondary prevention of CHD. Total weekly caloric expenditure in excess of 1,500 to 2,000 kcal may be necessary for this benefit. This level of activity and exercise requires approximately 4 to 6 hr per week of some combination

Table 3.12	Classification of Blood Pressure for Adults	
Category	Systolic (mm Hg)	Diastolic (mm Hg)
Normal	<120	<80
Prehypertension	120-139	80-89
Stage 1 hypertension	140-159	90-99
Stage 2 hypertension	>160	>100

From Van Horn 1997.

of structured exercise and increased lifestyle activity.[79] This has been supported recently by data showing that higher intensity, higher duration ("higher amount of exercise") exercise was more effective in changing lipoprotein concentration.[80]

It now appears that the efficacy of exercise in the prevention of CHD may be attributable, in part, to its effects on endothelial function. Acute and chronic exercise has positive effects on endothelial dysfunction in both larger conduit and smaller resistance arteries.[81,82] In both animals and humans, exercise and exercise training enhance vasodilation, improve endothelial dysfunction, and effect genetic expression of substances (endothelial nitric oxide synthase and other substances) that control endothelial function.[81,83]

A tool that may be useful in encouraging lifestyle activity and in progressive walking programs for patients is a step-counting pedometer. Walking has been shown to be related to reduced mortality rates from cardiovascular disease.[84-86] Programs using these pedometers have been successful in promoting the adoption and maintenance of physical activity among sedentary populations.[87] Secondary prevention programs should progress patients through levels of exercise and lifestyle activity (from sedentary to moderately active lifestyles through active, exercising lifestyles) using these tools. Combining structured exercise with increased lifestyle activity is often necessary to achieve the desired caloric output of 1,500 to 2,000 kcal or more per week.

Psychosocial Dysfunction

Psychosocial factors including depression, anger, hostility, and stress have all been shown to be related to increased mortality and morbidity rates.[88-90] It has also been shown that patients with depression and other confounding psychosocial stressors are less likely to adhere to programs of risk reduction and intervention, thus perhaps also negatively affecting mortality and morbidity secondary to the inability to follow such RF intervention.[90] Assessment of psychosocial function and status and referral to counseling and therapy when indicated and appropriate are among the recommended guidelines for Secondary Prevention programs by the AACVPR.[91]

There are few randomized, prospective trials using psychosocial intervention in CHD patients that show reduced morbidity and mortality. It has been shown that intervention with stress management techniques does decrease events in cardiac patients when compared with exercise training.[92-94] Treatment of chronic depression and other psychosocial stressors in patients with CHD is clearly indicated and should be recommended. (See chapter 4 for further discussion.)

Other Risk Factors

Studies suggest that more than 90% of CHD can be explained by traditional risk factors.[8] However, other factors may contribute to an increased risk for developing CHD. Some of these factors may be contributory, whereas others are physiological markers that may signal increased risk for CHD. As more data are collected and a more complete understanding of each of these factors is developed, some of them may be added to the list of established risk factors.

Genetics

The current expansion of genetic information related to the decoding of the human genome and burgeoning research associated with genetics is bringing a wealth of information about genetic connections to disease. Family history is informative, especially history of premature CHD in first-degree relatives. Williams[95] reported a 1.7 to 12.9 relative risk for CHD among those with a family history, defined as a male or female blood relative less than 55 years of age with a history of CHD. It appears that genetic risk may decline with age, but the attributable risk is highest from 55 to 74 years, when the prevalence of the disease is also highest.[95]

Phenotypes are strongly determined, genetic "measurable traits" for example, Lp(a). The genetic influence for Lp(a) is high in humans, but other lipoprotein types may be less significant. For example, the genetic influence of LDL cholesterol is less than 50%.[95] Identifying these highly abnormal traits in individuals with disease, especially in first-degree relatives, is important. It is estimated that 5% to 10% of CHD cases can be accounted for by monogenic disorders. However, many of these disorders are also magnified in the presence of lifestyle risk factors.

A gene may exist functionally in different forms, called polymorphisms or genotypes. Predisposition to CHD is probably associated with the interaction of these genotypes and the environment that is imposed on them (i.e., lifestyle). Lifestyle clearly affects prevalence of CHD in individuals, and genotype may represent the greatest amount of the genetic influence. Stampfer and colleagues[96] recently reported that 82% of CHD cases among 84,000 female nurses were attributable to a high-risk lifestyle. The Framingham study and others have shown that among persons with a family history of premature CHD, the risk is substantially reduced for those with an overall favorable risk profile, suggesting the effectiveness of preventive measures in persons with and without a positive family history.[6,97]

Heredity of disease can essentially be divided into two broad categories—(a) major monogenic diseases such as Huntington's chorea, LDL-receptor deficiency, cystic fibrosis, and Duchenne's muscular dystrophy, and (b) polygenic diseases that occur when multiple polymorphisms are inherited predisposing persons to a chronic disease such as CHD. Polygenic diseases result in "susceptibility" to a chronic disease such as atherosclerosis and type 2 diabetes mellitus, particularly when the genetic component is superimposed on environmental RFs such as obesity, physical inactivity, high-fat diet, or tobacco use.

In summary, the vast majority of CHD is caused by the interaction between genotype–phenotype (genetics) and RFs (environment). The prevailing theory is that multiple, common genotypes may have relatively small effects by themselves, but when high-risk lifestyles are superimposed, they account for the majority of atherosclerotic events. A recent study showed that classic, remedial risk factors are highly prevalent among patients with familial premature CHD.[98] The authors concluded that a "major contribution of genes acting in the absence of these traditional risk factors is unlikely."[98(p. 683)]

Thus, lifestyle and environmental factors exert a much greater influence on the risk of atherosclerosis than genetics. This understanding provides a powerful rationale for the aggressive lifestyle management of RFs in the secondary prevention of CHD.

Thrombogenesis

Several markers of thrombogenesis, such as elevated plasma levels of fibrinogen, Lp(a), factor VII, plasminogen activator inhibitor (PAI-1), and increased platelet aggregation, have been shown to be predictors of CHD-related events. Genetics, low levels of exercise, a high-fat diet, and increased triglycerides have all been documented to be associated with elevated plasma fibrinogen and increased clotting risk.[99] Controlled trials of both aspirin and anticoagulants in patients with CHD have shown significant benefits for both mortality and morbidity rates.[9] Exercise and diet have both been shown to favorably affect thrombogenesis, but neither has been shown in large, randomized, prospective clinical trials to affect morbidity and mortality rates specifically through the antithrombogenic effects. The ACC and the AHA consider low-dose (85 mg) or regular-dose (325 mg) aspirin to be considered standard practice for postmyocardial infarction patients, for patients with medically treated CHD, for patients post-coronary artery bypass graft (CABG), and for adult men and postmenopausal women.[3,33]

Postmenopausal Status

Hormone replacement therapy (HRT) has been a topic of some controversy for the past few years. The AHA recently recommended that HRT not be used in women with heart disease for purposes of secondary prevention of CHD because of the findings of a large, prospective study of HRT.[100,101] This statement, along with others, strongly recommends that previously established preventive therapies, including lifestyle approaches, be discussed, advised, and implemented as preventive measures in all women, including those with CHD.[100-102] However, postmenopausal women with elevated Lp(a) may benefit from HRT. Estrogen is known to decrease this highly atherogenic lipoprotein.[103] (See chapter 9 for further discussion.)

Endothelial Dysfunction

In persons without atherosclerosis, the predominant effect of endothelial activation and release of nitric oxide is vasodilation. Endothelial injury and denudation result in "dysfunction," which may be an initiating event in atherogenesis. In fact, endothelial dysfunction precedes the physical appearance of atherosclerosis on angiography.[104] Ludmer and colleagues[103] demonstrated paradoxical coronary vasoconstriction in "visually" normal coronary arteries of CHD patients in response to intracoronary acetylcholine. Rozanski and colleagues[104] recently compared finger blood flow responses to treadmill exercise in CHD patients and healthy volunteers. Fifty-three percent of the CHD patients demonstrated a progressive vasoconstriction, indicative of endothelial dysfunction, compared with none of the healthy participants. Although no randomized clinical trial has yet demonstrated a reduced risk for coronary events in CHD patients following treatment to improve endothelial dysfunction, several recent prospective studies have shown a significantly increased risk of future coronary events was independent of traditional risk factors in patients with and without CHD and endothelial dysfunction.[107,108]

Most traditional and nontraditional risk factors have been shown to be associated with impaired vascular endothelial function. Many of the risk factors initiate an inflammatory response within the vasculature that precedes endothelial dysfunction, which in turn precedes even the earliest stages of formation of atherogenic lesions.[109-111] Endothelial dysfunction is prognostic for myocardial infarction.[112-119] Numerous studies have demonstrated that intervention in these risk factors improves endothelial function.[120-124] The following box summarizes interventions that have been shown to attenuate endothelial dysfunction.

Both acute and chronic exercise positively affect endothelial dysfunction in persons with diagnosed CHD and other cardiovascular and metabolic disease.[125-132] Hambrecht and colleagues[121,122] demonstrated that aerobic exercise training improves endothelial dysfunction in CHD patients with and without left ventricular (LV) dysfunction. Others have shown that

Interventions Demonstrated to Improve Endothelial Dysfunction

- LDL lowering with pheresis
- LDL lowering by statins and other
- LDL lowering by low-fat diet
- ACE inhibitors and ACE II receptor blockers
- L-arginine
- Moderate alcohol intake
- Thermal therapy
- Purple grape juice
- Iron chelation

- Tea
- High monounsaturated fat diet
- Low-fat, high complex carbohydrate diet
- Folic acid
- Smoking cessation
- Antioxidant therapy
- Aerobic exercise training
- Weight loss

exercise training improves endothelial dysfunction in patients with DM and hypertension and in sedentary, middle-aged adults.[125-133] In secondary prevention of CHD, measures known to improve endothelial function should be initiated. These measures (see the box) coincide with RF interventions that most, if not all, CHD patients undertake.

High Sensitive C-Reactive Protein

High sensitive C-reactive protein (hs-CRP) is a marker of low-grade systemic inflammation that has been shown to predict both first and recurrent CHD events.[134-136] Recently, a study of patients with severe peripheral vascular disease demonstrated that hs-CRP is a strong predictor of MI during 6 months of follow-up.[137] In patients with known CHD, the European Concerted Action on Thrombosis and Disabilities Study (ECAT) showed that for each standard deviation increase in hs-CRP, there was a 45% increase in risk of MI or sudden death.[138]

Ridker and colleagues[139] recently published epidemiological data showing that CRP is a better predictor of CHD events than LDL and recommended screening for CRP level, perhaps in conjunction with LDL as a strong predictor of subsequent events. The American Heart Association and the Centers for Disease Control and Prevention recommended that hs-CRP be a recommended adjunct for risk stratification in persons in the 10% to 20% risk range for an event.[140] Thus, it appears that hs-CRP may be a useful prognostic marker for recurrent CHD events and should be considered for measurement and treatment in those with established disease. This consideration, however, raises the key question of whether lowering hs-CRP reduces the risk for recurrent event and, if so, what treatments are most effective. Aspirin, statins (as a class), and weight loss and physical activity have been shown to lower hs-CRP.[141] In secondary analyses of randomized trials, aspirin and statins have been associated with lowered hs-CRP and reduced risk of events.[137,141]

The results of specifically designed randomized clinical trials are needed to establish the role of treating hs-CRP in secondary prevention. There are no standardized guidelines for the measurement and treatment of hs-CRP. In addition, the specific roles of tobacco cessation, exercise, diet, weight loss, and other lifestyle factors are undetermined. Recently, physical activity and cardiovascular fitness have been shown to be positively correlated with decreased incidence of high hs-CRP in middle-aged and older men and women.[142,143] Fortunately, many of the standard therapeutic interventions including aspirin and statins are indicated for other purposes in those with known CHD.

Homocysteine

McCully[143] first reported an association between elevated homocysteine (Hcy) and atherosclerosis, and since that study, Hcy has been shown to be a relatively strong and independent risk factor for atherosclerotic cardiovascular disease.[144-146] Elevated Hcy is associated with endothelial dysfunction, increased arterial intimal wall thickness, arterial wall stiffening, and procoagulant activity.[147]

A major cause of hyperhomocysteinemia is vitamin deficiencies, particularly folic acid, B_6, and B_{12}. Recently several studies have shown that lowering Hcy reduces restenosis postpercutaneous coronary intervention, decreases signs and symptoms of ischemia, and improves endothelial dysfunction.[148-152] Although no definitive randomized controlled trial has demonstrated decreased morbidity and mortality following Hcy lowering, Rosenberg[152] suggested that Hcy should be measured in patients with known atherosclerosis and in those at high risk for vascular disease. Where indicated, appropriate treatment includes 400 to 1,000 μg of folic acid and B_6 and B_{12} if necessary to effectively lower Hcy.[153] For secondary prevention, Chai and Abrams have recommended treating the following patients with folate supplementation:[154]

- Smokers
- Patients with adverse CHD risk profile
- Patients with prior revascularization
- Patients with multivessel disease
- Patients with severe dyslipidemia

These recommendations seem reasonable in light of the efficacy, safety, and low cost of therapy.

Lipoprotein(a)

Prospective studies report a positive correlation between Lp(a) and CHD.[155] Lp(a) is known to accumulate in atherosclerotic lesions and appears to interact with hyperhomocysteinemia to promote a procoagulant state and thrombosis.[156,157]

It has also been suggested that Lp(a) may not be an independent risk factor but rather potentiates the effects of other lipid risk factors. LDL cholesterol and Lp(a) have been shown to act in the development of CHD, whereas other studies have shown that Lp(a) may counteract the beneficial effects of high HDL cholesterol.[158-160] The Atherosclerosis in Communities (ARIC) study suggested that Lp(a) is an independent risk factor for atherosclerosis and is associated with much higher risk ratios in Caucasian women.[161] Von Eckardstein and colleagues[161] showed that Lp(a) was especially predictive of CHD events among men with high LDL cholesterol, low HDL cholesterol, hypertension, or an overall high global risk for CVD.[162] Recently, the Heart and Estrogen/Progestin Replacement Study (HERS) showed a 17% to 21% increased risk for CHD among women in the highest quartile of Lp(a).[163]

Although routine screening of Lp(a) in either primary or secondary prevention is not recommended by any professional statement, some suggest measuring Lp(a) in patients with premature atherosclerosis and patients with a high global risk for a first or recurrent cardiac event.[155] Estrogen and niacin are the only agents that have been shown to effectively lower Lp(a). The effects of lifestyle changes such as diet, weight loss, and physical activity on Lp(a) are not well defined.

Until results from randomized clinical trials are complete, it is recommended that the focus of therapy be on global risk as determined by traditional risk factors. In patients with high levels of Lp(a) (>20 mg·dl⁻¹), targeted therapy with niacin or estrogen in postmenopausal women may be warranted.

Pattern B Dyslipidemia

Approximately 80% of patients who develop CHD have similar serum cholesterol levels as those who do not develop CHD.[164] Additionally, in secondary prevention trials of lipid lowering and reduction in CHD events, a large percentage of the patients in the treatment groups achieve a large reduction in blood cholesterol but still have recurrent coronary events. This is partially related to the fact that LDL is not one homogenous lipoprotein but a spectrum of heterogeneous particles.[164] Two major subspecies of LDL have been identified. In most healthy persons, the major subspecies is large and buoyant, whereas the smaller, dense LDL subspecies is generally present in small amounts.[164] The dense LDL subclass pattern, also referred to LDL pattern B, is a heritable trait.[164] Several studies have shown that this pattern is a powerful predictor of CHD risk, independent of triglycerides, HDL, LDL, and body mass index.[48,165] Angiographic studies of interventions in patients with documented CHD have shown that the patients who exhibited plaque regression had significantly greater reductions in dense LDL particles compared with those who showed progression.[166]

LDL pattern B trait is associated with elevated levels of triglycerides, very low density lipoproteins, and intermediate-density lipoproteins; decreased levels of HDL and insulin resistance; and enhanced postprandial lipemia.[164] In general, the higher the triglycerides and the lower the HDL levels, the greater the likelihood that the LDL particles are predominantly small and dense. Fifty percent of men with CHD have LDL pattern B trait characterized by a predominance of small, dense LDL particles.[164]

Physical training, weight loss, low-fat diet, nicotinic acid, and fibric acid derivatives are effective in improving LDL pattern B trait.[164] In one trial of lipid management in a lipid clinic–cardiac rehabilitation program, 52% of patients had LDL pattern B.[167] In this program, management of lipoprotein abnormalities was based on an algorithm that incorporated sophisticated lipid measurement and management.

In summary, the small, dense LDL pattern B appears to be the most common lipid disorder found in CHD patients. Many patients with CHD would benefit from more sophisticated measurement of lipid status. Fortunately, many of the standard recommendations for secondary prevention, such as exercise, diet, and weight loss, are effective in improving this condition.

Optimizing Secondary Prevention

Numerous studies show the relative ineffectiveness of traditional care in managing CHD risk factors.[168-176] These and other large-group studies of persons with known disease (including CHD, diabetes, and hypertension) show varying rates of poorly treated or untreated RFs. One recent report showed that approximately 31% of diagnosed hypertensive patients (~30% are undiagnosed), 12% of dyslipidemic patients (53% are undiagnosed), and 22% of diabetic patients (33% are undiagnosed) are adequately controlled to target as recommended by national standards and guidelines.[176]

Statements by the AACVPR, the Agency for Health Care Policy and Research (AHCPR), the AHA, and others call for aggressive management of traditional RFs including a recent call for a new paradigm–delivery model for cardiovascular rehabilitation (CVR) programs.[90,177-180] A model for risk stratification of patients entering CVR has been published and recommended in the AACVPR guidelines.[90,180] Optimizing secondary prevention requires the following:

1. Stratification of patients at entry for risk of disease progression
2. Assessment of readiness to improve each risk factor
3. Individually targeted therapy according to needs and readiness
4. Aggressive follow-up until treatment targets are achieved

A comprehensive, integrated approach to risk factor management is essential. Case management models have demonstrated superior outcomes with improving RFs, reducing or reversing disease progression, and preventing clinical events.[11,48,181-184] Two seminal case management trials (the Stanford Coronary Risk

Intervention Project [SCRIP] and MULTIFIT) demonstrated the efficacy of this method. With persistent and long-term follow-up (up to 3 years in SCRIP), results demonstrate markedly improved RF management, decreased progression of CHD, and reduced mortality and morbidity rates compared with usual care. Case management performed by allied health care professionals (RNs in this case) was used, and patients were managed to aggressive lipid, exercise, and medication regimen goals. Some of the pertinent results of SCRIP are summarized in table 3.13. Appendix C gives outcome goals according to major statements concerning risk factors from several different national organizations and groups. The end products are compliant patients, with changed behaviors (eating, activity, medication compliance), reduced RFs, and reduced events. Although reproducing clinical trial protocols in everyday clinical practice is challenging, it is a national imperative for CVR to develop and implement such comprehensive disease management programs.

Recently, an evidence-based, comprehensive CHD risk reduction program incorporating lifestyle management interventions (based on several behavior change theories including social learning, transtheoretical learning, and single concept learning) was shown to be efficacious.[183-185] This program uses a computerized patient management and tracking system and is delivered by nonphysician health care personnel (clinical exercise physiologists, registered dietitians, registered nurses) in a community setting and in a cost-effective manner. The results demonstrate comparable clinical

Table 3.13 Selected Results on Risk Factors From the Stanford Coronary Risk Intervention Project (SCRIP) Study

Variable	Risk reduction group	Usual care group
Total fat calories (%)	23.8	32.7
Saturated fat calories (%)	6.8	10.6
Dietary cholesterol (mg/day)	143.4	270.7
Tobacco use (%)	10.1	18.1
Exercising regularly (%)	90	70
% on lipid modifying medications	93.3	30.7
Body weight	−4%	+1%
Max exercise capacity (METs)	+1.7	+0.7
LDL cholesterol (mg·dl⁻¹)	−36	−6
HDL cholesterol (mg·dl⁻¹)	+5	+2
Triglycerides (mg·dl⁻¹)	−33	+2
SBP (mm Hg)	−1	+3
Fasting blood glucose (mg·dl⁻¹)	−3	+7
Total cardiac hospitalizations	25	44

Note. METs = metabolic equivalents; LDL = low-density lipoprotein; HDL = high-density lipoprotein; SBP = systolic blood pressure.
From Haskell et al. 1994.

outcomes, compared with either a contemporary cardiovascular rehabilitation program or a case management program supervised by a physician but case-managed by a nurse. In fact, all groups significantly improved most outcome measures. The community-based model and the contemporary CVR model demonstrated significantly increased functional capacity compared with the physician-supervised, nurse-managed model.[182-185] This model may be preferable in many settings, because it can be delivered in a variety of venues, including CVR programs, physician practices, worksites, health clubs, and in the home via electronic methods. In light of data showing that only 8% to 38% of patients with documented CHD enter traditional, exercise-based CVR (far fewer receive aggressive secondary prevention), this model may be of particular value in expanding patient access to an affordable and clinically effective secondary prevention program.[179,186]

A systematic review of randomized clinical trials (RCTs) of disease management programs in persons with documented CHD reported improved processes of care and better outcomes compared with usual care.[186] A total of 12 RCTs were identified and included in the review. Patients in disease management programs were more likely to be on efficacious medications including lipid-lowering agents, β-blockers, and antiplatelets. Rehospitalization rates were significantly lower in the interventions groups (risk ratio = 0.84, confidence interval 0.76-0.94). Most of the trials also reported enhanced quality of life and functional status and improved control of CVD risk factors. Finally, in a study comparing three groups treated with combined lipid-lowering drugs and lifestyle modification, those patients with the most aggressive changes in lifestyle (diet and exercise and weight loss) had significantly decreased events associated with their CHD as well as decreased perfusion abnormalities in follow-up positron emission tomography (PET) scans. Thus, the efficacy of aggressive lifestyle modification coupled with appropriate lipid-lowering therapy is confirmed.[187]

New, evolving models of secondary prevention must be incorporated into the current paradigm for cardiovascular rehabilitation services and programs. Usual care does not work. Traditional, exercise-based CVR programs are not as effective as either a case management model or an expanded model of lifestyle management and disease state management. It is incumbent on cardiovascular rehabilitation professionals to advocate aggressive, lifestyle management of as many risk factors as possible for the most efficacious results in secondary prevention of CHD. Specific implementations of intervention goals for individual risk factors are given in table 3.14. The most effective guidelines, treatments, behavioral modifications, and follow-up to reduce events are known. Implementation of those guidelines, treatments, and delivery models is a major task for cardiac rehabilitation and secondary prevention specialists.

Table 3.14   Specific Risk Factor Recommendations for Secondary Prevention

Risk factor	Recommendation
Smoking	Complete cessation of all tobacco use
Obesity	Isocaloric diet if BMI <25.0 Hypocaloric diet if BMI >25.0
Exercise	Weekly caloric expenditure ≥2,000 kcal Resistance training 2-3 days per week
Hypertension	BP <120/80 Sodium intake <1,500 mg·day^{-1}
Lipids	All lipids at ATP III goals
Diet	Fat = 15-25% of total calories SAFA <5% MUFA = 5-12% PUFA = 5-10% (omega-3 fatty acids) Cholesterol <150 mg·day^{-1} Include functional foods, e.g., stanols, increased soluble fiber
Stress	Acquire some kind of stress management skill and practice 5-7 days per week Therapy and counseling as indicated and required Remain socially connected, avoid isolation Control anger, hostility
Emerging risk factors	Assess CRP, Lp(a), and Hcy in premature CHD, or in absence of other major risk factors Recommend daily multiple vitamin tablet with B vitamins and folic acid

Note. BMI = body mass index; BP = blood pressure; ATP = Adult Treatment Panel; SAFA = saturated fats; MUFA = monounsaturated fats; PUFA = polyunsaturated fats; CRP = C-reactive protein; Lp(a) = lipoprotein a; Hcy = homocysteine. For patients with diabetes mellitus, management of both blood glucose (or HbA1c) and multiple risk factors is extremely important in reducing risk.

From Smith et al. 1995.

4

Psychosocial Issues and Strategies

Matthew L. Herridge, PhD, and John C. Linton, PhD

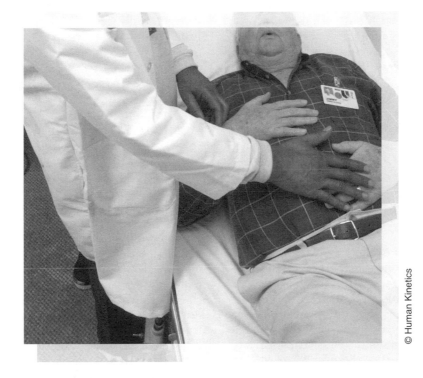

© Human Kinetics

There is an intimate connection between the mind and the heart. Depression, hostility, anxiety, and stress are implicated as strong predictors of health outcomes in patients with cardiovascular disease.[1-6] The patient's gender, age, social support, and factors such as motivation and self-efficacy may reduce or increase his or her psychological difficulties. A comprehensive cardiac rehabilitation program should offer individual participants a plan of care where all of these issues are considered. Patients should find a place where both their medical and psychological needs are understood and appropriate assistance is provided. It would be a mistake to underestimate the degree to which patients may look to you for this assistance. Early identification of participants' psychological needs can allow for multidisciplinary staff involvement with the first cardiac rehabilitation contact. Ideally, psychosocial screening of participants in cardiac rehabilitation should be completed on orientation. Cardiac rehabilitation staff should understand

the means of assessment for this important domain, and the coordination of treatment should be as seamless as possible.

An extensive body of research demonstrates that emotional states, personality patterns, behavior, social support, and cardiovascular reactivity likely interact with one another and affect the development and progression of heart disease. The mechanisms by which depression, anxiety, hostility, and stress may negatively influence cardiovascular functioning are complex, varied, and, in some cases, controversial. Ornish[7] posited a twofold process theory to best explain this relationship. First, chronic sympathetic nervous system activation creates a "toxic" cardiovascular climate.[7] Emotional difficulties have been shown to produce autonomic nervous system changes that can lead to decreased immune functioning, lipid level elevations, and changes in neurotransmitters. Individuals who are in a constant state of autonomic arousal caused by unbridled stress or poor coping are at increased risk for this toxic cardiac climate. A second line of research investigation has suggested that psychological problems can lead to reduced adherence to prescribed medical regimens as well as the pursuit of unhealthy behaviors such as the use of tobacco products, poor dietary habits, a sedentary lifestyle, and even substance abuse. For example, hostile individuals are more likely to smoke,[8] and depressed participants are less likely to complete lifestyle modification programs compared with those who are not depressed.[9]

The Ornish[7] comprehensive cardiac stabilization and heart disease reversal program emphasizes the critical value of stress management and relaxation training among the participants. Along with prescribing diet and exercise lifestyle modifications, this program requires that participants heighten their understanding of their psychological states. Managing stress and achieving a relaxation response are accomplished through guided practice at each program session. Ornish's data show that this facet of his program may well be pivotal in the treatment of heart disease. However, not every cardiac rehabilitation program uses the complete Ornish model; some may use other stress management and relaxation programs and techniques, and still others may not formally recognize stress management.

Many cardiac rehabilitation facilities focus largely on changes in diet and exercise tolerance as the benchmarks for success in their participants. However, whether or not the Ornish program is followed, the data strongly suggest that psychological factors contribute to overall recovery from a cardiac event. Therefore, it behooves every cardiac rehabilitation professional to consider psychological factors and arrange appropriate treatment for their patients.

GUIDELINES, 4TH EDITION

■ Chapter 8, pages 123-129

Psychosocial Evaluation

Cardiac rehabilitation participants present with a wide variety of personality styles and psychological reactions to their cardiac events. They have had unique medical experiences, whether it be a myocardial infarction, percutaneous coronary interventions, or coronary artery bypass graft surgery (CABG). Some participants have experienced no major cardiac events or procedures and are being treated medically to reduce the risk factors associated with cardiac events and procedures. Each person has a unique health history with the possibility of comorbid conditions such as diabetes or cancer. Each comes from a specific social stratum and has varying

degrees of social support. The cardiac rehabilitation staff should develop and implement a screening or assessment process to identify those participants who might be at risk for psychological complications, while neither overestimating nor underestimating problems in any given participant. The challenge is to balance the risk for false positives, that is, individuals who are seen as facing psychological problems who do not in fact have these problems, and false negatives, those who are experiencing psychological problems that are missed in the screening.

One danger in this population is to assume that because cardiac rehabilitation participants share a similar event background, they are homogeneous. In fact, although there are certain similarities and challenges, each participant is unique. The goal is to develop a general screening and assessment strategy that can be used for all cardiac rehabilitation patients, understanding that the goal is to cast a wide net that will capture most participant problems. Evaluation of psychological functioning may include general or specific screening questionnaires as well as focused questions asked during an orientation interview that might touch on behavioral health issues.

A large number of such psychological assessment instruments are available. Some focus on specific mental health difficulties such as depression, anxiety, or hostility. Others use a more general approach, assessing various domains of functional status that may include psychological functioning. Cardiac rehabilitation professionals are faced with various challenges when deciding what assessment tools to use. These challenges include participants' reading levels, the amount of time available to complete the instruments, and the validity and utility of the information gathered. Some cardiac rehabilitation professionals have even developed their own assessment instruments in response to these challenges.[10] Most cardiac rehabilitation staff prefer tools that can be administered by a variety of health care professionals, are completed and scored quickly and easily, and provide easily identified cutoff scores that indicate a need for further action. Some of the more commonly used instruments are found in table 4.1.

The results of this interview and assessment may lead to a consultation with a mental health professional or the staff member best equipped to deal with such problems. Although it is easy to defer to a mental health "expert," it can actually be a mistake in some cases. Patients may be resentful or defensive around behavioral health specialists, having a strong need to present themselves in a very favorable light. As in most medical settings, patients will first pick those with whom they feel familiar and comfortable to share important information or intimate personal thoughts or feelings. Therefore, professional cardiac rehabilitation staff should be trained to recognize psychological

Table 4.1 Selected Psychosocial Evaluation Instruments

Evaluation tool	Description
Medical Outcomes Study Short Form (MOS SF-36) Health Survey[29]	Generic health-related quality of life and functional status questionnaire assessing nine dimensions: physical functioning; role limitations attributable to physical health problems; bodily pain; social functioning; general mental health; role limitations attributable to emotional problems, vitality, energy, or fatigue; general health perceptions
Cook–Medley Hostility Questionnaire[30]	A 50-item questionnaire developed from the Minnesota Multiphasic Personality Inventory purported to measure cynical hostility
Center for Epidemiologic Studies—Depression Scale (CES-D)[31]	A 20-item easily scored depression scale evaluating current (within 1 week) functioning
Beck Depression Inventory (BDI)[32]	Popular 21-item self-report rating inventory measuring characteristic attitudes and symptoms of depression
Spielberger State–Trait Anxiety Inventory[33]	Evaluation of feelings of apprehension, tension, nervousness, and worry with two 20-item scales assessing state (current) and trait (chronic) anxiety
Beck Anxiety Inventory (BAI)[34]	Popular instrument measuring the severity of anxiety through psychological and cognitive symptoms of anxiety
Herridge Cardiopulmonary Questionnaire (HCQ)[10]	A 49-item pilot instrument assessing seven cognitive–behavioral variables that have consistently shown relationships to health outcomes and disease severity including hostility, depression, anxiety, stress, social support, self-efficacy, and motivation

problems in their patients, because these staff may be the gatekeepers who see these problems first and may be asked to remediate them without the assistance of the program's behavioral health specialist. If cardiac professionals believe that the presenting difficulties are beyond their level of expertise, they at least have developed a rapport that can ease the referral to a mental health professional.

The first weeks after a cardiac event are often considered to be the "magic moment" relative to behavioral change.[11] Patients are generally more motivated to make lifestyle changes at this time than any other, and cardiac rehabilitation offers a structure within which they can make these changes. Participation in cardiac rehabilitation often leads to improvement in overall psychological functioning. However, getting a patient to commit to begin the program is only the first step. To benefit, a participant must be able to maintain his or her involvement throughout the rehabilitation period. Therefore, the adherence of each patient for the duration of the program must be a primary focus and goal of cardiac rehabilitation staff. Because psychological and social functioning is a strong predictor of the level of compliance to treatment,[12] staff members must know how to assess each of their patients in this regard, aided by clinical pattern recognition as well as more formal screening tools.

Daly and colleagues[13] reviewed the literature relevant to participation and adherence in cardiac rehabilitation and summarized seven psychological issues possibly related to success. This outline is used in structuring the clinical lore pertaining to each area.

1. Self-efficacy: This reflects the degree to which patients believe they "have what it takes" to institute and maintain a lifestyle or behavior change.[14] It is valuable to ask about previous accomplishments, trying to determine if patients feel capable of understanding the program, if they are sufficiently literate to comprehend written material, and whether they feel that they have more control over their success than genetics and fate, for example.

2. Self-motivation: The cardiac health care professional must determine the patient's readiness for change.[15] Although one might assume patients are highly motivated because they have agreed to participate in cardiac rehabilitation, they could be there as a result of pressure from families or physicians, or for other reasons unrelated to their own need to change. There is always a dynamic balance between the push to make meaningful life changes and the urge to continue doing things that are familiar and unhealthy, but also very pleasurable. People are at a point along a continuum in this regard: Some are very motivated with

a clear plan of action, others have to be convinced that what they sacrifice will be worth the loss of favorite unhealthy habits, and some are still "on the fence." Determining a patient's motivation can be done either quickly through screening or slowly over time, as his or her motives and resistance become clear.

3. Self-esteem: Somewhat related to the first two factors, self-esteem refers to an individual's abiding sense of worth and value. Patients have developed this sense before any cardiac incident, and it follows them into the rehabilitation setting. However, they now have the cardiac event as part of their life experience. They may suddenly feel "old" or "worthless," that they cannot return to work or enjoy retirement, or that they are vulnerable to further illness. A dramatic decrease in self-esteem can lead to a loss of desire to engage in self-enhancing activities and can be a precursor to or covariate with depression. Because cardiac rehabilitation staff tend to be relatively young, professionally accomplished, in "the prime of life," and focused on personal fitness, developing empathy may be challenging.

4. Personality: Relatively fixed personality traits also predate the cardiac event and may contribute to the problem. Patients vary as to how much they value control over their lives and whether they will accept the need for change. Some listen well, whereas others are prone to hear only what already conforms to their beliefs and expectations. Some are extroverted and enjoy shared group experiences and discussions, whereas others are sensitive to threat, fear evaluation by others, and dislike any group activities. Some are followers who are happy just to be included, whereas others are extremely competitive and strive to be the "star" of the group. Some are hostile and require substantial education about toxic emotions.[16] Determining how to get the best from each personality type is the challenge. Personalities won't be changed substantially in a cardiac rehabilitation program, but each individual's strengths can be maximized if his or her style is understood and a plan of action unique to that participant is developed. Although programs are standardized, that does not mean that one size fits all. Good programs build on the diversity of their participants and adjust accordingly.

5. Depression: Much has been written about depression and cardiac events.[3, 4,17-23] The American Association of Cardiovascular and Pulmonary Rehabilitation recently commissioned a task force to examine the issue relative to cardiac rehabilitation participants. The task force concluded that a serious health risk exists for depressed participants based on a volume of empirical evidence. The task force report recommended that all cardiac rehabilitation participants be screened for clinical depression on entry into the program.[23] Even though the link between depression

and adverse health events is strong, the mechanism of this connection remains somewhat unclear. It may be that depression per se doesn't increase the chances for coronary artery disease or its exacerbation but rather predisposes one to engage in unhealthy behaviors that are more directly related to heart disease. Many patients are quite depressed before CABG and stenting and are also depressed immediately following a myocardial infarction (MI). However, in the cardiac rehabilitation phase, depression often decreases as the patient realizes that he or she has come through a trying time and now has a plan of action and social support. Depression and social isolation are often seen as connected. The attention and caring shown in rehabilitation may help reduce this isolation and therefore help some aspects of the depression.

Some patients are so depressed that their mood disorder becomes obvious. They appear sad, distressed, or withdrawn. Others are depressed but cover it well. Their depression may go undetected unless they are asked directly about their mood, sleep, appetite, concentration, and interest, by use of either screening tests or direct interviews. Many symptoms of a normal recovery from a cardiac incident mimic depressive mood. For example, patients may appear fatigued and admit to feeling vulnerable and somewhat less able to control their lives and their futures than before the incident. Therefore, trying to tell the difference between a normal pattern of recovery and depression in cardiac patients can be difficult. Because depression can interfere with one's adherence to a program, it is one of the more important facets of patient functioning and should be carefully assessed. Be particularly alert for signs of dramatic personality change, uncharacteristic hostility or bursts of anger, dramatic social withdrawal, and statements that patients cannot cope or that life is no longer worth living. Also be concerned if the dejection and sadness appear to last more than a few weeks and show no improvement over time. It can help to inform patients that depression frequently accompanies recovery from cardiac events, thereby increasing the chance that they will feel comfortable discussing depressive mood with staff.[24]

6. Anxiety: As with depression, some patients have a history of anxiety that predates their cardiac problems. But the threat of a major cardiac event can be dramatic and frightening, exacerbating existing anxiety and creating anxiety in those who did not have this problem before. On one hand, some apprehension and a heightened sense of vulnerability can counteract denial and help motivate patients to make necessary life changes. Staff members need to be sensitive to anxiety that goes beyond what is healthy given the realities of the patient's situation. Some patients will be overly sensitive to changes in their bodies during exercise, particularly those who have seldom exercised in the

Signs of Depression

- Low energy or restlessness
- Recurrent worry, regrets, somatic complaints, and thoughts of death
- Anhedonia—a diminished interest or loss of ability to experience pleasure
- Significant change in sleep, eating, and sexual drive habits
- A recurring sense of being overwhelmed by current stressors
- Self-blame and self-criticism
- Poor concentration and memory
- Suicidal thoughts

past and have limited experience in how their bodies have felt when physically challenged. Others may feel fragile and may both overestimate the threat of their problem and underestimate their ability to cope or the program's ability to help them. They may fear being alone, driving, or traveling away from their health care providers. These may even believe that they are in an alien situation, becoming hypervigilant while feeling unprepared to deal with any threat. Patients who "sensitize" will show their anxiety by appearing tense, apprehensive, and perhaps pale and sweaty. They will look frightened or insecure and will look to staff for frequent reassurance. Those who "repress" will more likely keep these feelings to themselves and put on a face of calm and confidence. You will need to know your patients well enough that you can calm those who are excessively anxious and draw out those who are suffering in silence, because both need reassurance but ask for it in different ways. Some patients show their anxiety by being stiff and disagreeable, whereas others become overly compliant. Again, getting to know how your patients really feel will help you best channel their anxiety away from suffering and direct it to problem solving and developing self-confidence in their new roles.

A final consideration is the patient's socioeconomic status. Williams[25] suggested that a common factor which the various psychological and behavioral risk factors for the development and exacerbation of cardiovascular disease tend to be associated with is low socioeconomic status (SES). This factor may *increase the effect* of the other psychosocial risk factors.

> It is becoming increasingly evident that lower SES, rather then being simply one among a list of other psychosocial risk factors, may be, in fact, a 'master' risk factor that contributes to increased levels of the other risk factors.
>
> Redford B. Williams[25(p. 662)]

Williams noted that, along with low SES, depression and social isolation "confer a poorer prognosis." The mechanism by which these psychosocial risk factors harm cardiovascular health is through continuation of specific unhealthy behaviors. For example, individuals who are depressed, socially isolated, and poorly motivated with low self-efficacy are more likely to drop out of cardiac rehabilitation, continue to eat in an unhealthy manner, and maintain a sedentary lifestyle.

It must be emphasized again, however, that each participant is unique. Although demographic variables and SES seem to predict future cardiovascular risk and adherence, the participant's beliefs about his or her health status also play a large role. The health

Common Anxiety Presentations

- Fear of being alone
- Worry about traveling away from immediate medical care
- Preoccupation with visceral feedback and its meaning
- Panic attacks
- Excessive need for reassurance during exercise

belief model (figure 4.1) offers another psychosocial approach for examining the participant's cognitions and understanding of his illness. One interpretation of this model focuses on the need to examine three particular perceptions of the participant: (a) Does the individual have a sense of vulnerability? (b) Does the individual have confidence that he or she can succeed? (c) Has the individual experienced a personally motivating event to begin change? By answering these questions, cardiac rehabilitation staff can better predict who may need more attention and assistance facing the challenge of rehabilitation and risk attenuation. The likelihood of taking the recommended action is dependent on the result of an equation comparing the perceived benefit of the change versus the perceived barriers. These questions can be integrated into the orientation interview along with asking the participant to complete the psychological questionnaires chosen for the department.

Patients are only in cardiac rehabilitation a few hours each week and spend most of their time at home. Thus, the significant others of cardiac rehabilitation participants can play an important role in their adjustment. These significant others are often the mediators of the patient's life change, from diet and exercise modification to stress management. O'Farrell and colleagues[26] found that a large percentage of spouses of cardiac rehabilitation participants met criteria for distress. The most common concerns were for the patient's treatment, recovery, and prognosis, the heightened moodiness of the patient, worries about money and the patient's ability to return to work,

sexual concerns, and the patient's apathy and resultant need for the spouse to assume a greater role in the marriage. Distressed spouses reported less intimacy in their marriages, poorer family functioning, and symptoms of tension, poor sleep, and feeling easily hurt. Younger spouses reported more distress than older spouses. The most common maladaptive coping style among distressed spouses was disengagement, where they emotionally withdrew from the situation and did only what was necessary.

It is wise to ask each patient about his or her social support system and, in particular, about any intimate connections as found in marriage or long-term relationships. This will allow staff to understand what support resources are available away from the rehabilitation setting. Some family members may attend cardiac rehabilitation sessions with the patient. This can reflect a mature effort to be educated about the process to better support the patient, or it might suggest that the patient and the family member have consciously or unconsciously agreed that the patient will abdicate all responsibility for changes to them. Often this is the spouse, usually the wife, who then assumes the liability if the patient eats the wrong things, stops exercising, skips medication doses, or becomes depressed, hopeless, or hostile. Clearly, this arrangement is to be avoided. Again, the overarching goal is to reduce negative and maladaptive emotions while increasing the patient's sense of self-reliance. It may be prudent to consider the distress of spouses or significant others as well, because this can have a substantial impact on the patient's ability to successfully complete the program

SENSE OF VULNERABILITY?

Yes   No

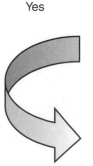

CONFIDENCE?

Yes   No

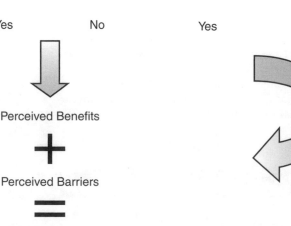

Perceived Benefits

+

Perceived Barriers

=

Likelihood of Change

MOTIVATING EVENT?

Yes   No

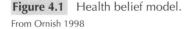

Figure 4.1   Health belief model.

From Ornish 1998

and to begin long-term adherence to the life changes that you have introduced.

Psychosocial Interventions

Providing appropriate psychological assistance for participants in need is a challenge faced by many cardiac rehabilitation programs. Most programs do not have the luxury of having a mental health professional on staff who can provide immediate consultation services. However, most programs can maintain a consultative relationship with an outpatient mental health professional. This liaison may assist the program in three ways: (a) by addressing staff concerns about general and specific psychological concerns or presentations by participants, (b) by providing individualized treatment or referrals for treatment for participants as needed, and (c) by providing group psychoeducational presentations to participants. If the liaison is recognized as a "familiar face" by the participants, there is a much greater likelihood that they will follow-up with the liaison individually as the situation may warrant. Williams[25] stated that group settings have particular strengths in regard to behavior change compared with individualized treatment. Participants learn from each other as well as the instructor or facilitator. They also benefit through the social support offered by such a setting. Thus, even general cardiac rehabilitation education classes may be of powerful benefit to participants' psychological functioning.

A standardized plan of care may prove beneficial for participants with specific psychological needs. The first step is referral to the liaison. As stated previously, however, not all participants will be comfortable or compliant with a referral to a mental health professional. Most mental health issues are still initially addressed and treated through primary care physicians. Many participants will be more comfortable speaking to their physician than a psychologist or counselor. If a participant in need of psychological services refuses or is noncompliant with referral to the liaison, that participant should next be referred to his or her physician. However, some participants may not comply with this approach either and may need another type of motivation.

As with any effort aimed at encouraging behavior change, cardiac rehabilitation staff must often balance the need to support with the need to confront. Particularly difficult participants may be those using denial as their primary coping mechanism or those with a strong external locus of control (a belief that luck, fate, or other people control what happens to them). Depressed participants may have a sense of hopelessness, and anxious patients may feel a strong need to avoid any confirmation of a problem. Whatever the reason for noncompliance with a referral, participants can be approached in a collaborative manner and still be asked direct, open-ended questions. By addressing the participant's specific concerns in a direct but supportive manner, the cardiac professional may minimize barriers such as denial and an external locus and move the participant closer to taking action. Suggested questions are as follows:

- What do you see as your biggest challenge in regard to improving your health?
- How have you been able to successfully change unhealthy behaviors in the past?
- How have things changed for you since your cardiac event or diagnosis?
- What kind of concerns do you have about meeting with a counselor, psychologist, or mental health professional?
- How can we assist you best in meeting your goals?

General psychological functioning concerns are not the only issues that participants may struggle with, however. Occasionally, patients and their partners ask questions about sexual relations following cardiac events. Some physicians educate patients proactively about sex by either discussion or the use of written material. Others physicians do not, and if the patient and partner do not feel comfortable asking the physician, they wait until cardiac rehabilitation to ask. Some staff feel comfortable answering such questions, but most programs have a particular staff member who assumes the role of sexuality "coach" and is willing to keep up to date on literature and patient education material with regard to sexuality in this population. This is perhaps the best approach, and it reduces the likelihood of uncomfortable staff or patient misinformation. Information in regard to sexual functioning following a cardiac event is often hard to obtain, and typically there is no clear consensus of medical advice. Patients and their partners have a need to return to a sense of intimacy and security between them, but they also fear precipitating another cardiac event during sex. Naturally each case is unique, but it is probably safe to say that most patients and partners worry more about the effects of sexual exertion than they need to. Using everyday terms that are appropriate to the case at hand, such as, "if you can climb two flights of stairs then you can have sexual relations without a problem," is preferred over scientific explanations and statistics. Sex is important to patients of all ages, so the program staff should be prepared to answer questions about sex as comprehensively as those in all other areas. But again, be sure that the staff person fielding these questions is knowledgeable, and refer to the patients' physicians as needed for additional information about sexual functioning.

Promoting Adherence

Working with cardiac rehabilitation participants is a mixture of science and art. In the effort to promote adherence with dietary, exercise, tobacco, and psychological recommendations, staff may need to use a variety of innovative and idiosyncratic methods. Miller and Rolnick[27] described a strategy for helping people change called motivational interviewing. There are five principles that make up the approach: (a) be empathic, (b) create cognitive dissonance (helping participants see the discrepancy between their goals and their actual behavior), (c) avoid arguing, (d) "roll" with resistance, and (e) reinforce self-efficacy. By keeping these five principles in mind when interacting with participants, cardiac rehabilitation staff can help participants make lifestyle change for the short-term and increase confidence to aid in long-term adherence. Sometimes mistakes can be made when staff become either too pushy or too nurturing.

Another strategy for increasing adherence over the long-term was reviewed and then revised by Goldstein and colleagues[28] and is described as the Five As. Adapted from Miller and Rolnick's[27] motivational interviewing program, this approach emphasizes a structured plan of action for health care providers that encompasses these actions: address the agenda, assess, advise, assist, and arrange follow-up. You must ask about the participants' agenda first. What are their goals? Why are they here? Second, you must assess the participants' knowledge, emotions, and readiness to make changes in their lifestyles. Advising the participants is next and depends on their responses to questions about their agenda, knowledge, and emotions in regard to the behavior in question. Fourth, you must now assist the patient in the appropriate manner. The motivational interviewing approach described here may be appropriate, or if the participant is ready to begin change, goal setting may begin. Finally, appropriate follow-up can be scheduled and completed. This may be designed to fit your program's resources and schedule. After cardiac rehabilitation participation is completed, long-term adherence can often be dramatically improved simply with a brief follow-up meeting or phone call.

Daly and colleagues[13] offered specific suggestions for improving participation and adherence in cardiac rehabilitation. Cardiac rehabilitation programs should be advertised as "multiple risk reduction programs" and should not focus on only exercise and diet change. This may help participants accept the idea that they are changing "for life" and not just for 12 weeks. Developing collaborative relationships with physicians so that they validate the patient's participation and effort for improvement can also be very valuable. Tailoring the program for each individual is also a long-term investment in adherence. Along these same lines, participants with risk factors for nonadherence should be targeted early for help and intervention. These risk groups include older individuals, women, and those with low self-efficacy, motivation, and social support (see table 4.2).

Table 4.2	Assessment Domains and Relationship to Adherence
Assessment domain	**Relationship to adherence**
Depression	−
Anxiety	−
Anger, frustration, hostility	−
Stress	−
Self-efficacy	+
Motivation	+
Social support	+
Female	−
Older	−

Summary

Research suggests that psychosocial factors and cardiovascular reactivity interact to affect the development and progression of heart disease. In addition, psychological problems can lead to reduced adherence to treatment and the pursuit of unhealthy behaviors. Cardiac rehabilitation patients should be screened for psychological status, and cardiac rehabilitation program staff should have defined short-term and long-term strategies available for psychological interventions when needed. Patient support systems and intimate relationships should also be assessed, and cardiac rehabilitation program staff should be aware that partners of patients may suffer significant distress as a result of the patient's cardiac disease. A collaboration model involving a mental health professional is the preferred approach for assessing and intervening on psychological issues.

PART II

Role of Exercise in Heart Disease

Exercise and the Coronary Heart Disease Connection

Ray W. Squires, PhD, and Larry F. Hamm, PhD

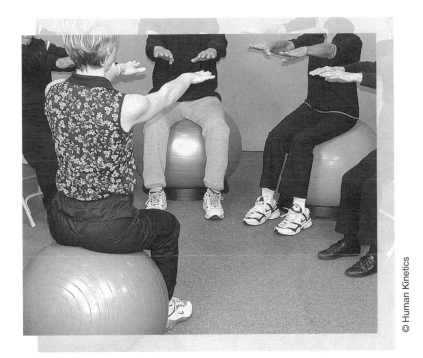

© Human Kinetics

A sedentary lifestyle has been established as a major modifiable coronary risk factor by the American Heart Association.[1] Unfortunately, approximately 70% of U.S. adults are sedentary or underactive, and almost one half of America's young people (aged 12-21 years) are not physically active on a regular basis.[2] The reasons for this observation are closely related to industrialization, automation, and the resultant decreased requirement for occupational, household, and leisure-time physical activity over the past many decades. The need to walk, climb stairs, perform energy-requiring chores around the house, or engage in physical activity in the workplace has dramatically decreased for the vast majority of persons. In the 21st century, individuals must make a conscious choice to be physically active.

The definitions of *physical activity, exercise,* and *cardiorespiratory fitness* are important in this discussion. The 1996 National Institutes of Health Consensus Conference on Physical Activity and Cardiovascular Health defined *physical activity* as "bodily movement produced by skeletal muscles that requires energy expenditure and produces progressive health benefits."[3(p. 3)] Physical activity is informal in nature and structure and may include everyday activities such as walking, bicycling, and stair climbing (for transportation) as well as household or yard tasks and low-intensity sports such as golf. Physical activity occurs within the structure of the requirements of usual daily living. *Exercise* (or exercise training), on the other hand, was defined as "planned, structured, and repetitive bodily movement done to improve or maintain one or more components of physical fitness."[3(p. 3)] It is characterized by periodic formal workouts involving sustained moderate- to high-intensity effort. It usually involves specific clothing (such as footwear) and equipment (as present in fitness facilities) and is usually not an absolutely necessary part of the daily routine. *Cardiorespiratory fitness* is defined as the capacity to take in and process oxygen for the production of energy for physical activity via aerobic metabolism. This is the component of physical fitness most associated with coronary risk. Cardiorespiratory fitness is directly related to performance of habitual exercise training but is also affected by genetic potential,[4] age, and gender as well as by underlying chronic diseases that affect the cardiorespiratory systems, nervous system, blood, and skeletal muscle.

The purpose of this chapter is to summarize and discuss the role of exercise and physical activity in the prevention of coronary heart disease (CHD). The following topics are included for this purpose:

- Observational (epidemiologic) data concerning the relationship of occupational and leisure-time physical activity to coronary risk
- Studies evaluating the relationship of cardiorespiratory fitness or change in cardiorespiratory fitness and coronary risk
- Data addressing the results of exercise training in persons with established CHD in terms of future coronary events
- The risks of acute exercise
- Potential mechanisms for the cardioprotective effects of physical activity and exercise

GUIDELINES, 4TH EDITION

- Chapter 6, page 72
- Chapter 8, pages 113-123
- Chapter 9

Observational Data

An inherent limitation of observational (epidemiological) studies is selection bias. Individuals may be sedentary because of undetected pathology or active because of better general health. However, investigations of either occupational or leisure-time (recreational) physical activity and coronary risk provide valuable information based on very large groups of subjects.

Studies that are limited to occupational physical activity are concerned with quantifying the amount of physical activity that occurs during the performance of job duties. Most studies of this type will report occupational physical activity in categories (e.g., most, moderately, and least active). Because occupational physical activity has decreased over recent years and is currently at relatively low levels in developed countries, researchers have more recently focused on studying the relationship between leisure-time physical activity and cardiovascular disease and

other chronic diseases. This type of physical activity is limited to activity engaged in by persons during discretionary time occurring outside of work, domestic chores, and activities for daily living. Examples of this type of activity include recreational sports, competitive sports, walking, jogging, and cycling.

Occupational Physical Activity

Several investigations have demonstrated an inverse relationship between amount and intensity of job-related physical activity and coronary risk. The following three studies are illustrative of this finding.

A very large population of U.S. railroad workers (191,609 men, age range 30-64 years) were evaluated by Taylor and associates.[5] Physical activity at work was determined by job class: sedentary clerks, more active switchmen, and most active section men. There was no attempt to control for potential confounding variables. Death caused by atherosclerosis was more frequent for clerks (relative risk 2.03) and switchmen (relative risk 1.46) when compared with the more physically active section men.

Morris and colleagues[6] studied 667 male London double-decker bus drivers and conductors (age range 30-69 years) for a 5-year interval. Physical activity on the job was assessed by specific work duties: The drivers were sedentary whereas the conductors moved about the buses collecting fares. The incidence of CHD was much lower for the more physically active conductors than for the drivers (age-adjusted relative risk of 1.8).

Paffenbarger and colleagues[7] followed 6,351 San Francisco longshoremen, aged 35 to 74 years, for 22 years. Physical activity was defined by specific job requirements and categorized as light (1.5-2.0 kcal·min^{-1}, 1.3-1.8 metabolic equivalents [METs] for a 70-kg person), moderate (2.4-5.0 kcal·min^{-1}, 2.0-4.3 METs), or heavy (5.2-7.5 kcal·min^{-1}, 4.4-6.4 METs). Death attributable to coronary heart disease was inversely associated with job energy expenditure (relative risk 1.7 in moderate and 1.8 in light categories compared with the heavy category).

Leisure-Time Physical Activity

Numerous investigators have studied the association between the amount and intensity of leisure-time physical activity and CHD end points. The most well-known study in this group is the Harvard Alumni Study of Paffenbarger and associates.[8] Beginning in 1962 and continuing until 1978, 16,936 men were followed for a variety of end points including first myocardial infarction (MI), cardiovascular death, and CHD death. An index of physical activity in kcal·week^{-1} was estimated for each subject based on self-reported physical activity, including number of blocks walked, stairs climbed, and participation in vigorous exercise. Among the findings of the study was an inverse relationship between amount of habitual activity and first MI (age-adjusted relative risk 1.64 for men with <2,000 kcal·week⁻¹ vs. men with >2,000 kcal·week⁻¹). Interestingly, having participated in athletics as a young person was not associated with a lower risk unless there was evidence of current physical activity. After adjustment for age, smoking, and hypertension, there was a significant dose response. Figure 5.1 shows the dose-response relationship as well as the cardioprotective advantage of vigorous exercise over less vigorous activity.

In 1977, a second physical activity questionnaire was administered to the Harvard Alumni cohort. A subgroup of 12,516 survivors without documented coronary heart disease were followed until the end of 1993.[9] End points included development of a first MI, angina pectoris, coronary revascularization, and coronary death. After adjustment for age and multiple well-established coronary risk factors, subjects expending more than 1,000 kcal·week⁻¹ experienced an approximately 20% lower coronary event risk than subjects who expended less than 1,000 kcal·week⁻¹. The strongest reductions in coronary risk were for total energy expenditure and vigorous exercise. A third questionnaire was given to 7,307 Harvard Alumni Study subjects in 1988 and included questions regarding the frequency and duration of each episode of physical activity.[10] Follow-up until the end of 1993 revealed that after adjustment for total energy expenditure, duration of each exercise episode no longer had an independent effect on coronary risk. As long as the total energy expenditure was similar, longer exercise sessions did not have a greater effect on risk reduction.

Morris and colleagues[11] studied 17,944 British male civil servants, aged 40 to 64 years, for an average of 8.5 years. Baseline levels of physical activity were assessed by a unique 48-hr recall of leisure-time physical activity. Vigorous activities were defined as requiring at least 7.5 kcal·min⁻¹ (6.4 METs for a 70-kg person). During follow-up there were 1,138 coronary events (fatal and nonfatal first MI). The age-adjusted relative risk of a coronary event for men reporting nonvigorous exercise versus those reporting vigorous activity was 2.2.

The Nurses Health Study enrolled 72,488 women, aged 40 to 65 years, who were initially free of CHD.[12] Habitual patterns of physical activity, including walking, cycling, jogging, swimming, racket sports, calisthenics, aerobics, stairs climbed, and walking pace, were collected in 1986 and updated in 1988 and 1992. After 8 years of follow-up, 645 coronary events (MI, coronary death) occurred. There was a graded, inverse relationship between physical activity and coronary events. Multivariate adjusted relative risk for the most active versus the least active quintile of the population was 0.66 (34% lower risk). Walking amount was inversely associated with risk. Vigorous exercise resulted in a 30% to 40% reduction in coronary events. Sedentary subjects who became active enjoyed a lower risk than subjects who remained inactive.

The Women's Health Study included 39,372 health professionals who were at least 45 years of age and free of CHD at baseline.[13] Levels of physical activity, including walking, pace of walking, flights of stairs climbed, and sporting activities, were assessed. After an average follow-up interval of 5 years, 244 cases of CHD occurred (MI, coronary revascularization, coronary death). A 25% reduction in risk (multivariate relative risk of 0.75) was found for the most active (>1,500 kcal·week⁻¹) compared with the least active (<200 kcal·week⁻¹) quartiles of subjects. Time spent walking was more important in risk reduction than

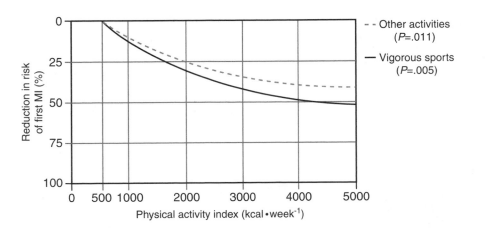

Figure 5.1 Exercise and physical activity in reducing the risk of a first myocardial infarction: the Harvard Alumni Study.

was pace of walking. For women with coronary risk factors (obesity, smoking, hypercholesterolemia), physical activity was also protective. Subjects who walked 1 hr per week had one half of the risk of those who did not walk.

Cardiorespiratory Fitness and Coronary Death

When estimated with maximal graded exercise testing, cardiorespiratory fitness has been shown to be inversely related with cardiovascular risk. The following are examples of investigations, some that included both genders as well as younger and older subjects. An important limitation of these studies is that genetic potential plays a central role in cardiorespiratory fitness, independent of habitual exercise.[4]

Blair and associates[14] studied patients at the Aerobics Center in Dallas, TX who had an initial evaluation including a maximal treadmill exercise test. Middle-aged men (n = 10,224) and women (n = 3,120) were categorized by fitness level (low, moderate, high) based on treadmill exercise performance and were followed for an average of 8 years. The coronary death rate decreased dramatically with increasing fitness level for both genders (table 5.1). However, there were relatively few coronary deaths in this population of rather young subjects (66 for men, 7 for women). Blair also assessed the effects of improvement in cardiorespiratory fitness on coronary risk with subjects at the Aerobics Center.[15] A large cohort of men (n = 9,777, age range 20-82 years) underwent two maximal treadmill exercise tests at a mean interval of 4.9 years. The subjects were followed for an average of 5.1 years. There were 87 cardiovascular deaths during follow-up. Relative to subjects who remained unfit, subjects who

improved their fitness category experienced an age-adjusted relative risk of 0.48 (52% reduction in risk; 95% confidence interval 0.31-0.74).

A cohort of 1,960 Norwegian men (age range 40-59 years) underwent maximal graded exercise testing and were followed for an average of 16 years.[16] Eighty-seven cardiovascular deaths occurred. After extensive statistical control of potential confounding factors, a strong inverse relationship between cardiorespiratory fitness and risk was found. Compared with men in the lowest fitness quartile, the relative risks for quartiles 2, 3, and 4 were 0.59, 0.45, and 0.41, respectively.

Two studies involving all residents of Olmsted County, Minnesota, who underwent maximal treadmill exercise testing in the late 1980s, provide additional insight into the relationship of cardiorespiratory fitness and coronary risk. Roger and colleagues[17] followed 1,452 men and 741 women who had treadmill exercise tests in 1987 and 1988 for 6.3 ± 2.0 years. Cardiovascular end points included cardiac death, nonfatal MI, and congestive heart failure. A total of 160 cardiovascular end points occurred during follow-up (106 in men, 54 in women). After multivariate adjustment, peak treadmill workload in METs was the only variable associated with the outcome measures. For each 1 MET increment in cardiorespiratory fitness, cardiac events were reduced by 25%, with a similar effect for both genders. Using similar methods, Goraya and associates[18] followed 3,107 Olmsted County residents who underwent maximal treadmill exercise testing in 1987 to 1989 for a median of 6.0 years. Both genders were included, and 514 of the subjects were over 65 years of age. For each 1 MET increase in cardiorespiratory fitness, cardiovascular events were reduced by 14% and 18% for younger and older (>65 years) subjects, respectively.

Myers and colleagues[19] reported on exercise capacity in a mixed sample of 6,213 men without and with CHD. Exercise testing was performed for a variety of clinical reasons. During the follow-up period (mean = 6.2 years), age-adjusted peak METs (1 MET = 3.5 $ml \cdot kg^{-1} \cdot min^{-1}$) was the strongest predictor of mortality during the follow-up.

In two studies by Kavanagh and colleagues,[20,21] measured peak oxygen uptake ($\dot{V}O_2$peak) during graded exercise testing was found to be a strong independent predictor of subsequent mortality in patients with documented CHD. In one study involving 12,169 men referred to a cardiac rehabilitation program, measured $\dot{V}O_2$peak less than 15 $ml \cdot kg^{-1} \cdot min^{-1}$ at entry into the program was predictive of both cardiac and overall mortality during the follow-up (mean = 7.9 years). Specifically, measured $\dot{V}O_2$peak of less than 15, 15 to 22, and greater than 22 $ml \cdot kg^{-1} \cdot min^{-1}$ resulted in multivariate adjusted hazard ratios of 1.00, 0.62, and 0.45, respectively, for cardiac mortality.[20]

Table 5.1	Rates of Coronary Death by Fitness Level: The Aerobics Center Study	
	Males	**Females**
N	10,224	3,120
Age (mean years)	41.5	40.8
Follow-up (years)	8	8
CORONARY DEATH RATE[a] BY FITNESS LEVEL		
Low	24.6	7.4
Moderate	7.8	2.9
High	3.1	0.8

[a]Per 10,000 person-years.

Adapted from Blair 1989.

The second study by Kavanagh and associates[21] involved 2,380 women with CHD. Measured $\dot{V}O_2$peak of 13 ml·kg^{-1}·min^{-1} or more on an initial exercise test resulted in a 50% decrease in cardiac mortality ($p = .001$) during the follow-up (mean = 6.1 years). When the authors analyzed $\dot{V}O_2$peak as a continuous variable, women in this study demonstrated a 10% reduction in cardiac mortality for each 1 ml·kg^{-1}·min^{-1} advantage.

Exercise Training in Established Coronary Disease

Research indicates that exercise training can reduce coronary end points for patients with documented coronary disease. These data are the result of both observational and randomized, controlled studies. Because exercise training is a core component of cardiac rehabilitation programs, health care professionals working in cardiac rehabilitation must be familiar with and understand the documented effects of exercise training in persons with established coronary disease.

Observational Data

In the Harvard Alumni Study, reviewed previously in this chapter, a subset of 782 subjects of the entire 16,936-person cohort had documented CHD at the beginning of the study.[8] Over a follow-up interval of approximately 12 years, the more physically active subjects (expended >2,000 kcal·week^{-1} in leisure-time physical activity) experienced a 30% lower coronary event rate than less active subjects with coronary dis-

ease (figure 5.2). The beneficial effect persisted after statistical adjustment for smoking, blood pressure, body weight, family history of CHD, and age.

In the British Regional Heart Study, 772 of the 5,934 men in the cohort had documented CHD.[22] A baseline assessment of habitual physical activity, including intensity of activity, was performed. After 5 years of follow-up, 131 deaths had occurred (94 from cardiovascular disease). Compared with inactive subjects, persons who performed light, moderate, or vigorous exercise experienced a substantially lower all-cause and cardiovascular mortality (table 5.2). These results were similar for younger and older (>65 years of age) subjects.

Randomized Trials

Kallio and colleagues[23] randomized 301 men and 74 women with a history of MI to a comprehensive rehabilitation program (exercise training, dietary and smoking cessation advice, psychosocial counseling) or to a control group. Compared with the control group, the intervention group experienced an improvement in habitual physical activity, blood lipids, and blood pressure. The 3-year cumulative mortality rate was 18.6% in the intervention group versus 29.4% in the control group ($p = .02$). The difference was primarily the result of a reduction in the incidence of sudden cardiac death in the intervention group (5.8% vs. 14.4%, $p < .01$). The rate of nonfatal reinfarction was similar for both groups.

Hamalainen and associates[24] reported 10-year follow-up data for these same subjects. No organized intervention occurred after the first 3 years of the study. At 10 years, the incidence of sudden cardiac death was less for the intervention group (12.8% vs. 23.0%, $p = .01$). Cardiac mortality was also lower for intervention subjects (35.1% vs. 47.1%, $p = .02$). The

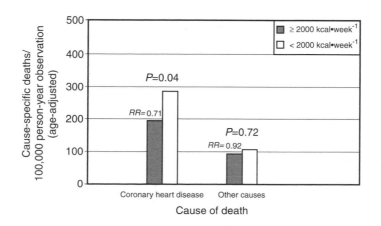

Figure 5.2   Physical activity and death rates in coronary heart disease patients in the Harvard Alumni Study. RR = Relative risk.

Table 5.2   Cardiovascular Mortality by Activity Level in the British Regional Heart Study

	CARDIOVASCULAR MORTALITY	
Activity level	Age-adjusted RR	Fully-adjusted RR[a]
Inactive or occasional	1.00	1.00
Light	0.33	0.38
Moderate	0.39	0.50
Moderate to vigorous	0.49	0.61

Note. RR = relative risk.

[a]Adjusted for age, smoking, social class, self-rated health status, diabetes, and history of myocardial infarction and stroke.

Adapted from Meyers 2002.

largest difference in mortality was observed during the first year of the investigation when β-blocker use was similar for both groups.

Meta-Analyses

Although there are many randomized, controlled trials of cardiac rehabilitation including exercise training, no other studies besides the two previously discussed have provided evidence for a statistically significant reduction in coronary risk. Many of these trials have been plagued by insufficient numbers of subjects to achieve adequate statistical power and by subject dropouts and crossovers. Investigators have pooled data from the various trials (meta-analysis) to partially overcome these limitations and to determine pooled estimates of benefits.

In 1989, O'Connor and colleagues[25] performed a meta-analysis of 22 randomized trials of exercise training and standard risk factor intervention of varying intensity resulting in a total sample of 4,554 post-MI patients. Compared with control subjects, patients who were randomized to the exercise intervention experienced a reduction in total mortality, cardiovascular mortality, and fatal reinfarction of 20%, 22%, and 25%, respectively.

A recent expanded meta-analysis by Jolliffe and associates[26] was published in the Cochrane Database. The authors searched electronic databases for appropriate randomized trials from the earliest date until the end of 1998. They included studies with both genders and included subjects with diagnoses of MI, coronary bypass surgery, percutaneous revascularization, angina pectoris, and angiographically documented coronary atherosclerosis. All accepted trials used exercise training as a component of the intervention. End points included mortality, morbidity, health-related quality of life, and standard coronary risk factors. A total of 32 trials were included in

their analysis with 8,440 subjects. A 31% reduction (relative risk 0.69) in cardiac mortality for intervention subjects was found. There was no effect on nonfatal myocardial infarction.

Risks During Acute Exercise

Previous sections of this chapter have provided clear evidence for the cardioprotective effects of regular physical activity or exercise training. However, during an acute bout of exercise, the risk of sudden cardiac death or MI is transiently increased.[27] Acute exertion may trigger a cardiac event in a susceptible individual. Coronary atherosclerosis is the major underlying pathology in exercise-related sudden death or acute MI in adults. Mittleman and colleagues[28] interviewed 1,228 survivors of acute MI. In approximately 5% of cases, heavy exertion apparently triggered the infarction.

The annual incidence of exercise-related cardiac arrest in previously healthy persons is 5.4/100,000[2]. The incidence is 56 times higher than that at rest for sedentary men and 5 times higher for physically active men.[29] The risk of MI during exercise is 2 to 6 times higher than at rest.[27]

Even highly trained endurance athletes are not immune from exercise-associated cardiac death, although the risk is extremely low. In a survey of 215,413 marathon runners, four deaths were documented during running (prevalence of 0.002%).[30] Three of the four deaths were attributable to previously undetected coronary atherosclerosis.

Survey data from the 1980s are available regarding the incidence of cardiac events in patients with CHD who exercise under supervision in cardiac rehabilitation programs.[31] The rates per 1,000,000 patient-hours of exercise for cardiac arrest, acute MI, and cardiac death were 8.9, 2.4 and 1.3, respectively.

Mechanisms of Exercise-Associated Cardiac Risk

What mechanisms are responsible for the transient increase in cardiac risk during an acute bout of exertion? Although not completely understood, the following are accepted as reasonable mechanisms:

- Hemodynamic stress may result in rupture and subsequent thrombus formation in a high-risk coronary plaque. Burke and associates[32] reported autopsy evidence of this type of occurrence in 68% of cases of sudden cardiac death associated with exertion. Plaque rupture and thrombosis may also result in acute MI.

- Myocardial ischemia is an important contributor to malignant ventricular arrhythmia. In patients with coronary atherosclerosis, an acute bout of exercise may cause constriction of diseased coronary segments, unlike the usual exertion-related vasodilation of healthy coronary arteries. This increases the likelihood of the development of ischemia. The reasons for this paradoxical coronary vasoconstriction include excessive sympathetic nervous system activation, endothelial dysfunction, and platelet aggregation.[33]

- Autonomic nervous system imbalance (autonomic dysfunction), with inappropriate activation of the sympathetic division and diminished parasympathetic activation, may result in ventricular arrhythmia independent of myocardial ischemia.[34]

Potential Mechanisms of Exercise Benefit

The evidence is clear that habitual physical activity is beneficial in reducing the risk of coronary heart disease. The precise mechanisms resulting in the benefit are not fully understood. Does exercise training result in structural improvements in the coronary arteries? Can habitual physical activity favorably modify risk factors? Can it change the usual progressive course of coronary atherosclerosis? Does it reduce myocardial ischemia or alter the anatomy of the coronary circulation? The following discussion highlights many of the potential reasons for the cardioprotective effect of exercise.

Structural Improvements in Coronary Arteries

Habitual physical activity may result in structural adaptations of the epicardial coronary arteries such as the following:

- Increased cross-sectional area of the lumen[35]

- Improved capacity for vasodilation, probably resulting from enhanced endothelial function[36]

- Potential increased collateral circulation in patients with ischemic left ventricular dysfunction[37]

Improvement in Coronary Risk Factors

Exercise or physical activity may reduce the severity of several common modifiable risk factors:

- Hypertension
- Adverse blood lipid profile
- Obesity
- Psychosocial stress

Observational data from the Harvard Alumni Study are consistent with the concept that habitual exercise appears to reduce the chances of developing *hypertension*.[38] Regular exercise may modestly lower blood pressure in hypertensive patients and in individuals with blood pressure in the normal range by an average of 6 to 9 mm Hg for both systolic and diastolic pressures.[39]

Regular exercise results in modest improvements in the *blood lipid profile*. A meta-analysis revealed an average reduction in total cholesterol of 7 to 13 mg·dl^{-1}, low-density (LDL) cholesterol of 3 to 11 mg·dl^{-1}, and triglycerides of 14 to 22 mg·dl^{-1}.[40] High-density lipoprotein (HDL) cholesterol increased by an average of 2 mg·dl^{-1}. There is marked interindividual variability in the effect of exercise training on blood lipids.

The role of exercise in augmentation of *HDL cholesterol* deserves further comment. HDL appears to be an extremely important factor in reducing atherothrombotic risk.[41] It has various coronary protective effects that include antioxidant, anti-inflammatory, and antithrombotic properties; it is profibrinolytic and plays a pivotal role in reverse cholesterol transport from the arterial wall to the liver. Although the effects of exercise in increasing HDL cholesterol appear modest, it is generally accepted that for each 1 mg·dl^{-1} increase, coronary risk is reduced by 2% to 3%.

Obesity is a particularly important risk factor. The prevalence of obesity has increased by 61% since 1991. The Behavioral Risk Factor Surveillance System report for the year 2000 indicated that 19.8% of the U.S. adult population were obese (body mass index [BMI] ≥30).[42] The prevalence of overweight (BMI ≥25) was 56.4% (increase of 45% since 1991). Obesity is an independent coronary risk factor and is also associated with other potent factors such as glucose intolerance and type 2 diabetes mellitus, hypertension, dyslipidemia, and a sedentary lifestyle. Excess abdominal subcutaneous adipose tissue is strongly associated with abnormal glucose metabolism and dyslipidemia.[43]

Obesity (as well as many other established risk factors) also results in impaired endothelial function, an early occurrence in the pathogenesis of atherosclerosis. It is associated with the inflammatory marker C-reactive protein as well as a variety of other proinflammatory cytokines such as tumor necrosis factor-α and interleukin-6.[44,45]

Exercise, in adequate amounts, is effective as part of a comprehensive approach to reduce fat weight in obesity. McGuire and colleagues[46] studied differences in obese subjects who were successful in maintaining an average 37-lb (16.7-kg) weight loss over 7 years compared with subjects who were not successful.[46] For subjects who maintained the weight loss, the average number of weekly sessions of physical activity was higher (8.4 vs. 5.5) as was the number of strenuous exercise sessions each week (2.8 vs. 1.8). The American College of Sports Medicine recommends 200 to 300 min·week^{-1} of exercise for long-term weight loss and control,[47] more than the typical amount of physical activity recommended for general health benefits. Exercise training also reduces abdominal fat to a greater extent than gluteal or femoral fat in obese men.[43] In the Aerobics Center Longitudinal Study, more than 5,000 men and women underwent three treadmill exercise tests (between 1970 and 1994) and were followed for an average of 7.5 years.[48] Subjects who increased fitness from one treadmill test to the next, presumably by increasing habitual exercise, attenuated the usual age-related increase in body weight. In obese subjects, weight loss of more than 9 kg has been shown to substantially reduce C-reactive protein as well as proinflammatory cytokines (tumor necrosis factor-α and interleukin-6, for example).[44,45]

Symptoms of *depression* consistently improve with habitual physical activity.[49] Physically active persons appear to be at lower risk for the development of depression, and patients with documented depression may demonstrate improvement with exercise training. In patients with documented coronary heart disease, exercise has been shown to improve anxiety, emotional distress, and depression.[50]

Attenuation of Metabolic Syndrome

Patients who have a clustering of three or more of the following risk factors have the "metabolic syndrome."[51]

- Abdominal obesity (waist circumference >102 cm for men, >88 cm for women)
- Hypertriglyceridemia (>150 mg·dl^{-1})
- Low HDL cholesterol (<40 mg·dl^{-1} for men, <50 mg·dl^{-1} for women)
- Hypertension (≥130/85)
- High fasting blood glucose (≥110 mg·dl^{-1})

The metabolic syndrome is closely linked to the generalized metabolic disorder of insulin resistance (impaired normal actions of insulin). The prevalence of this syndrome increases with age and is approximately 22% for the U.S. adult population (similar prevalence for men and women). The causes of the metabolic syndrome for the overwhelming majority of patients are an improper diet and too little physical activity. It is closely linked to insulin resistance. First-line therapy for the metabolic syndrome is increased physical activity and weight reduction.[52,53]

Improved Glucose Metabolism and Reduced Risk for Type 2 Diabetes Mellitus

Persons who perform exercise training have a lower plasma insulin concentration and improved insulin sensitivity compared with sedentary individuals.[54] With cessation of regular training, insulin concentration and sensitivity return to levels observed in sedentary persons.

Unfortunately, with the increasing prevalence of obesity and overweight as discussed previously, the prevalence of type 2 diabetes mellitus in adults has also increased and is now 7.3% (an increase of 49% since 1991).[42] Exercise and proper nutrition have been shown to improve glucose metabolism and to prevent the onset of type 2 diabetes mellitus. A 1-year program of exercise and diet change resulted in an average weight loss of 10 kg and resulted in a decrease in fasting blood glucose and insulin concentrations.[45] In another study comparing lifestyle intervention including exercise with drug therapy (metformin) in persons with impaired glucose tolerance, the lifestyle intervention resulted in the greatest reduction in the incidence of diabetes developing during the nearly 3 years of follow-up.[55]

Table 5.3.	Weekly Exercise Amount and the Risk of Developing Type 2 Diabetes: Nurses' Health Study	
Weekly exercise duration (hr)	**Relative risk**
<0.5	1.0
0.5-1.9	0.89
2.0-3.9	0.87
4.0-6.9	0.83
≥7.0	0.71

Adapted from Hu 2000.

In the Nurses' Health Study, subjects who performed more than 30 min of exercise per week experienced a much lower relative risk of developing diabetes over the 16 years of follow-up (table 5.3).[56] The Diabetes Prevention Study was a randomized, controlled trial of an intervention of exercise and diet in 552 middle-aged men and women with impaired glucose tolerance but not type 2 diabetes mellitus.[57] After 3 years, intervention subjects had lost an average of 3 to 4 kg and experienced a 58% reduction in the incidence of diabetes (diabetes occurred in 11% of intervention subjects vs. 23% of controls).

Improved Autonomic Nervous System Function

Autonomic dysfunction, defined as a sustained increase in sympathetic activity and a decrease in parasympathetic activity, is associated with increased coronary risk and mortality.[34] Clinical indicators of autonomic dysfunction include the following: resting heart rate greater than 90 beats·min⁻¹, inability to achieve 85% of age-predicted maximal heart rate during graded exercise testing, abnormally slow heart rate recovery after maximal exercise (failure to decrease heart rate >12 beats·min⁻¹ during the first minute of recovery), and decreased heart rate variability (failure to change heart rate by ≥10 beats·min⁻¹ during 1 min of slow deep breaths). Autonomic dysfunction may result in endothelial dysfunction, coronary vasospasm, left ventricular hypertrophy, and malignant ventricular arrhythmias.

Exercise transiently increases sympathetic tone and reduces parasympathetic activity. Exercise training results in a favorable decrease in sympathetic activity and an increase in parasympathetic tone in both healthy subjects[58] and in patients with coronary disease.[59]

Improved Endothelial Function

Endothelial dysfunction occurs in response to exposure to coronary risk factors and is an early and late player in atherogenesis.[60] The following abnormalities may result:

- Impaired vasodilation, increased vasospasm
- Increased permeability to lipoproteins and other blood constituents
- Increased adhesion of platelets, glycoproteins

Endothelial dysfunction may result in reduced myocardial perfusion and plaque rupture leading to acute coronary syndromes of unstable angina, acute myocardial infarction, and sudden cardiac death.[61] Exercise training improves measures of endothelial function (endothelial-dependent vasodilation) in patients with coronary atherosclerosis.[62-64]

Reduced Progression of Coronary Atherosclerosis

Exercise training, in sufficient amounts, appears to slow the progression of, or even modestly reverse, coronary atherosclerosis. A 1-year randomized, controlled trial of supervised, moderate-intensity exercise and a low-fat diet without the use of lipid-lowering medication was performed in approximately 60 subjects.[65] Angiographically determined progression of disease occurred in 45% of controls and 10% of exercise subjects. A modest degree of regression of disease was found in 28% of exercisers versus 6% of controls. Figure 5.3 shows that partial regression of coronary atherosclerosis was present only in patients who expended an average of 2,200 kcal·week⁻¹or more in exercise (approximately 5-6 hr of moderate-intensity exercise per week).

Decreased Thrombosis Risk

Acute exercise results in a transient activation of the coagulation system resulting in an increased risk of thrombosis.[66] However, exercise training results in a

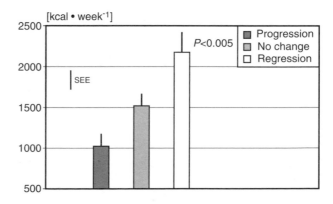

Figure 5.3 Energy expenditure per week and changes in angiographic coronary lesion morphology over 1 year.

decrease in thrombotic risk by the following mechanisms.[67-69]

- Reduced fibrinogen concentration
- Reduced platelet aggregation
- Decreased plasminogen activator inhibitor-1 (PAI-1)
- Increased endogenous tissue plasminogen activator (t-PA)

Improvement of Myocardial Ischemia

Exercise training may improve exercise-induced myocardial ischemia by decreasing myocardial demand and improving oxygen delivery to the heart.[70-72] As seen in figure 5.4, for a standard submaximal exercise intensity, after training, the rate–pressure product is reduced (lower myocardial oxygen requirement). This enables the patient to perform a higher intensity of physical activity before exceeding the ischemic threshold. This assumes that the ischemic threshold is relatively constant.

Data indicate that the rate–pressure product at the ischemic threshold is increased by training, independent of changes in other risk factors or anti-ischemic medications, suggesting that myocardial blood supply has improved.[73] Exercise-induced myocardial ischemia, measured by exercise thallium perfusion imaging and without alteration in the rate–pressure product, has been shown to improve by 54% and 34% after training.[71,72]

Summary

The data presented in this chapter demonstrate that habitual exercise and physical activity consis-

tently reduce overall coronary risk by a substantial amount. Although it is clear that an acute bout of exercise transiently increases the risk of a coronary event, the absolute risk is very small. The data for primary prevention are observational in nature, and randomized trials have not been performed because of logistical and ethical constraints. Occupational as well as leisure-time activities are cardioprotective. Cardiorespiratory fitness is inversely related to coronary risk. Investigations for secondary prevention include both observational and randomized trials. Individual trials were generally underpowered to detect differences in mortality and reinfarction, but meta-analyses have consistently demonstrated a powerful protective effect.

The data are consistent with the concept that the greater the total energy expenditure in physical activity or exercise, the lower the coronary risk. Most of the data suggest that higher-intensity activity is more protective than lower-intensity activity.

The potential mechanisms responsible for the cardioprotective action of exercise and physical activity are not completely understood but include improvement in the classic coronary risk factors, reduction in autonomic nervous system and endothelial cell dysfunction, reduced thrombosis and increased fibrinolysis, less progression and possible modest regression of coronary atherosclerotic lesions, and a reduction in myocardial ischemia. All of this information provides a solid evidence base for the use of exercise training as part of a comprehensive approach to primary and secondary prevention of coronary heart disease.

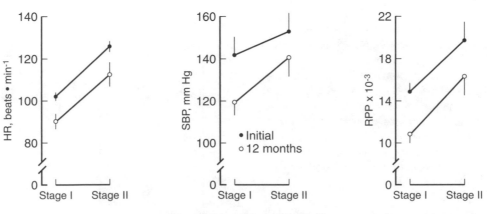

Figure 5.4 Effects of 12 months of exercise training on heart rate (HR), systolic blood pressure (SBP), and the rate–pressure product (RPP) at stages 1 and 2 of the Bruce treadmill exercise testing protocol. All variables were significantly lower ($p<0.01$) aftr training.

Cardiovascular and Exercise Physiology

Jonathon N. Myers, PhD

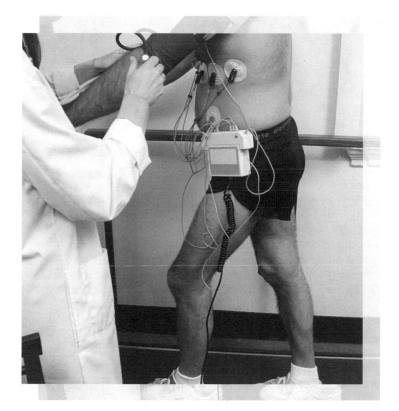

Although cardiac rehabilitation encompasses physical, psychosocial, vocational, and educational components, at its foundation rests the fact that a program of regular exercise results in cardiovascular and other physiological adaptations that will enable the patient to more readily return to normal activities of daily living and will limit the effects of the illness. The field of cardiac rehabilitation developed several decades ago as research led to recognition that bed rest after a myocardial infarction was associated with numerous deleterious physiological effects (see the sidebar)[1-3] and that regular exercise was associated with many physiological benefits. Regular exercise training improves exercise capacity, relieves symptoms in many patients, enhances the capacity to perform daily activities, and improves cardiovascular morbidity and mortality rates.[4,5] Thus, allied health professionals must understand the physiology underlying acute and chronic responses to exercise.

Acute Physiological Responses to Exercise

The acute response to exercise involves the transformation of chemical energy bound in the muscle into mechanical energy, which permits the individual to perform work. The transformation of chemical energy into mechanical energy requires the complex integration of the cardiovascular and pulmonary systems, which provide gas exchange between the muscle cells

GUIDELINES, 4TH EDITION

- Chapter 6, pages 72-84

Physiological Consequences of Prolonged Bed Rest

1. Loss of muscle mass, strength, and endurance
2. Decreased plasma and blood volume
3. Decreased ventricular volume
4. Increased hematocrit and hemoglobin
5. Diuresis and natriuresis
6. Venous stasis
7. Bone demineralization
8. Increased heart rate at rest and submaximal levels of activity
9. Decreased resting and maximum stroke volume
10. Decreased maximum cardiac output
11. Decreased maximum oxygen uptake
12. Increased venous compliance
13. Increased risk of venous thrombosis and thromboembolism
14. Decreased orthostatic tolerance
15. Increased risk of atelectasis, pulmonary emboli

and the atmosphere. Ultimately, the body is able to perform work because energy for muscular contraction is produced by cellular respiration. Cellular respiration is the process by which the body breaks down fuels with the aid of oxygen to generate energy. Exercise largely depends on the oxidation of carbohydrates and fat for the regeneration of adenosine triphosphate (ATP), which is required to sustain muscle contraction. The exercising muscles consume oxygen in the mitochondria and produce chemical energy in the form of ATP, with carbon dioxide (CO_2) as the major by-product. This aerobic process is called oxidative phosphorylation, and it provides the major source of chemical energy needed during sustained exercise. In addition to oxidative phosphorylation, ATP can be generated for muscle contraction through two other systems: the ATP-phosphocreatine (ATP-PCr) system and the glycolytic system. The ATP-PCr system is called on for short bursts of activity lasting less than 15 s. Energy released by the breakdown of PCr is not used directly to accomplish cellular work but rather to rebuild ATP to maintain a constant supply. The glycolytic system involves the production of energy through the breakdown of glucose (glycolysis). In this process, glucose or glycogen is broken down to pyruvic acid via glycolytic enzymes. When this process occurs with inadequate oxygen supply, pyruvic acid is converted to lactic acid. This process for energy production is inefficient relative to oxidative phosphorylation; 1 mol of glycogen yields 3 mol of ATP during glycolysis, whereas 1 mol of glycogen yields 39 mol of ATP during oxidative phosphorylation. In addition, the lactic acid produced during nonoxidative glycolysis can limit exercise by stimulating ventilation and inhibiting further steps in glycolysis. Early lactate accumulation in the blood and its consequences limit exercise in many patients with heart disease.

Cardiopulmonary Response

Although virtually all of the body's physiological and metabolic systems function in a coordinated manner to provide energy to the exercising muscle, the cardiopulmonary system has a particularly critical role in the acute response to exercise. The cardiovascular system responds to exercise with a series of adjustments that ensure the following:

1. Active muscles receive blood supply that is appropriate to their metabolic needs.
2. Heat generated by the muscles is dissipated.
3. Blood supply to the brain and the heart is maintained.

These adjustments require a major redistribution of cardiac output along with a number of local metabolic changes. The magnitude by which the basic hemodynamic and metabolic variables change from rest to a moderately high level of exercise is illustrated in figure 6.1. Exercise capacity is determined by a central component (cardiac output) that describes the capacity of the heart to function as a pump and by peripheral factors (arteriovenous oxygen difference) that describe the capacity of the lung to oxygenate the blood delivered to it and the capacity of the working muscle to extract this oxygen from the blood. Figure 6.2 outlines the factors that affect cardiac output and arteriovenous oxygen difference. Exercise capacity can be limited in patients with cardiovascular or pulmonary disease by one or several of these links in the chain that deter-

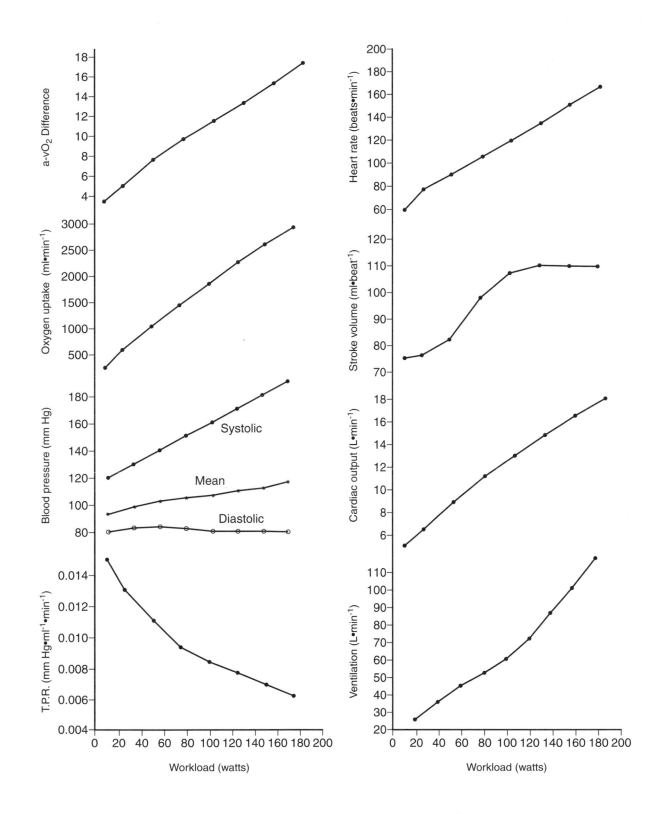

Figure 6.1 Response of basic hemodynamic and metabolic variables from rest to a moderately high level of exercise in the upright position.

Reprinted from *Primary Care,* Vol. 28, J. Myers, The physiology behind exercise testing, pgs. 5-28, Copyright 2001, with permission from Elsevier.

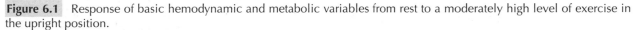

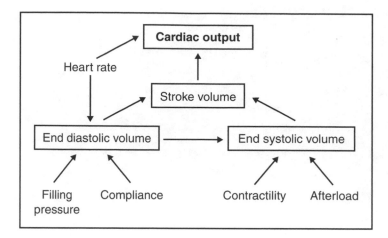

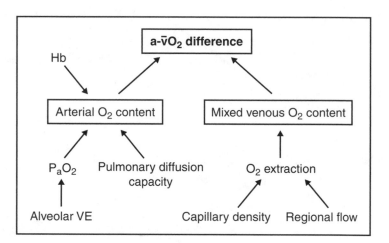

Figure 6.2 Central and peripheral determinants of maximal oxygen uptake. $(a\text{-}\bar{v})O_2$ difference = the difference between arterial and venous oxygen; Hb = hemoglobin; $\dot{V}_E$ = minute ventilation; P_AO_2 = partial pressure of alveolar oxygen.

Adapted, by permission, from J. Myers and V.F. Froelicher, 1991, "Hemodynamic determinants of exercise capacity in chronic heart failure," *Annals of Internal Medicine* 115: 337-386.

mine oxygen supply to the tissues. In the following, the major central and peripheral factors are discussed relative to the acute response to exercise.

Central Factors

Central factors refer to the changes that must occur acutely within the heart to adequately meet the increased metabolic demands of the body during exercise. Generally, these factors include those that influence the capacity of the heart to receive blood from the venous side of the circulatory system and eject blood into the arterial circulation. This will determine the ability of the body to deliver oxygen to the metabolically active skeletal muscles. Specific central factors include heart rate, stroke volume, filling pressure, ventricular compliance, contractility, afterload, and ventricular volume.

Oxygen Uptake The usual measure of the capacity of the body to deliver and use oxygen is the maximal

oxygen uptake ($\dot{V}O_2$max), which can be expressed by the Fick principal:

$$\dot{V}O_2\text{max} = \text{maximal cardiac output} \times \text{maximal arteriovenous oxygen difference}$$

Oxygen uptake increases linearly with increasing work and increases 5 to 20 times from its resting value. This is accomplished by a two- to threefold increase in heart rate and an approximate 50% increase in stroke volume, resulting in an increase in cardiac output ranging from 2 to 5 times. Maximal oxygen uptake may reach levels as high as 4 to 5 L·min^{-1} in young, fit individuals, commensurate with an increase in the resting metabolic rate of 15 to 20 times. Because $\dot{V}O_2$max is related to body weight, it is commonly adjusted for weight in kilograms; normal values for healthy adults generally range from 25 to 50 ml·kg^{-1}·min^{-1}. Increases in cardiac output are paralleled by increases in ventilation, such that ventilation and perfusion are appropriately matched in the lung. Cardiac output must closely match ventilation in the lung to deliver oxygenated blood to the working muscle. $\dot{V}O_2$max can also be expressed by the maximal amount of ventilation moving into and out of the lung and by the fraction of oxygen in this ventilation that is extracted by the tissues:

$$\dot{V}O_2 = \dot{V}_E \times (F_IO_2 - F_EO_2)$$

where $\dot{V}_E$ is minute ventilation and F_IO_2 and F_EO_2 are the fractional amounts of oxygen in the inspired and expired air, respectively (the equation shown is a bit oversimplified because it makes several assumptions). Thus, the physiological response to exercise requires the integration of cardiac, pulmonary, and peripheral components.

Total body oxygen uptake and myocardial oxygen uptake are distinct in their determinants and in the way that they are measured or estimated (table 6.1). Total body or ventilatory oxygen uptake is the amount of oxygen that is extracted from the inspired air as the body performs work. Myocardial oxygen uptake is the amount of oxygen consumed by the heart muscle. This distinction is important because patients with coronary artery disease are frequently limited in activity by myocardial oxygen demand and not by total body oxygen uptake. The determinants of myocardial oxygen uptake include intramyocardial wall tension (left ventricular pressure × end-diastolic volume), contractility, and heart rate. Myocardial oxygen uptake is estimated with reasonable accuracy by the product of heart rate and systolic blood pressure (double product or rate–pressure product).[6] This relationship between myocardial oxygen demand and double product is valuable clinically because stable exercise-induced angina often occurs at the same myocardial oxygen demand (double product), and thus it is one physiological variable that is useful when evaluating therapy.

Heart Rate The initial hemodynamic response to exercise is an increase in heart rate. With the onset of exercise, sympathetic outflow to the heart and systemic blood vessels increases, whereas vagal outflow decreases. Of the two major components of cardiac output, heart rate and stroke volume, heart rate is responsible for most of the increase in cardiac output during exercise, particularly at higher levels. Heart rate increases linearly with workload and oxygen uptake. Increases in heart rate occur primarily at the expense of diastolic and not systolic time. Thus, at very high heart rates, such as might be observed in a patient with atrial fibrillation, diastolic time may be so short as to preclude adequate ventricular filling.

The heart rate response to exercise is influenced by several factors, including age, the type of activity, body position, fitness, presence of heart disease, medications, blood volume, and environment.[7] Of these, perhaps the most important is age; a decline in maximal heart rate occurs with increasing age. This appears to be attributable to intrinsic cardiac changes rather than to neural influences. There is a great deal of variability around the regression line between maximal heart rate and age; thus, age-related maximal heart rate is a relatively imprecise index of maximal effort.[7,8]

Stroke Volume The product of stroke volume (the volume of blood ejected per heart beat) and heart rate determines cardiac output. Stroke volume is equal to the difference between end-diastolic and end-systolic volumes. Thus, a greater diastolic filling (preload) will increase stroke volume. Alternatively, factors that increase arterial blood pressure will resist ventricular outflow (afterload) and result in a reduced stroke volume. Normal values for stroke volume are roughly 75 ml·beat^{-1} at rest, although highly trained individuals may have values as high as 100 ml·beat^{-1}. During exercise, stroke volume increases up to approximately 50% to 60% of an individual's maximal exercise capacity, after which increases in cardiac output are attributable to further increases in heart rate (figure 6.1). The extent to which increases in stroke volume during exercise reflect an increase in end-diastolic volume or a decrease in end-systolic volume can vary considerably and depends on ventricular function, body position, and intensity of exercise.

In addition to heart rate, end-diastolic volume (and therefore stroke volume) is determined by two other factors: *filling pressure* and *ventricular compliance*.

Filling Pressure The most important determinant of ventricular filling is venous pressure.

Table 6.1	**Physiologic Determinants of Myocardial and Total Body (Ventilatory) Oxygen Consumption**	
Myocardial oxygen consumption	Heart rate × systolic blood pressure
	Determinants include wall tension (left ventricular pressure × volume), contractility, and heart rate.
Ventilatory oxygen consumption ($\dot{V}O_2$)	External work performed, or cardiac output × (a-v̄)O_2difference[a]

[a]The arteriovenous oxygen difference, or (a-v̄)O_2 difference, is approximately 15 to 17 ml O_2·100 ml^{-1} blood at maximal exercise in most individuals; therefore, $\dot{V}O_2$ max provides an approximate estimate of cardiac output.

The degree of venous pressure is a direct consequence of venous return. The Frank–Starling mechanism dictates that, within limits, all of the blood returned to the heart will be ejected during systole. As the tissues demand greater oxygen during exercise, venous return increases, which increases end-diastolic fiber length (preload), resulting in a more forceful contraction. Venous pressure increases as exercise intensity increases. Over the course of a few beats, cardiac output will equal venous return.

Several other factors affect venous pressure and, therefore, filling pressure during exercise. These include blood volume, body position, and the pumping action of the respiratory and skeletal muscles. A greater blood volume increases venous pressure and, therefore, end-diastolic volume by making more blood available to the heart. Because the effects of gravity are negated, filling pressure is greatest in the supine position. In fact, stroke volume generally does not increase from rest to maximal exercise in the supine position. The intermittent mechanical contraction and relaxation of the skeletal muscles during exercise also enhance venous return. Last, changes in intrathoracic pressure, which occur with breathing during exercise, facilitate the return of blood to the heart.

Ventricular Compliance Compliance is a measure of the capacity of the ventricle to stretch in response to a given volume of blood. Specifically, compliance is defined as the ratio of the change in volume to the change in pressure. The diastolic pressure–volume relation is curvilinear; that is, at lower end-diastolic pressures, large changes in volume are accompanied by small changes in pressure and vice versa. At the upper limits of end-diastolic pressure, ventricular compliance declines; that is, the chamber becomes stiffer as it fills.

Contractility End-systolic volume is influenced largely by two factors: contractility and afterload. Contractility describes the forcefulness of the heart's contraction. Increasing contractility reduces end-systolic volume, which results in a greater stroke volume and thus cardiac output. This is precisely what occurs with exercise in the normal individual; the amount of blood in the ventricle that is ejected with each beat increases, owing to an altered cross-bridge formation. Contractility is commonly quantified by the *ejection fraction* (stroke volume ÷ end-diastolic volume × 100), which is the percentage of blood ejected from the ventricle during systole as measured by radionuclide, echocardiographic, or angiographic techniques. Despite its wide application as an index of myocardial contractility, ejection fraction has been repeatedly shown to correlate poorly with exercise capacity (figure 6.3).[8-11]

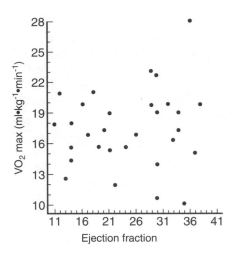

Figure 6.3 The relationship between resting left ventricular ejection fraction and maximal oxygen uptake in patients with chronic heart failure ($r = .13$, not significant). Numerous studies have confirmed that the relationship between exercise capacity and left ventricular function is poor.

Reprinted from *American Heart Journal,* Vol. 124, J. Myers et al., Ventilatory mechanisms of exercise intolerance in chronic heart failure, pgs. 710-718, Copyright 1992, with permission from Elsevier.

Afterload Afterload is a measure of the force resisting the ejection of blood by the heart. Increased afterload (or aortic pressure, as is observed with chronic hypertension) reduces ejection fraction and increases end-diastolic and end-systolic volumes. During dynamic exercise, the force resisting ejection in the periphery (total peripheral resistance) is reduced by vasodilation as a result of the effect of local metabolites on the skeletal muscle vasculature. The chemical factors that exert local vasodilatory effects on the vessels include decreased pH, increased partial pressure of carbon dioxide (PCO_2), and increased lactic acid concentration. Thus, despite even a fivefold increase in cardiac output among normal individuals during exercise, mean arterial pressure increases only moderately.

Ventricular Volume Response to Exercise Results of studies evaluating the volume response to exercise have varied greatly. The volume response to exercise depends on the presence and type of disease, the method of measurement (radionuclide or echocardiographic), the type of exercise (supine vs. upright), and the exercise intensity (submaximal vs. maximal). In general, the response from upright rest to a maximal level of exercise is an increase in end-diastolic volume and a decrease in end-systolic volume. End-diastolic volume increases through enhanced venous return and filling pressure. This stretches myocardial fibers, causing a more forceful contraction (the Frank-Starling mechanism), which decreases end-systolic volume. Within physiological limits, end-diastolic volume increases progressively as exercise intensity increases. The volume response to exercise among patients with cardiovascular disease differs somewhat from people with healthy hearts depending on the limits imposed by the disease. For example, most studies using echocardiography to study the volume response to upright exercise in patients with cardiovascular disease (CVD) have shown that the percentage (though not absolute) increase in end-diastolic volume is greater compared with that in people with healthy hearts, and end-systolic volume may actually increase slightly from resting values at near-maximal effort.

Peripheral Factors

With exercise, blood flow is directed away from the inactive tissues to the active skeletal muscle. In the skeletal muscle, oxygen uptake depends on capillary density, diffusion, muscle fiber distribution, and the oxidative potential of the muscle fibers. Oxygen extraction by the tissues during exercise reflects the difference between the oxygen content of the arteries and the oxygen content of the veins (see the sidebar). During exercise, this difference widens as the working tissues extract greater amounts of oxygen; venous oxygen content reaches very low levels, and a $\dot{V}O_2$ difference may be very high with exhaustive exercise. Some oxygenated blood always returns to the heart, however, as smaller amounts of blood continue to flow through metabolically less active tissues that do not fully extract oxygen. Generally, a-$\dot{V}O_2$ difference does not explain differences in $\dot{V}O_2$ max between subjects who are relatively homogeneous. That is, a-$\dot{V}O_2$ difference is generally considered to widen by a relatively fixed amount during exercise, and differences in $\dot{V}O_2$ max

have been historically explained by differences in maximal cardiac output. However, many patients with cardiovascular and pulmonary disease exhibit reduced $\dot{V}O_2$ max values that can be attributed to a combination of central and peripheral factors.

Arterial Oxygen Content Arterial oxygen content is related to the partial pressure of arterial oxygen, which is determined in the lung by alveolar ventilation and pulmonary diffusion capacity and in the blood by hemoglobin content. In the absence of pulmonary disease, arterial oxygen content and saturation generally remain similar to resting values throughout exercise, even at very high levels. This is true even among most patients with severe CVD or chronic heart failure. Patients with pulmonary disease, however, often neither ventilate the alveoli adequately nor diffuse oxygen from the lung into the blood normally, and a decrease in oxygen saturation during exercise is one of the hallmarks of this disorder. Arterial hemoglobin content is also usually normal throughout exercise. Naturally, a condition such as anemia would reduce the oxygen-carrying capacity of the blood, as would any condition that shifts the O_2 dissociation curve leftward, such as reduced 2,3 diphosphoglycerate, PCO_2, or temperature.

Venous Oxygen Content Venous oxygen content reflects the capacity to extract oxygen from the blood as it flows through the muscle. It is determined by the amount of blood directed to the muscle (regional flow) and by capillary density. Muscle blood flow increases in proportion to the increase in work rate and, thus, the oxygen requirement. The increase in blood flow is brought about not only by the increase in cardiac output but also by a preferential redistribution of the cardiac output to the exercising muscle (table 6.2); greater than 85% of the total cardiac output may be redistributed to

Oxygen Content

At rest:

- Arteries—18 to 20 ml O_2 per 100 ml blood
- Veins—13 to 15 ml O_2 per 100 ml blood
- (a-$\bar{v}$)O_2 difference—4 to 5 ml O_2 per 100 ml blood
- O_2 extraction—approximately 23%

During intense exercise:

- Arteries—18 to 20 ml O_2 per 100 ml blood
- Veins—4 to 6 ml O_2 per 100 ml blood
- (a-$\bar{v}$)O_2 difference—14 to 16 ml O_2 per 100 ml blood
- O_2 extraction—greater than 85%

Table 6.2	Distribution of Cardiac Output at Rest and During Strenuous Exercise	
Tissue	Rest (%)	Strenuous exercise (%)
Bone	5	1
Coronary	5	5
Skin	5	2
Brain	15	4
Kidneys	20	1
Liver	25	2
Muscle	20	85
Lungs	100	100

Note: Percentages reflect typical fractions of the total cardiac output directed toward each of tissues over a given period of time.

the skeletal muscle at high levels of exercise. A reduction in local vascular resistance facilitates this greater skeletal muscle flow; systemic vascular resistance decreases two- to threefold during exercise. In turn, locally produced vasodilatory mechanisms, and possibly neurogenic dilation caused by higher sympathetic activity, mediate the greater skeletal muscle blood flow. A marked increase in the number of open capillaries reduces diffusion distances, increases capillary blood volume, and increases mean transit time, facilitating oxygen delivery to the muscle.

Pulmonary Ventilation Minute ventilation ($\dot{V}_E$) is the volume of air taken into and out of the lungs, expressed in liters per minutes. It is determined by the product of respiratory rate and the volume of air exhaled with each breath (tidal volume). At rest, $\dot{V}_E$ is typically 6 to 10 L·min^{-1} and may increase to levels greater than 150 L·min^{-1} during maximal exercise in healthy, athletic individuals. At lower levels of exercise, $\dot{V}_E$ increases largely by increasing tidal volume, whereas at higher levels of exercise $\dot{V}_E$ is augmented by a higher respiratory rate. $\dot{V}_E$ increases linearly with oxygen uptake at low and moderate levels of exercise. At higher exercise intensities, however, $\dot{V}_E$ increases out of proportion to $\dot{V}O_2$. This is caused by the buffering of accumulating lactate in the blood, the by-product of which is CO_2, which further drives $\dot{V}_E$. The specific intensity at which this occurs is critical to both an athlete's performance and the capacity of the patient with heart disease to sustain daily activities.

Despite the important role of the pulmonary system in sustaining endurance exercise, maximal exercise is generally not limited by ventilatory factors unless pulmonary disease is present. A "breathing reserve" exists, such that only 60% to 80% of total breathing capacity is used with maximal effort. This is one of the major reasons why maximal exercise is generally thought to be limited by circulatory, and not pulmonary, factors.

Perturbation of the Exercise Response in CVD

Exercise intolerance can be caused by an abnormality in one or several of the cardiopulmonary or peripheral factors that determine peak $\dot{V}O_2$; such abnormalities are common in the presence of heart or lung disease. A low peak $\dot{V}O_2$ fundamentally reflects a lower than normal maximal cardiac output response to exercise. When left ventricular dysfunction is present (which can be caused by CHF, valvular disease, or exercise-induced ischemia), a low stroke volume underlies the reduction in cardiac output. To compensate, heart rate increases and $(a-\bar{v})O_2$ difference widens at comparatively low work rates. Low blood flow conditions influence biochemical changes in muscle such that

1. creatine phosphate levels are reduced,
2. phosphate and lactate concentrations are higher, and
3. pH values are reduced.

Heightened lactate levels can limit exercise by increasing ventilation and limiting further steps in glycolysis, which lead to fatigue. In patients with CVD, muscle biopsy studies have demonstrated reduced activity of aerobic enzymes and fiber atrophy.[12,13] Reductions in the activity of enzymes of the citric acid cycle in the leg muscles correlate with increases in femoral venous lactate during exercise,[13] suggesting that lactate production is related to a reduction in oxidative phosphorylation.

Normally, ventilation closely matches cardiac output in the lung in order to deliver oxygenated blood to the working muscle. The matching of ventilation and cardiac output is determined by the ratio of alveolar ventilation to lung perfusion. Some patients with abnormal cardiac output responses to exercise (e.g., patients with chronic heart failure) or abnormal diffusion in the pulmonary vasculature (e.g., patients with chronic lung disease) have a mismatching of ventilation to perfusion, breathe inefficiently, and exhibit exercise intolerance caused by shortness of breath. Patients with poor cardiac output responses to exercise often exhibit a heightened ventilatory response that parallels the degree of ventricular dysfunction. This hyperventilatory response is related both to lactic acidosis in the blood and to inefficient pulmonary gas exchange caused by inadequate pulmonary blood flow (poor ventilation–perfusion matching).[14-16] There is also recent evidence that augmented ergoreflex sensitivity (afferent fibers present in the skeletal muscle that are sensitive to metabolic changes during muscular work) contributes to hyperventilation in these patients.[17] This is often compounded by a characteristic rapid, shallow respiration because of reduced breathing capacity, an effort to reduce the work of breathing, or both.

Adaptations to Exercise Training

Regular exercise increases work capacity; hundreds of studies have documented a greater exercise capacity among active persons than among sedentary individuals in cross-sectional analyses or by comparing groups after a period of training. In general, patients with cardiovascular disease are equally able to benefit from exercise training as are healthy individuals, although some of the specific mechanisms for the training response differ. Improving exercise tolerance through a training program has numerous benefits, including a better capacity to sustain daily activities, an improvement in the rate of return to work, and an improvement in quality of life,[4,5,18] and studies have shown that both nondiseased people[19,20] and patients with CVD[20,21] with a higher exercise capacity have a significantly better survival rates.

The magnitude of the improvement in exercise capacity with training varies widely, generally ranging from 5% to 25%, but increases as large as 50% have been reported. The degree of change in exercise capacity depends primarily on the individual's initial state of fitness, but it is also affected by age and the type, frequency, and intensity of training. $\dot{V}O_2$ max may be as low as 10 to 15 ml·kg^{-1}·min^{-1} in patients with severe CVD, and values as high as 80 to 90 ml·kg^{-1}·min^{-1} have been observed among elite endurance athletes. The cardiovascular, hemodynamic, ventilatory, and metabolic adaptations to training are summarized in table 6.3 and reviewed in the following.

Cardiovascular Adaptations

Many animal studies have demonstrated significant morphologic changes with training, including myocardial hypertrophy with improved myocardial function, increases in coronary artery diameter, and increases in the myocardial capillary to fiber ratio. However, although the literature is replete with such studies among animals,[2] these adaptations have been difficult to demonstrate in humans.[8] The major cardiovascular morphologic outcome of a training program in healthy humans is probably an increase in cardiac size (left ventricular mass and chamber size), but this appears to occur primarily in younger subjects (e.g., <30 years) and is unlikely to be an adaptation observed in patients with CVD undergoing rehabilitation. In young,

Table 6.3. Physiologic Adaptations to Exercise Training in Humans

Morphologic adaptations	• Myocardial hypertrophy
Hemodynamic adaptations	• Decreased peripheral vascular resistance
	• Increased end-diastolic volume
	• Increased maximal and submaximal stroke volume
	• Increased maximal cardiac output
	• Decreased heart rate for any submaximal workload
Metabolic adaptations	• Increased mitochondrial volume and number
	• Greater muscle glycogen stores
	• Enhanced fat utilization
	• Enhanced lactate removal
	• Increased enzymes for aerobic metabolism
	• Increased maximal oxygen uptake
Ventilatory adaptations	• Increased maximal ventilation
	• Reduced ventilation at matched submaximal workloads
	• Delay in ventilatory threshold
	• Increased strength of respiratory muscles in selected patients (with specific respiratory muscle training)

healthy subjects, stroke volume increases at rest and throughout exercise after a period of exercise training. Evidence suggests that this adaptation is attributable more to increases in preload and possibly to local adaptations that reduce peripheral vascular resistance than it is to increases in myocardial contractility. A larger left ventricular end-diastolic volume after training has the effect of augmenting stroke volume via the Frank–Starling mechanism, increasing cardiac output and thus maximal oxygen uptake.

There is evidence that training improves left ventricular end-diastolic compliance (the capacity of the ventricle to stretch in response to a given volume of blood). Although comparisons between athletic and nonathletic populations have shown better compliance in athletes,[22,23] recent evidence suggests that regular exercise may improve compliance in at least some patients with congestive heart failure (CHF). This has been demonstrated by more rapid ventricular relaxation and improved Doppler filling patterns after 2 to 6 months of rehabilitation in patients with dilated cardiomyopathy.[24,25] This is a potentially important adaptation because diastolic dysfunction is more widely recognized than in the past, having a prevalence of at least 40% in patients with a diagnosis of CHF.[25] These patients exhibit an increased resistance to left ventricular filling and increased end-diastolic *and* end-systolic volumes, although ejection fraction is often normal.

Hemodynamic Adaptations

Hemodynamic changes after training include reductions in heart rate at rest and any matched submaximal workload, a reduction in total peripheral resistance (TPR) during exercise, increases in blood volume, enhanced vascular tone, enhanced vasodilatory capacity, and a better redistribution of the available blood flow. Maximal heart rate is unchanged or may be slightly reduced after a program of training. Resting heart rate frequently is reduced after training, which is attributable to enhanced parasympathetic tone. Heart rate is reduced at any matched submaximal workload after training. For the patient with coronary artery disease, the latter is one of the most important adaptations to exercise. Because heart rate closely parallels myocardial oxygen uptake, daily activities can be performed with less demand on the heart muscle, and angina symptoms are frequently lessened.

$\dot{V}O_2max$ has been demonstrated to be highly correlated to total blood volume; an increase in blood volume after training contributes both to the capacity to sustain a higher stroke volume during exercise and to an increase in the total cardiac output. In addition, fit subjects may have a greater capacity to redistribute blood flow toward the working muscles and away from nonexercising tissue. Over the last decade, a great deal of research has been directed toward studying the capacity and limitations of the vasculature to dilate in response to various stimuli in patients with heart disease. Exercise is an important stimulus for vasodilation, and the capacity to vasodilate is an important mechanism to increase blood flow to the working muscle. It is well established that patients with heart disease (particularly chronic heart failure) have abnormal vasodilatory capacity, which contributes to limiting perfusion to the muscle during exercise.[26] In recent years, numerous studies have demonstrated that the capacity for the peripheral vasculature to dilate in response to various stimuli, including exercise, is enhanced after training.[27,28]

Data from cross-sectional studies demonstrate that fit individuals have a greater skeletal muscle capillary density than sedentary subjects, and advances in histochemical techniques have permitted the demonstration of increases in the number of capillaries and higher capillary-to-fiber ratios after training.[29-31] Many of the skeletal muscle adaptations to training are reversible with deconditioning.[33] Both the total number and the density of capillaries (total number per gram of tissue) increase, on the order of 5 to 10%, with training.[32,33] This increases the surface area for capillary diffusion and increases red blood cell transit time. Both of these mechanisms provide a greater opportunity for oxygen and metabolite exchange in the tissues.

Metabolic Adaptations

It is often suggested that in patients with heart disease, the major physiological effects of training occur in the skeletal muscle. The metabolic capacity of the skeletal muscle is enhanced through increases in mitochondrial volume and number and oxidative enzyme content. The oxidative breakdown of fuels and the production of ATP depend on the action of mitochondrial oxidative enzymes, which catalyze the breakdown of nutrients to form ATP. Key enzymes such as succinate dehydrogenase and citrate synthase are significantly enhanced by training. These adaptations enhance perfusion and the efficiency of oxygen extraction, resulting in a widening of the $(a-\bar{v})O_2$ difference. Perhaps more important than the effect these enzymes have on peak $\dot{V}O_2$ is their effect on substrate utilization. These changes lead to a glycogen-sparing effect, which permits a higher intensity of exercise to be performed for a longer period of time. This is related to both a shift in the substrate used (e.g., a relatively greater use of fat vs. carbohydrate) and an increase in the lactate threshold, permitting a higher intensity of sustained exercise before the accumulation of lactate and subsequent metabolic acidosis and hyperventilation. Lactate accumulation in the blood is disadvantageous because it causes metabolic acidosis (which leads to hyperventilation) and can inhibit critical steps in the energy-producing processes in the mitochondria. The extent to which training reduces lactate production or enhances its removal is not clearly established, but reduced blood lactate is one of the important benefits of a training program. This is particularly true for patients who exhibit early lactic acidosis in response to exercise, such as severely deconditioned patients or those with chronic heart failure.

Ventilatory Adaptations

Resting pulmonary function, including vital capacity and flow rate (such as forced expiratory volume in 1 s, or FEV_1), generally does not change with training. In addition, because the respiratory system usually does not limit exercise (unless significant pulmonary disease is present), it is generally thought that there is little to be gained by training in terms of the respiratory system. However, a number of noteworthy adaptations to training increase the efficiency of the pulmonary system.

Maximal ventilation can increase substantially after training, to a degree that parallels the increase $\dot{V}O_2$peak. Tidal volume and respiratory rate increase by roughly equal amounts. Minute ventilation is reduced for any given workload or any given $\dot{V}O_2$, which is expressed by the ratio between $\dot{V}_E$ and carbon dioxide production (VCO_2) (figure 6.4). This is an important adaptation in that many patients who have had a myocardial infarction, those with chronic obstructive pulmonary disease (COPD), or those with congestive heart failure (CHF) exhibit dyspnea as their chief complaint. The major mechanism for the reduction in submaximal ventilation is a reduction in blood lactate for any given work rate after training, although better matching of ventilation to perfusion in the lung, more efficient breathing patterns, and alterations in skeletal muscle receptor activation may contribute.[34]

Respiratory muscles are a key modulator of the sensation of dyspnea, and researchers have hypothesized that training directed specifically to condition the respiratory muscles would attenuate exertional dyspnea and improve exercise tolerance, particularly in those limited by dyspnea.[35] In CHF, respiratory muscle training consisting of deep breathing at maximal sustainable respiratory capacity, resistive breathing, and strength training three times weekly for 3 months improved maximal sustainable respiratory capacity, maximal voluntary ventilation, respiratory muscle strength, peak $\dot{V}O_2$, and 6-min walk time.[34] In addition, a number of investigators have used ventilatory muscle training in efforts to improve pulmonary function, alleviate dyspnea, improve exercise tolerance, or all three in patients with COPD.[36-38] These studies have varied in terms of training protocols, intensity, and duration, but all have demonstrated to one extent or another that training targeted to these muscles can improve ventilatory capacity in patients with COPD. These findings in both CHF and COPD underscore a pulmonary component to exercise performance in selected patients. The improvements in submaximal and maximal exercise performance may result from an improvement in respiratory muscle strength, an increased ventilatory capacity, or desensitization to dyspnea. Although data in this area remain sparse, results of these studies suggest that training directed specifically to the respiratory muscles favorably affects exercise tolerance among patients who exhibit breathing limitations.

Summary

Acute exercise is an important medium with which to assess the physiology underlying cardiovascular and pulmonary disease. Documenting the physiological response to acute exercise is useful for determining the presence and extent of disease, for developing an individualized exercise program, and for stratifying risk in individuals with or suspected of having disease. Studies performed since the late 1960s have documented the many beneficial physiological changes that occur with rehabilitation. Although there are important central (cardiac) changes that occur with exercise training, the most important adaptations in the patient with cardiovascular or pulmonary disease occur in the periphery. These include skeletal muscle metabolic changes such as increases in mitochondrial volume

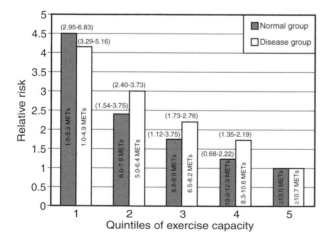

Figure 6.4 Age-adjusted relative risks of all-cause mortality by quintiles of exercise capacity among nondiseased subjects and patients with cardiovascular disease. The subgroup with the highest exercise capacity (quintile 5) is the referent group. For each quintile, the range of values for exercise capacity represented appears within each bar; 95% confidence intervals for the relative risks appear above each bar.

and number, increases in oxidative enzyme content of the muscle, and a shifting of substrate utilization. Hemodynamic changes that occur in response to training include reductions in heart rate at rest and any matched submaximal workload, a reduction in TPR during exercise, increases in blood volume, enhanced vascular tone, enhanced vasodilatory capacity, and a better redistribution of the available blood flow. These adaptations allow the individual to become more efficient in producing, delivering, and using energy for muscular work and alleviating symptoms associated with various cardiovascular and pulmonary conditions. Exercise training has also been demonstrated to improve cardiovascular morbidity and mortality rates in patients who have sustained a myocardial infarction.

Exercise Prescription

Barry A. Franklin, PhD, and Adam T. de Jong, MA

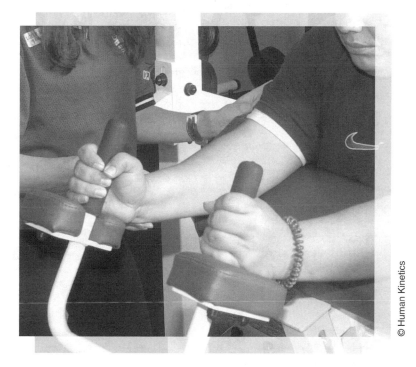

© Human Kinetics

E xercise training is widely recognized as an important component in comprehensive interventions aimed at the primary and secondary prevention of coronary heart disease (CHD). Secondary prevention involves patients with residual left ventricular dysfunction or exertion-induced symptomatic or asymptomatic myocardial ischemia, stable congestive heart failure, pacemaker, or implantable cardioverter defibrillators and those who have undergone coronary artery bypass graft surgery or angioplasty.[1] Physicians and allied health professionals who prescribe exercise for such patients must consider the patient's age, gender, clinical status, medications, related medical problems, habitual physical activity, musculoskeletal integrity, and, most importantly, the results derived from a progressive exercise tolerance test.[2]

This chapter reviews the physiological and clinical bases for the prescription of exercise in persons with and without CHD, with specific reference to the types of exercises and activities; the prescribed inten-sity, frequency, and duration of training; and the rate of progression. In addition, the value of upper-body and resistance training is discussed, along with specific prescriptive guidelines. Two case studies are also provided in appendix D, including clinically relevant data, treadmill test results, and the corresponding exercise prescriptions. Recommendations for exercise prescription for the inpatient, highlighting the value of orthostatic or gravitational stress (i.e., intermittent sitting or standing) during the bed rest stage of hospital convalescence,[3] are described elsewhere.[1]

GUIDELINES, 4TH EDITION

- Chapter 8, pages 114-123
- Chapter 9, pages 139-140
- Appendixes I, K, & M

Mode

The most effective exercises for physical conditioning use large muscle groups, are maintained continuously, and are rhythmic and aerobic in nature. These are commonly referred to as endurance exercises. Other exercise modalities often used in exercise-based primary and secondary prevention programs include calisthenics, particularly those involving sustained total body movement; flexibility and stretching exercises; resistance training; and recreational games. Recent research studies have shown that a lifestyle approach to physical activity (e.g., household chores, walking, gardening) can be as effective as a traditional exercise program.[4,5]

Endurance Exercise

Activities that evoke the greatest increase in aerobic capacity have certain characteristics, including alternately contracting and relaxing the muscles, especially in large muscle groups, that qualify the exercise as an endurance or cardiorespiratory activity. Examples include walking, jogging (in place or moving), running, stationary or outdoor cycling, swimming, skipping rope, rowing, climbing stairs, stepping on and off a bench, and cross-country skiing. A useful approach to endurance activity prescription is to identify a prescribed heart rate range for training,[6] using perceived exertion as an adjunctive intensity modulator.

Walking has several advantages over other forms of exercise during the initial stage of a physical conditioning program. Investigations in individuals with and without heart disease have shown that brisk walking on a flat surface, if undertaken at moderate speeds (e.g., 3-4 mph, or 4.8-6.4 km·hr^{-1}), can achieve an exercise intensity that is sufficient to induce a training effect, conservatively defined as 70% of the measured maximal heart rate.[7,8] Walking offers an easily tolerable exercise intensity and causes fewer musculoskeletal and orthopedic complications than jogging or running.[9] Moreover, it is a "companionable" activity that requires no special equipment other than a pair of well-fitted athletic shoes. Walking in water[10] or with a backpack[11] offers additional options for those who wish to reduce body weight and fat stores, improve cardiorespiratory fitness, or both.

Recreational games provide participants with recreational opportunities after the conditioning phase, and such activities often enhance compliance. However, game rules should be modified to maximize participant success and decrease the energy cost and heart rate response to play. For example, a volleyball game that allows one or more bounces of the ball per side facilitates longer rallies, provides additional fun, and reduces the intensity level of play. Through such modifications, the exercise professional can minimize skill requirements and competition and emphasize the primary objective of the activity, which is increased physical activity and enjoyment of the game itself. Heart rates should be monitored periodically.

Flexibility

Properly selected stretching exercises should be incorporated into the fitness program to develop and maintain range of motion. These exercises should stretch the major muscle groups, especially the low back and posterior thigh regions to reduce the risk of chronic low back pain. At least four repetitions per muscle group should be performed for a minimum of 2 to 3 days per week.[12] Two regimens, static and proprioceptive neuromuscular facilitation, are commonly recommended. Static stretches should be held for 10 to 30 s. Proprioceptive neuromuscular facilitation techniques, which consist of alternating 6 s of isometric muscle contraction with 10 to 30 s of passive, assisted stretching movements, have been shown to be superior to static or ballistic exercises in increasing flexibility.[13]

Resistance Exercise

Resistance exercise training involves activities that use low- to moderate-repetition movements (i.e., 8-15 repetitions) against resistance or fixed loads to increase muscular strength and endurance. For individuals without contraindications, the prescribed intensities generally approximate 50% of the maximal voluntary contraction.[14] Three common types of equipment are available to accommodate different types of training and different resistance training goals: free weights (e.g., barbells or dumbbells), multistation machines, and selectorized devices. Body weight (calisthenics), rubber band devices, pulley weights, dumbbells or wrist weights, barbells, or weight machines can be generally adapted for older, more frail individuals or those with left ventricular dysfunction.[15]

Lifestyle

Over the last decade, researchers have reexamined the scientific evidence linking a sedentary lifestyle with a variety of chronic diseases (see chapter 5). These analyses suggest that the intensity or dosage of exercise needed to achieve health-related benefits is probably less than that required to improve cardiorespiratory fitness. Accordingly, frequent bouts of moderate-intensity exercise—for example, 3 to 6 metabolic equivalents (METs; 1 MET = 3.5 ml O_2·kg^{-1}·min^{-1})—interspersed throughout the day may be as effective in improving health as a single bout of vigorous exercise, provided that the daily caloric cost is comparable.[16,17] Moreover, if a significant portion of the energy expenditure is performed above a minimum or threshold intensity, that is, above 60% to 70% of the measured maximal heart rate,[18,19] a corresponding increase in aerobic capacity would be expected to occur.

Two key terms in this discussion are exercise and physical activity. Physical activity is bodily movement that is the result of the contraction of skeletal muscles resulting in a substantial increase in energy expenditure. Exercise is a subcategory of physical activity involving planned, structured, and repetitive body movement done to improve or maintain one or more components of physical fitness (set of attributes required to perform physical activity).[20]

Several randomized trials have shown that a lifestyle approach to physical activity among previously sedentary adults can be effective and has similar effects on aerobic fitness, body composition, and coronary risk factors compared with a traditional structured exercise program.[4,5] These findings have important implications for public health, suggesting a wider range of choices of physical activity and potentially greater flexibility in scheduling. Thus, health and fitness professionals should consider broadening their clients' exercise prescriptions from the traditional frequency, intensity, duration, and modes of training that are associated with structured programs, to encourage them to increase physical activity in daily living as well. The Activity Pyramid (figure 7.1) has been suggested as a model to facilitate this objective.[21]

Intensity

The prescribed exercise intensity should be above a minimal level required to induce a "training effect" yet below the metabolic load or aerobic requirement that evokes abnormal clinical signs or symptoms. For example, myocardial ischemia can alter depolarization, repolarization, and conduction velocity, triggering threatening ventricular arrhythmias which, in extreme cases, may be the harbingers of ventricular tachycardia or fibrillation. Accordingly, the target heart rate for endurance exercise should be set safely below ($\geq$10 beats·min^{-1}) the ischemic electrocardiographic or anginal threshold,[1] or in the case of a transient myocardial perfusion abnormality without concomitant ST-segment depression or anginal symptoms, at the minimal or threshold intensity for aerobic training.

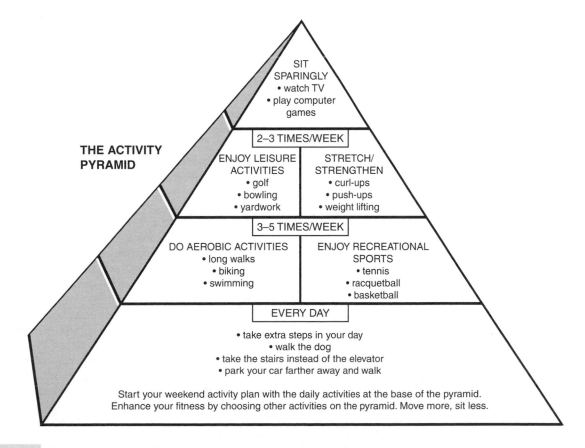

Figure 7.1 The Activity Pyramid.

Considerable evidence suggests that the threshold intensity for improving cardiorespiratory fitness increases in direct proportion to the pretraining $\dot{V}O_2$max or the level of habitual activity.[6] The American College of Sports Medicine (ACSM) recommends an intensity of exercise corresponding to between 55% and 90% of maximum heart rate (HRmax) or between 40% and 85% of the heart rate reserve (HRR) to improve cardiorespiratory fitness.[12] The HRR is the difference between HRmax and resting heart rate (HRrest). Presumably, the threshold or minimal effective intensity for training previously sedentary or deconditioned individuals would correspond to the low end of these ranges, that is, 55% to 65% HRmax or 40% to 50% HRR.

Determining Oxygen Consumption Reserve

Although it was traditionally believed that a given percentage of the HRR corresponded to the same percentage of the $\dot{V}O_2$max, recent studies have shown that HRR more closely approximates the same percentage of the oxygen consumption reserve (%$\dot{V}O_2$R).[22,23] The latter is the difference between $\dot{V}O_2$max and resting oxygen consumption. This concept relates HRR to a level of metabolism or an aerobic requirement that starts at a resting level (i.e., 1 MET), rather than from zero. An additional advantage is increased accuracy in calculating a target $\dot{V}O_2$ from an HRR prescription, especially for low-fit patients, and in establishing training workloads for this cohort.[24]

To calculate the target $\dot{V}O_2$ (T$\dot{V}O_2$) based on $\dot{V}O_2$R, the following equation is used, which has the same format as the HRR calculation of the target heart rate using the calculation by Karvonen and colleagues[25]:

$$T\dot{V}O_2 = (\dot{V}O_2max - \dot{V}O_2rest)\ (\text{exercise intensity}) + \dot{V}O_2rest$$

In this equation, $\dot{V}O_2$rest is 3.5 ml $O_2 \cdot kg^{-1} \cdot min^{-1}$ (1 MET), and the exercise intensity is as low as 40% (for extremely unfit or deconditioned persons) to 85%, according to the most recent ACSM position stand.[12] Intensity is expressed as a decimal in the equation. For example, what is the T$\dot{V}O_2$ at 40% of $\dot{V}O_2$R for a patient who completes stage 1 of the Bruce treadmill protocol, corresponding to approximately 5 METs or 17.5 ml $O_2 \cdot kg^{-1} \cdot min^{-1}$?

$$T\dot{V}O_2 = (17.5 - 3.5)\ (0.40) + 3.5 = (14.0)\ (0.40) + 3.5$$
$$= 5.6 + 3.5 = 9.1\ \text{ml}\ O_2 \cdot kg^{-1} \cdot min^{-1}\ \text{or}\ 2.6\ \text{METs}$$

This value is 30% higher than the T$\dot{V}O_2$ derived from the traditional method of calculation (i.e., 40% of 17.5 ml $O_2 \cdot kg^{-1} \cdot min^{-1}$ = 7.0 ml $O_2 \cdot kg^{-1} \cdot min^{-1}$ or 2 METs). Smaller proportional errors in target $\dot{V}O_2$ or MET levels would occur with more fit patients.

Once an appropriate T$\dot{V}O_2$ (MET) level is identified, a corresponding work rate may be calculated through the use of metabolic equations or by selecting an activity with an appropriate aerobic requirement from published tables.[26] Nevertheless, the corresponding heart rate and perceived exertion should be used as adjunctive intensity modulators.

What is the minimal effective training intensity to improve cardiorespiratory fitness in individuals with and without cardiovascular disease? To answer this question, Swain and Franklin[18] translated the training intensities in previous studies to % $\dot{V}O_2$R units to determine threshold intensities for improving cardiorespiratory fitness among healthy subjects with varied baseline $\dot{V}O_2$max values. Only those studies that directly measured pre- and posttraining $\dot{V}O_2$max and used low to moderate intensities (i.e., ≤60% $\dot{V}O_2$max) were included for analysis. Results indicated that individuals who begin training with an aerobic capacity greater than 40 ml·kg^{-1}·min^{-1} or 11 METs can expect improvements in $\dot{V}O_2$max by using training intensities of at least 45% $\dot{V}O_2$R, provided that a sufficient training frequency and duration are used. This relative intensity approximates 69% HRmax. In contrast, individuals with baseline aerobic capacities below 40 ml·kg^{-1}·min^{-1} can obtain improvements in $\dot{V}O_2$max with training intensities as low as 30% of $\dot{V}O_2$R or 60% HRmax. A similar analysis of 23 training studies in coronary patients found no evidence of a threshold but recommended that 45% of $\dot{V}O_2$R should be considered the minimal effective intensity for eliciting improvements in cardiorespiratory fitness in this population.[19] The reason for the higher relative $\dot{V}O_2$R in coronary patients than low-fit healthy people (45% vs. 30%) may be that the latter are more likely to achieve a true $\dot{V}O_2$max during exercise testing, whereas coronary patients often do not. The recommended minimum intensity of 45% $\dot{V}O_2$R for coronary patients, which was based on their peak oxygen uptake, would probably be much lower if their true $\dot{V}O_2$max were known.

Establishing the Target Heart Rate

To attain a desired metabolic load for exercise training, one must either measure the oxygen uptake directly or have an equivalent index for it. Because heart rate and oxygen uptake are linearly related during dynamic exercise involving large muscle groups, a predetermined training or target heart rate (THR) has become widely adopted as an indicator of exercise intensity.[27]

The THR concept has several important advantages in controlling exercise intensity and modulating cardiac demands. For example, a THR (e.g., 120-132 beats·min^{-1}), established during peak or symptom-limited exercise testing, can be applied outside the exercise training environment to assess the relative cardiac demands of varied physical tasks. The THR has a built-in regulator for improvements in fitness, enabling the patient to maintain the same relative intensity throughout an exercise program. As the patient becomes more fit, the work rate on the treadmill or cycle ergometer must be slowly increased to compensate for the conditioning bradycardia elicited by training; the THR initially achieved by a given level of effort can later be reached by greater energy expenditure. THR also provides for extremes in environmental conditions. For example, in hot or humid weather less work is required to achieve a specific THR,[28] even though the work of the heart (myocardial oxygen uptake) remains unchanged. The subject who is taught to monitor THR can also detect new arrhythmias (e.g., premature ventricular beats, atrial fibrillation) and should be advised to reduce the training intensity and seek medical advice when unusual rhythm irregularities are noted.

Training heart rates for cardiorespiratory conditioning are commonly determined by one of three methods from data obtained during graded exercise testing to volitional fatigue or the appearance of adverse signs or symptoms[1]: (a) using a plot of heart rate versus oxygen consumption or work rate data; (b) using a fixed percentage of the HRmax; and (c) using the HRR method. Regardless of the method, the goal should be to maintain an average heart rate (during the endurance phase) close to the midpoint of the prescribed range.

■ Heart Rate Versus $\dot{V}O_2$ Regression Method

The first method involves identifying the steady-state heart rates that occurred during a series of progressive oxygen uptake or MET levels during a progressive exercise test (figure 7.2). This technique allows one to prescribe an appropriate THR below the point of adverse signs and symptoms and is especially well suited to patients with low fitness levels or a blunted heart rate response to exercise (e.g., secondary to β-blockade).

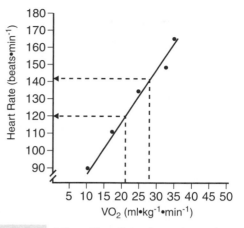

Figure 7.2 A line of best fit has been drawn through the data points on this plot of heart rate and oxygen consumption data observed during a maximal exercise test in which $\dot{V}O_2$max was measured at 35 ml·kg⁻¹·min⁻¹ (10 METs) and maximal heart rate was 165 beats·min⁻¹. A target heart rate range was determined by finding the heart rates that correspond to 60% and 80% of $\dot{V}O_2$max. For this individual, 60% of $\dot{V}O_2$max was approximately 21 ml·kg⁻¹·min⁻¹, and 80% of $\dot{V}O_2$max was approximately 28 ml·kg⁻¹·min⁻¹. The corresponding target heart rates are approximately 119 and 141 beats·min⁻¹.

■ Percent of HRmax

One of the oldest methods of establishing the THR, initially promulgated by the American Heart Association, uses a fixed percentage (e.g., 70-85%) of the measured HRmax.[29] This method has been shown to yield remarkably similar regressions of %$\dot{V}O_2$max on %HRmax (i.e., 57-78% $\dot{V}O_2$ ~ 70-85% HRmax),[30] encompassing the anaerobic or ventilatory threshold (figure 7.3),

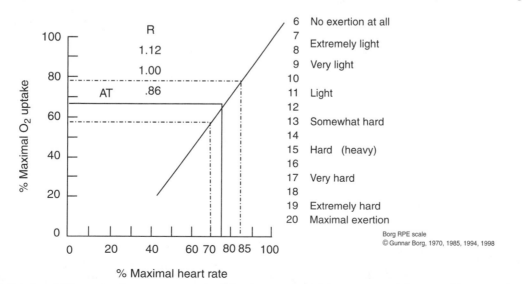

Figure 7.3 Relationships among the percentage of maximal oxygen uptake, percentage of maximal heart rate, respiratory exchange ratio (R), anaerobic threshold (AT), and Borg's rating of perceived exertion (RPE) scale. The AT falls within the optimal intensity for exercise training (57-78% $\dot{V}O_2$max), corresponding to 70% to 85% of maximal heart rate.

RPE scale: Reprinted, by permission, from G. Borg, 1998, *Borg's Perceived Exertion and Pain Scales* (Champaign, IL: Human Kinetics) 47.

regardless of the subject's age, gender, aerobic fitness, body weight, and fat stores; the muscle groups involved; the exercise testing modality; the presence or absence of coronary disease; or the use of cardiac medications.[31,32] Percent of HRmax is also simple to compute. For the individual who achieves a peak heart rate of 160 beats·min[-1] during exercise testing, the THR range is 112 to 136 beats·min[-1].

■ Heart Rate Reserve Method

The final method of establishing the THR is the maximal heart rate reserve method of Karvonen et al.,[25] which requires reliable measurements of resting (standing) and peak or maximal heart rate:

$$THR = (HRmax - HRrest) \times 0.40 \text{ to } 0.85 + HRrest$$

For example, a patient who achieved 6 METs during a graded exercise test, with resting and maximal heart rates of 70 and 140 beats·min[-1], respectively, who wanted to exercise at two-thirds of his aerobic capacity (4 METs), would have a prescribed THR as calculated:

$$THR = (140 - 70) \times 0.67 + 70 = 117 \text{ beats·min}^{-1}$$

Although this THR would approximate an aerobic requirement of 4 METs, the actual energy expenditure would, according to recent studies,[22,23] more closely reflect the %$\dot{V}O_2R$, or 4.35 METs.

A comparison of the second and third prescriptive methods, using standardized training intensities (i.e., 70% and 85%) with varied resting heart rates, is shown in table 7.1. The straight percentage method yielded the lowest training heart rates which, regardless of the resting heart rate, were approximately 20 and 10 beats·min[-1] below those calculated by the heart rate reserve method at the 70% and 85% relative intensities, respectively. In contrast, target heart rates for the heart rate reserve method increased slightly as a function of the resting heart rate.

Determining Exercise Intensity Without a Preliminary Exercise Test

Although the ACSM suggests peak or symptom-limited exercise testing as an essential screening component in exercise programs for middle-aged and older adults (men ≥45 years, women ≥55 years), for those at increased risk for cardiovascular events (e.g., two or more major risk factors or one or more signs or symptoms of coronary heart disease), and for those with known cardiac, pulmonary, or metabolic disease, especially when vigorous exercise (>60% $\dot{V}O_2$max) is contemplated,[1] this recommendation has been increasingly challenged in recent years. A Consensus Group from the American Heart Association and the Ameri-

Table 7.1   Comparison of Target Heart Rates Calculated by Percent of Maximum Heart Rate (HRmax) and Heart Rate Reserve Methods Using Varied Resting Heart Rates

			RESTING HEART RATE					
			60 beats·min[-1]		70 beats·min[-1]		80 beats·min[-1]	
	PERCENT OF HRmax		HEART RATE RESERVE METHOD					
HRmax (beats·min[-1])	70%	85%	70%	85%	70%	85%	70%	85%
100	70	85	88	94	91	96	94	97
110	77	94	95	103	98	104	101	106
120	84	102	102	111	105	113	108	114
130	91	111	109	120	112	121	115	123
140	98	119	116	128	119	130	122	131
150	105	128	123	137	126	138	129	140
160	112	136	130	145	133	147	136	148
170	119	145	137	154	140	155	143	157
180	126	153	144	162	147	164	150	165
190	133	162	151	171	154	172	157	174

Note. Calculated for common maximal heart rates for middle-aged and older adults with and without heart disease, using both the percent of maximal heart rate and heart rate reserve methods at two relative intensities (i.e., 70% and 85%), with three different resting heart rates (60, 70, 80 beats·min[-1]) used in the latter calculations.

can College of Cardiology categorized routine exercise stress testing before the initiation of a vigorous exercise program in healthy men older than 45 and women older than 55 as a class 2B recommendation, that is, a situation where the usefulness and efficacy are not well established.[33] Similarly, Gill and colleagues[34] argued that any policy (e.g., the need for routine exercise testing) that further deters a large number of older persons from participating in an exercise program may cause more harm than good. Others have emphasized that exercise tests are limited in their ability to detect future cardiac events, because acute myocardial infarctions often occur at the site of previously nonobstructive atherosclerotic plaques.[35,36] Consequently, insurance carriers have increasingly questioned the need for routine exercise testing as a screening procedure for exercise training.

Over the last few years, an escalating number of patients have been referred to outpatient cardiac rehabilitation programs without an entry low-level or symptom-limited exercise stress test. McConnell[37] suggested that four types of clinically stable patients might be referred to an exercise-based cardiac rehabilitation program without a baseline exercise test:

1. Patients with extreme debilitation (general muscular weakness and low endurance) who may not be able to achieve an adequate level of cardiac stress

2. Patients with orthopedic or other clinically relevant exercise limitations, such as arthritis, amputation, or neuromuscular dysfunction

3. Patients limited by concomitant pulmonary disease and shortness of breath

4. Patients whose exercise test may not provide any new information of diagnostic or prognostic value

Consequently, a reasonable approach is needed for safely and effectively exercising these patients and others who have not had an exercise test before program entry.

An initial exercise prescription for patients with no preliminary exercise stress test is shown in table 7.2.[38] Prescribing exercise intensity in this situation by using a training heart rate equal to the resting heart rate plus 20 beats·min^{-1} (HRrest + 20) or at an RPE equal to 11 to 13 (as used in table 7.2) was studied by Joo and colleagues.[39] Results showed that there was a considerable difference in the actual energy expenditure using these two forms of intensity prescription, as well as significant interpatient variability. The mean measured $\dot{V}O_2$ during walking using the HRrest + 20 method versus the RPE 11 to 13 method was 10.9 and 16.3 ml·kg^{-1}·min^{-1} and the average percent of $\dot{V}O_2R$ was 41.8 and 71.0, respectively. In addition, high-risk patients (see figure 5.1 on page 63 in the *Guidelines*) exercising according to HRrest + 20 tended to exceed 85% $\dot{V}O_2R$, whereas

Table 7.2   Guidelines for Exercise Prescription for Cardiac Patients Without an Entry Exercise Stress Test

Component	Initial recommendations
Warm-up and cool-down	Mode: Low-level aerobic exercise, stretching Duration: 5-10 min
Aerobic exercise	Mode: Treadmill (1.0-2.5 mph or 1.6-4.0 km·hr^{-1}; 0% grade), leg ergometer (25-50 W; dependent on patient's body weight), Air-Dyne (0.5-1.0 kp), arm ergometer (<25 W), stairs Intensity: HRrest + 20 beats·min^{-1}; RPE = 11-13 Frequency: 1-2 times per day; 5 days per week Duration: MI and CABG: 30-45 min [a]
Flexibility	Mode: Stretching, ROM exercises Frequency: 5 days per week Duration: 5-10 min
Muscular conditioning and resistance training	Mode: All major muscle groups; 8-10 exercises Number of sets: 1 Repetitions per set: 10-15 Frequency: 2 days per week Duration: 10-20 min

Note. HRrest = resting heart rate; RPE = rating of perceived exertion; MI = myocardial infarction; CABG = coronary artery bypass graft surgery; ROM = range of motion.

[a]For patients who can tolerate more than 5 min, allow up to 10 min on each exercise mode for a cumulative exercise duration of 30-45 min.

Adapted from Pollock and Gomes 1999.

low-risk patients tended to exercise at an intensity less than 50% $\dot{V}O_2R$. These data emphasize that these methods should be used with caution.

In patients without an entry exercise test, a period of continuous electrocardiographic monitoring is highly recommended, progressing the program by monitoring the heart rate, rhythm, and perceived exertion responses, with close observation of associated symptomatology. If ischemic ST-segment depression is noted, this should be compared with the baseline resting electrocardiogram (ECG) and, if appropriate, confirmed with 12-lead electrocardiographic monitoring during a simulated exercise session.

Pharmacologic stress testing is commonly used to detect myocardial ischemia in patients with physical limitations that may compromise the predictive accuracy of an exercise test, including those with neurologic, vascular, or orthopedic impairment of the lower extremities. If pharmacologic findings are negative for myocardial ischemia, the highest heart rate obtained can be used as a guide to determine the initial THR. When pharmacologic stress tests yield abnormal results, other complementary methods (e.g., symptoms, perceived exertion, electrocardiographic telemetry monitoring) should be used in conjunction with conservative heart rate guidelines to determine the exercise intensity.

One study compared the rehabilitation outcomes in 229 post–myocardial infarction and coronary artery bypass outpatients who had undergone preliminary exercise testing with 271 matched coronary patients who did not.[40] Program prescription and progression for the former group involved conventional intensities (70-85% HRmax, RPE 11-14); the latter group (n = 271) initiated training at approximately 2 to 3 METs and, in the absence of abnormal signs and symptoms, progressed using heart rate and perceived exertion. The program lasted 12 weeks, and all patients underwent continuous electrocardiographic telemetry monitoring for the first 3 to 6 weeks. Both groups showed similar physiological improvements and there were no cardiovascular events in either group.

Frequency

Although improvements in cardiorespiratory fitness and body composition generally increase as a function of the frequency of training, the ACSM recommends training 3 to 5 days per week to facilitate this objective.[12] In contrast, our experience demonstrated that two exercise sessions per week were as effective as three per week during a 5-week early (phase II) cardiac rehabilitation program in 50 low-risk male patients recovering from acute myocardial infarction.[41] Training regimens of two and three sessions per week produced similar increases in treadmill time and directly mea-

sured aerobic capacity and decreases in heart rate at a standard submaximal workload.[41] Moreover, studies in healthy, middle-aged men suggest that the additional aerobic benefits of five training sessions per week appear to be minimal, whereas the incidence of lower extremity injuries increases abruptly.[42]

Given that the current *health benefit* recommendation is to accomplish a moderate amount of physical activity on all or most days of the week,[43] patients may want to increase the number of days per week that they are physically active and engage in regular exercise.

Duration

The duration of exercise required to elicit a significant training effect should, according to the ACSM, approximate 20 to 60 min of continuous or intermittent aerobic activity.[12] Considerable evidence suggests that the exercise duration varies inversely with the intensity[44]; thus, moderate-intensity activity for middle-aged and older adults, which approximates 40% to 59% $\dot{V}O_2R$ or 3 to 6 METs, should be conducted over a longer period of time ($\geq$30 min/session) and, conversely, individuals training at hard to very hard intensities should train 20 min or longer.[12,16] Moreover, numerous studies have shown that exercise can be accumulated in multiple short bouts (minimum of 10-min bouts conducted throughout the day), yielding similar improvements in selected health and fitness variables, provided that the total volume of training (kilocalorie expenditure) is comparable.[45] For some patients, short, accumulated exercise bouts may fit better into a busy schedule than a single long bout.

Using an "exercise prescription form" is an ideal way of documenting your exercise recommendations to the patient (figure 7.4); however, the prescription should be regularly updated (e.g., every 6-12 months).[46] This is especially important when medications are altered that may potentially change the prescribed heart rate for training. For example, if β-blocker therapy is decreased or discontinued, repeat exercise testing is often recommended to screen for threatening ventricular arrhythmias, ischemic ST-segment depression, or anginal symptoms that may now be provoked at higher heart rates. Unfortunately, repeat exercise testing during the course of outpatient cardiac rehabilitation is seldom, if ever, covered by insurance companies. In contrast, if the β-blocker dosage is increased, simply note the reduced heart rate response at the patient's usual training work rates and establish this as the "revised" target heart rate, using perceived exertion as an adjunct intensity guide. Finally, interrelationships among the frequency, intensity, and duration may permit a subthreshold level in one variable to be partially or totally compensated for by increases in one or both of the others.[44]

MD _____

Name _____ Age _____ Starting Date _____

Clinical Status: Normal

Arrhythmia Angina CABG CHD HTN MI PTCA VR _____

Note

- This prescription is valid only if you remain on the same medications (type and dose), and you are in the same clinical status as on the day your exercise test was conducted.

Contraindications

- Angina at rest, fever, or illness
- Temperature and weather extremes (below 30 °F or more than 80° with high humidity)

Activities to avoid

- Sudden strenuous lifting or carrying
- Exertion that leads to holding your breath

Exercise type

- Aerobic types of exercise that are continuous, dynamic, and repetitive in nature

Frequency

- _____ times/day _____ days/week

Duration

- Total duration of exercise session: _____ min

To be divided as follows

- Warm-up: (light flexibility and stretching routine) _____ min
- Aerobic training: _____ to _____ min
- Cool-down: (slow walking and stretching) _____ min

Intensity

Target heart rate: _____ to _____ beats/min

_____ to _____ beats/10 sec

Perceived exertion should not exceed "somewhat hard"

Re-evaluation

Your next exercise test is due: _____

Call our office to schedule an appointment. Phone: _____

Exercise Physiologist: _____

Figure 7.4 Exercise prescription form used at William Beaumont Hospital, Royal Oak, Michigan. CABG = coronary artery bypass graft; CHD = coronary heart disease; HTN = hypertension; MI = myocardial infarction; PTCA = percutaneous transluminal coronary angioplasty; VR = valve replacement.

From William Beaumont Hospital, Royal Oak, Michigan.

Rate of Progression

The recommended rate of progression in a physical conditioning program depends on several variables, including the individual's level of habitual physical activity, functional capacity, age, orthopedic and musculoskeletal status, comorbid conditions (e.g., obesity, diabetes), and activity goals and preferences. Nevertheless, activity progression can be facilitated by gradual increases in the components of the exercise prescription, that is, intensity, frequency, and duration of training. Using a prescribed heart rate range (i.e., target heart rate zone) provides a built-in regulator for improvements in fitness. As the patient becomes more fit, the work rate on a given exercise device must be subtly increased over time to maintain the prescribed heart rate range.

The recent release of the Institute of Medicine report[47] on dietary guidelines, which calls for 60 min of physical activity each day, twice the recommendation of the ACSM and the Centers for Disease Control[12] as well as the U.S. Surgeon General,[43] confounds previous recommendations on the appropriate rate of activity progression. Many experts believe that by increasing the duration to 60 min of moderate intensity physical activity per day, the report has the potential to raise doubt among sedentary persons that 30 min a day, or shorter bouts of physical activity such as three 10-min walks, provide any health benefit. Because this cohort includes 40 to 50 million U.S. adults, it would seem that the latter recommendation (i.e., 30 min of exercise per day) is a more realistic starting point,[12,43] and this message needs to be reinforced. For healthy individuals and coronary patients at low risk for recurrent cardiac events, the endurance component of the exercise prescription has three stages of progression: initial, improvement, and maintenance (table 7.3).[1] In contrast, moderate- to high-risk cardiac patients may, over time, require more attenuated gradations in exercise dosage.

Initial Stage

The initial phase of conditioning should begin with a low total volume of exercise and include only modest increases in frequency, intensity, and duration over the first month. The first week of training might consist of three sessions at a moderate intensity for only 15 to 20 min of continuous or intermittent activity (minimum of 10-min bouts accumulated throughout the day). For most previously sedentary middle-aged and older adults, the initial intensity might range from 2 to 4 METs, corresponding to walking on level ground at 1.5 to 3.5 mph (2.4-5.6 km·hr^{-1}). Although the aforementioned duration and frequency are less than those recommended by the U.S. Surgeon General[43] (i.e., 30 min of moderate intensity activity on most, and preferably all, days of the week), they are generally well-tolerated by the novice exerciser with little or no discomfort or muscle soreness.

Improvement Stage

Presumably, the preceding stage prepares the body, from both a cardiorespiratory and a musculoskeletal perspective, to undertake more aggressive increases in the training stimulus that occurs during the improvement stage. This stage, which includes months 2 through 6, begins with three to four exercise sessions

---

Table 7.3   Training Progression for Healthy Participants and Low-Risk Cardiac Patients During Endurance Exercise Regimens

Program stage	Week	Exercise frequency (sessions/week)	Exercise intensity (%HRR)[a]	Exercise duration (min)
Initial stage	1	3	40-50	15-20
	2	3-4	40-50	20-25
	3	3-4	50-60	20-25
	4	3-4	50-60	25-30
Improvement stage	5-7	3-4	60-70	25-30
	8-10	3-4	60-70	30-35
	11-13	3-4	65-75	30-35
	14-16	3-5	65-75	30-35
	17-20	3-5	70-85	35-40
	21-24	3-5	70-85	35-40
Maintenance stage	24+	3-5	70-85	30-60

[a]HRR = heart rate reserve; it is recommended that low-risk cardiac patients train at the lower end of these ranges.

Adapted from ACSM 2002.

per week, 25 to 30 min per session, at moderate to hard exercise intensity. This duration, however, pertains only to the endurance or stimulus phase and does not include the recommended warm-up or cool-down periods. Depending on the individual's progress, there are systematic increases in the frequency (up to five sessions per week), intensity (up to 85% HRR or $\dot{V}O_2R$), and duration (up to 40 min per session) of training at 6 months (table 7.3). Flexibility and resistance training are also emphasized during this stage,[12,15] along with recreational games and lifestyle activities,[4,5] to complement the structured, endurance exercise routine.

Maintenance Stage

The goal of this stage of training is the long-term maintenance of improved cardiorespiratory fitness developed during the improvement stage. The focus of the program, however, should be directed at specific additional health fitness goals that have not yet been achieved (e.g., attainment of ideal body weight and relative body fatness). For the most part, the frequency, intensity, and duration remain unchanged from those used at the conclusion of the improvement stage. Of course, if a person increases any of these aspects of the exercise prescription during the maintenance phase, additional health fitness benefits will accrue.

The concept of achieving caloric thresholds may have particular relevance during the maintenance stage, because many of the health benefits of physical activity have been linked to a given exercise dosage, expressed as kilocalories per week. According to the ACSM, individuals should be encouraged to move toward the attainment of 150 to 400 kcal of energy expenditure per day in physical activity or structured exercise, preferably at the upper end of this range during the maintenance stage of training. One study in patients with CHD, which included a low-fat, low-cholesterol diet, showed that a minimum of ~1,500 kcal·week^{-1} of leisure-time activity may halt the progression of coronary disease, whereas regression may be achieved with an energy expenditure of ~2,200 kcal·week^{-1}.[48] For the 80-kg patient, these goals would require walking 16 and 24 miles (25.7 and 38.6 km) per week or running 11 and 16 miles (17.7 and 27.7 km) per week, respectively.

Training Specificity

The physiological adaptations to exercise training appear to be largely specific to the muscle groups that have been trained. Clausen and colleagues[49] demonstrated that leg training elicited a substantial conditioning bradycardia during submaximal leg exercise but not during arm exercise. Conversely, arm training resulted in an attenuated heart rate response to arm exercise but not to leg exercise. Similar "muscle-specific" adaptations have been shown for blood lactate[50] and pulmonary ventilation,[51] suggesting that a significant portion of the training response derives from peripheral rather than central changes, including cellular and enzymatic adaptations that increase the oxidative capacity of chronically exercised skeletal muscle.[52]

The limited degree of crossover of training benefits from one set of limbs to another appears to discredit the general practice of prescribing exercise for the legs alone. Many occupational and leisure-time activities require arm work to a greater extent than leg work. Consequently, patients who rely on their upper extremities should be counseled to train the arms as well as the legs, with the expectation of attenuated cardiorespiratory and hemodynamic responses to both forms of effort.

Although upper-body exercise for cardiac patients traditionally has been contraindicated, at a given heart rate, arm exercise elicits no greater incidence of dysrhythmias, ischemic ST-segment depression, or angina pectoris than does leg exercise.[53] Moreover, it appears that the upper extremities respond to aerobic conditioning in the same qualitative and quantitative manner as the lower extremities, showing comparable relative decreases in the submaximal rate–pressure product and increases in peak power output and $\dot{V}O_2$peak for both sets of limbs when the same exercise training intensity, frequency, and duration are used for the arms and legs.[54]

Arm Exercise Prescription

Some cardiac rehabilitation patients may have a preexisting disability that precludes lower-extremity or weight-bearing exercise, whereas others may want to return to occupational or recreational activities that require significant use of the arms. For these patients, it is appropriate to incorporate arm exercises into their rehabilitation programs. In formulating an arm exercise prescription, you must establish the training intensity, specifically the exercise training heart rate, the workload that will achieve this heart rate, and the appropriate training equipment or modalities.[55]

Mode

Specially designed arm ergometers (i.e., Monarch Rehab Trainer or Bilateral Arm Trainers) or combined arm and leg ergometers are commonly recommended for upper-extremity training. For many years, we have used the Playbuoy exerciser for dynamic upper-extremity exercise in our cardiac rehabilitation program.[56] The device, a swimming pool buoy that is shuttled back and forth between two partners on waxed ropes attached to handles, is lightweight, inexpensive, and particularly applicable to gymnasium programs. Our studies in men with documented CHD showed that the aerobic requirements of the device were compatible with arm training, corresponding to mean values of 1.5, 2.0, and 3.0 METs at progressive work rates.[57]

Other equipment suitable for upper-body training includes rowing machines, weight training devices, elliptical trainers, wall pulleys, light dumbbells, ladder climbing apparatuses, shoulder wheels, and cross-country simulators. A metronome can be used with some of these devices to vary the rate of movement or work intensity. Walking while pumping handheld 1- to 3-lb (0.45- to 1.36-kg) weights can also be used for simultaneous training of the upper extremities, eliciting significantly greater increases in heart rate, oxygen consumption, and caloric expenditure over conventional walking at comparable speeds.[58] Indeed, walking while pumping handheld weights has been shown to evoke oxygen consumption levels comparable to that of slow jogging.

Selected occupational and leisure-time pursuits, like gardening, raking, and wood sawing, can also provide upper-body exercise, as can varied sport and recreational activities, such as canoeing, swimming, and cross-country skiing. Specific precautions should be taken during the latter, particularly with cardiac patients, as heart rates are frequently inordinately high and do not correspond with ratings of perceived exertion.[59]

Intensity

Because the arm and leg regressions of the percentage of relative oxygen uptake ($\%\dot{V}O_2max$) on relative heart rate ($\%HRmax$) are nearly identical, a given percentage of HRmax during arm exercise (i.e., 70-85%) results in a percentage of arm $\dot{V}O_2max$ comparable to that of leg exercise (i.e., 57-78% $\dot{V}O_2max$).[60] Moreover, the heart rate–oxygen uptake relation that is determined during a progressive treadmill test can be generalized to combined arm and leg exercise when the intensity approximates 70% $\dot{V}O_2max$.[61] This has particular applicability to ergometers that use the arm levers and leg pedals simultaneously.

Although the prescribed heart rate for arm training ideally should be based on the results of a progressive exercise test of the upper extremities, this may not always be feasible. Research indicates that a slightly lower maximal heart rate (3-23 beats·min⁻¹; mean, 11 beats·min⁻¹) is generally obtained during arm exercise compared with leg exercise testing.[55] Consequently, an arm exercise prescription based on a maximal heart rate obtained during treadmill testing or leg ergometry may result in an inappropriately high target heart rate for arm training. We have found that the prescribed heart rate for leg training should be reduced by about 10 beats·min⁻¹ for arm training, using perceived exertion as an adjunctive intensity modulator.

In establishing the work rate that will achieve the target training heart rate, it is important to reemphasize the contrasting physiological responses to submaximal and maximal arm and leg exercise. Maximal work rates and $\dot{V}O_2max$ are generally lower for arm than leg exercise. At a given submaximal work rate, however, heart rate, systolic blood pressure, minute ventilation, oxygen uptake, rate–pressure product, and perceived exertion are greater for arm than for leg exercise.[55] Consequently, work rates appropriate for leg training, expressed as kilogram meters per minute (kg·m·min⁻¹) or watts (1 W ~ 6 kg·m·min⁻¹), will have to be decreased for arm training. In our experience, work rates approximating 50% to 66% of those used for leg training are generally appropriate for arm training.[55,62] Thus, a workload of 300 kg·m·min⁻¹ for leg training would be reduced to 150 to 200 kg·m·min⁻¹ for arm conditioning, with the expectation of comparable (or slightly lower) heart rates and perceived exertion ratings. These findings suggest that work rates for arm training can be reasonably estimated from those used during leg training, obviating the need for a peak or symptom-limited arm ergometer evaluation.

Resistance Training

It has been demonstrated that resistance training can safely and effectively increase weight-carrying tolerance and skeletal muscle strength, improve cardiovascular function, favorably modify coronary risk factors, and enhance psychosocial well-being in stable coronary patients.[15] Because increased muscle mass correlates with an increased basal metabolic rate, it complements aerobic training, increased lifestyle activity, and caloric restriction for weight control. Weight training has also been shown to attenuate the heart rate and systolic blood pressure responses to a given submaximal load,[63] which may reduce myocardial demands during daily activities such as carrying groceries or lifting moderate to heavy objects. There are also intriguing data to suggest that strength training can increase muscular endurance, despite modest to no improvement in $\dot{V}O_2max$.[64,65]

Contraindications

Contraindications to traditional resistance training, defined as using weight loads that are greater than 50% of the maximal voluntary contraction,[14] are similar to those used for the aerobic component of adult fitness or cardiac exercise programs. These include the following:

- Unstable angina
- Uncontrolled hypertension (systolic blood pressure ≥160 mm Hg or diastolic blood pressure ≥100 mmHg)

- Uncontrolled dysrhythmias

- A recent history of congestive heart failure that has not been evaluated and effectively treated

- Severe valvular disease

- Left ventricular outflow obstruction (e.g., hypertrophic cardiomyopathy with obstruction)[15]

Moreover, moderate to good left ventricular function and reasonable cardiorespiratory fitness (>5 or 6 METs) without signs or symptoms of myocardial ischemia or threatening ventricular arrhythmias have been suggested as additional participation criteria for traditional resistance training.[66] Nevertheless, even patients, especially elderly patients, who do not meet these criteria can often participate in more modest regimens, using calisthenics, rubber band devices, pulley weights, dumbbells, wrist weights, or combinations of these.[15]

Prescriptive Guidelines

Single-set resistance training programs performed a minimum of two times a week are recommended over multiset programs, especially among middle-aged and older novice exercisers, because these programs are highly effective in improving muscular strength and endurance, less time consuming, and less likely to result in injury or soreness.[67] Although greater frequencies of training and more sets may be used, the additional gains are usually small.[12] Such regimens should include 8 to 10 different exercises (figure 7.5) at a load that permits 8 to 12 repetitions per set for healthy young and middle-aged participants and 10 to 15 repetitions per set at a lower relative resistance for cardiac patients and healthy older participants.[1,12,15,46] The rationale for the increased repetition range at a lower relative effort for older subjects and those with coronary disease is prevention of musculoskeletal and cardiovascular complications.

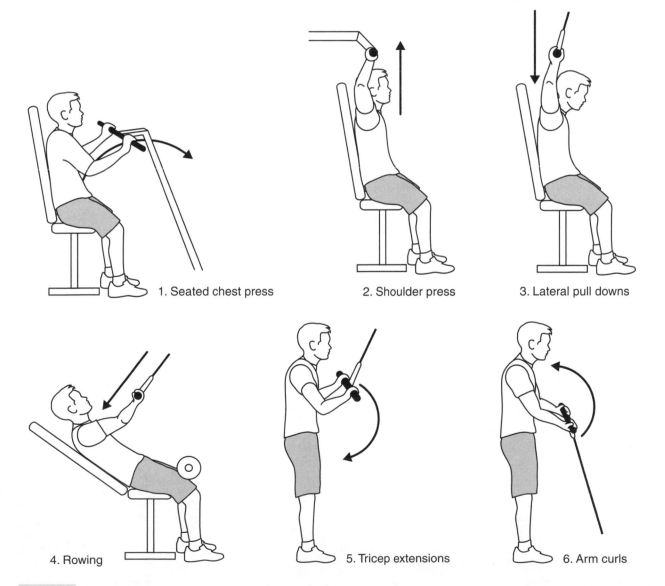

1. Seated chest press   2. Shoulder press   3. Lateral pull downs

4. Rowing   5. Tricep extensions   6. Arm curls

Figure 7.5 Exercises that are commonly used in a resistance training program. Ideally, such regimens should include 8 to 10 different exercises.

Electrocardiography in Heart Disease

Shu-Fen Wung, PhD, RN

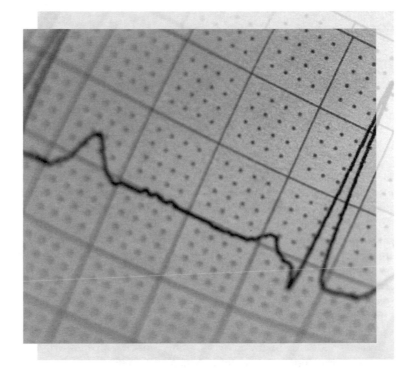

Chapter Intent

Interpretation of an electrocardiogram (ECG) is limited to licensed physicians, and there are published standards for the minimum knowledge a physician should possess to make interpretations.[1] However, other health care professionals (e.g., exercise physiologists, nurses, therapists) working in cardiac rehabilitation need to have adequate knowledge of the ECG to understand ECG information contained in medical reports, recognize changes in a patient's current ECG recording to a previous recording, and, most important, recognize significant or dangerous arrhythmias that may occur during monitored exercise training. These ECG skills are necessary to ensure a safe environment in the cardiac rehabilitation program.

The electrocardiogram (ECG) is a graphic recording of cardiac electrical activity. Electrical signals can be inscribed onto grid paper consisting of small and large squares. The width of each square represents time; a large square is 0.2 s and a small square is 0.04 s, or 40 ms. The height of each square represents voltage; a large square is 0.5 mV or 5 mm, and a small square is 0.1 mV or 1 mm. The 12-lead ECG is also standardized for accurate measurement of voltage (figure 8.1). The standard speed for recording an ECG is 25 mm·s^{-1}.[2]

The impulse normally begins in the pacemaker cells that are located in the sinoatrial (SA) node. These SA nodal cells typically depolarize between 60 and 100

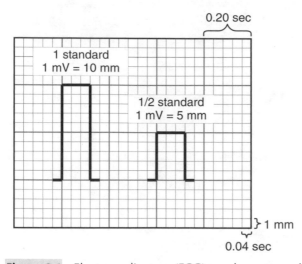

Figure 8.1 Electrocardiogram (ECG) graph paper and standardization.

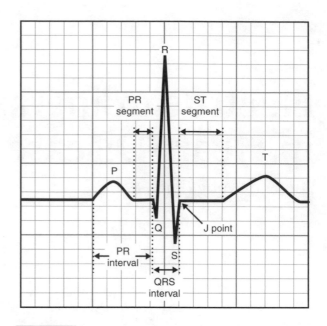

Figure 8.2 Electrocardiogram (ECG) waveforms, segments, and intervals.

beats·min[-1]. The impulse from the SA node proceeds in a leftward direction toward the left atrium and inferiorly toward the atrioventricular (AV) node. The primary function of the AV node is to slow the conduction of the impulse to allow sufficient time for atrial contraction during ventricular filling. The impulse then conducts down the bundle of His, the bundle branches, and the Purkinje fibers into the ventricles. Because the His–Purkinje system is a subendocardial structure, the impulse in the ventricles is conducted from endocardium to epicardium.

The ECG waveforms and intervals are illustrated in figure 8.2. The *P wave* represents the depolarization of atria and is normally small and smoothly rounded, less than 2.5 mm in voltage and less than 0.12 s in duration. Normal atrial activation results in an upright P wave in leads I, II, aVL, aVF, and V_4 through V_6 and negative P wave in lead aVR. P waves can be positive, negative, or biphasic in leads III and V_1 through V_3. During exercise, normal responses include a significant increase in P-wave magnitude in inferior leads (II, III, and aVF) but not in P-wave duration.[3]

The *PR segment* begins with the end of the P wave and ends with the onset of the QRS complex. The PR segment should be isoelectric, meaning it is neither positive nor negative. The *PR interval* reflects atrial depolarization plus the normal delay at the AV node. It begins at the beginning of the P wave and ends with the onset of the QRS complex. The normal PR interval is 0.12 to 0.20 s. If AV conduction is prolonged, the PR interval will increase beyond 0.20 s. During exercise, the PR segment usually shortens and slopes downward in inferior leads.[3]

The *QRS complex* represents depolarization of the ventricles. All upright deflections of the QRS complex are called *R waves*; a second upright deflection is *R'*. An uppercase *R* may be used when the positive deflection is greater than 5 mm, whereas a lowercase *r* is used when the positive deflection is 5 mm or less. An initial downward deflection of the QRS complex is called the *Q wave*, if preceding the R wave, or the *S wave*, if following the R wave. *Monomorphic* QRS means that the QRS complexes have a consistent pattern indicating a single site of impulse origin. *Polymorphic* QRS means that the QRS complexes have multiple QRS shapes indicating multiple sites of impulse origin. The QRS duration measurements can vary across different ECG leads; therefore, durations of QRS complexes should be measured with more than one lead, and the widest QRS measurement, often found in lead V_1 or V_2, is the most accurate.[4] The upper normal value for QRS duration is less than 0.12 s.[5,6] At maximum exercise, the R wave normally decreases in amplitude and the S wave increases in depth.[3]

The *ST segment* starts at the J point (the junction at the end of the QRS complex) and ends at the beginning of the T wave. ST segment deviation is usually measured at 60 or 80 ms following the J point, called J + 60 or J + 80 ms. When the ventricular rate is fast (>130 beats·min[-1]), a J + 60 ms is suggested to determine the extent of ST-segment deviation.[3] The ST, PR, and TP segments should be isoelectric. The QRS complex and the ST segment represent a time when the ventricles are in an absolute refractory period and are not responding to any stimulation. Normally, the J point is depressed during maximum exercise and gradually returns toward preexercise values in recovery. J-point depression during exercise is more common in the elderly.[3]

The *T wave* represents repolarization of the ventricles. The polarity of the T wave is generally the same as the preceding QRS complex. T waves are positive in leads I, II, aVL, aVF, and lateral precordial leads V_4 through V_6 and negative in lead aVR. T- wave polarity can vary in leads III and V_1 through V_3. Usually, the T-wave amplitude is gradually decreased in all leads during early exercise and begins to increase at maximal exercise.[3]

GUIDELINES, 4TH EDITION

- Chapter 5, pages 64-67
- Chapter 6, pages 75-76
- Chapter 11, pages 198-199

Electrodes and Leads

To understand the morphologic appearance of a given waveform on the ECG, we need to understand the basic principals between the electrode locations and the direction of electrical impulse. Briefly, when the direction of depolarization travels toward a positive electrode, an upward deflection is recorded. When the direction of depolarization travels away from a positive electrode, a downward (negative) deflection is recorded. When the direction of depolarization is perpendicular to a positive electrode, a small equiphasic (equally positive and negative) deflection or a straight (isoelectric) line is recorded (figure 8.3).

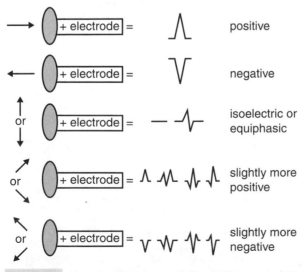

Figure 8.3 Impulse direction and the resultant waveform relative to the positive electrode.

The standard 12-lead ECG includes three bipolar limb leads (I, II, III), three augmented unipolar limb leads (aVR, aVL, aVF), and six unipolar precordial leads (V_1-V_6). Each of the 12 leads records cardiac electrical activity from its unique location.

- Bipolar Limb Leads

  Bipolar limb leads consist of two electrodes placed on two different limbs. One electrode serves as the exploring or positive electrode and the other serves as a reference (negative) electrode (figure 8.4). The left arm (LA), right arm (RA), and left leg (LL) electrodes form the *Einthoven triangle*. The right leg (RL) electrode serves as a ground electrode to stabilize the ECG signals and does not contribute to the ECG waveforms.

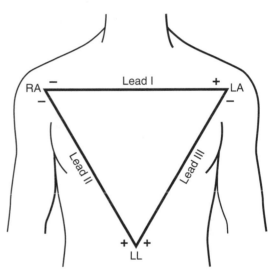

Figure 8.4 Bipolar limb leads. Lead I records the electrical potential difference between the LA (positive electrode) and the RA (negative electrode). Lead II records the potential difference between the LL (positive electrode) and the RA (negative electrode). Lead III records the potential difference between LL (positive electrode) and LA (negative electrode). LA = left arm; RA = right arm; LL = left leg.

- Augmented Unipolar Limb Leads

  Unipolar leads record the electrical potential at the positive electrode site in relation to a reference point (zero electrical potential), known as the *Wilson central terminal*. This terminal averages the input from LA, RA, and LL electrodes and lies at the center of electrical field of the heart. The positive electrode is the RA electrode for lead aVR, the LA electrode for lead aVL, and the left foot electrode for lead aVF. When the Wilson central terminal is used as the

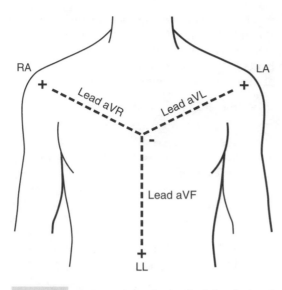

Figure 8.5 Augmented unipolar limb leads. Lead aVR records the electrical potential difference between the RA (positive electrode) and the mean output from the LA and the LL (reference point). Lead aVL records electrical potential difference between the LA (positive electrode) and the mean output from the RA and the LL (reference point). Lead aVF records the electrical potential difference between the LL (positive electrode) and the mean output from the RA and the LA (reference point). LA = left arm; RA = right arm; LL = left leg.

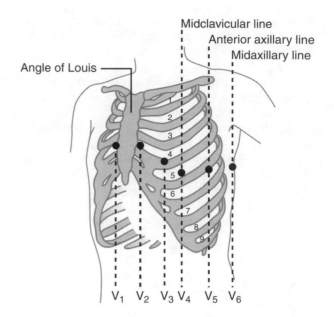

Figure 8.6 Unipolar precordial leads. Six standard precordial leads are placed on the chest according to the following anatomic landmarks: V_1 at the fourth intercostal space (ICS) and the right sternal border; V_2 at the fourth ICS and the left sternal border; V_3 midway between leads V_2 and V_4; V_4 at the fifth ICS and midclavicular line; V_5 at the anterior axillary line at the same level as lead V_4; and V_6 at the midaxillary line at the same level as V_4.

Reprinted, by permission, from B.J. Drew, University of California School of Nursing, San Francisco. © B.J. Drew.

reference point, the ECG amplitudes on these unipolar limb leads are small because the same electrode is included in both the exploring and the reference input. Thus, the reference potential was mathematically modified to augment approximately 50% of ECG amplitude. In the modified reference system, the negative input consists of the mean potentials from only two of the three limb electrodes (figure 8.5). For example, for lead aVR, the exploring electrode is on the RA and the reference electrode is the mean output from LA and LL. The letter *a* in front of each unipolar limb lead indicates augmentation.

- Unipolar Precordial Leads

  The *unipolar precordial leads* record the electrical potential at each precordial site (positive electrode) in relation to the Wilson central terminal (zero electrical potential). Accurate placement of precordial leads on the chest is crucial because slight alterations in the position of one precordial electrode can significantly distort the appearance of the cardiac waveforms and may have a significant influence on the diagnosis (figure 8.6).[7]

Supraventricular Arrhythmias

An *arrhythmia* is any cardiac rhythm other than a normal sinus rhythm.[8] An arrhythmia can be either sinus or ectopic in origin. It can be regular or irregular. An arrhythmia may be caused by a disturbance in impulse formation or conduction, either at an abnormal rate or from a site other than the sinus node. Arrhythmia can occur during exercise or during the recovery period and may range in severity from benign to life threatening. A detailed discussion of all exercise-induced arrhythmias is beyond the scope of this chapter; thus, only selected exercise-related arrhythmias will be discussed here.

Premature Atrial Contractions

A premature atrial contraction (PAC) originates from a focus in the atria outside the SA node and creates an early beat and a distorted P wave, called a P' wave (figure 8.7). The PAC normally conducts through the

II   Premature P' wave

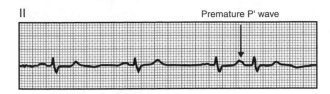

Figure 8.7 A premature atrial contraction (PAC) with a right bundle branch block and left atrial enlargement. Premature atrial contraction is characterized by a premature P' wave with a PR interval exceeding 0.12 s (the fourth beat below). The P'-wave morphology is different from that of the sinus P waves and indicates a different focus of origin than the sinus node. This premature P' wave is at the tail end of the preceding T wave, thus altering the shape of the T wave. The QRS complex of this PAC is identical to the preceding QRS complexes.

AV junction; therefore, the impulse is often conducted with a narrow QRS complex that is identical to the sinus-conducted beats. A nonconducted PAC occurs when a PAC originates very early and the AV junction is still refractory to conduct another impulse to the ventricles; the QRS is absent. Supraventricular premature beats induced by exercise are observed in 4% to 10% of normal individuals and up to 40% of patients with heart disease.[9]

Supraventricular tachycardia (SVT) refers to tachyarrhythmias (>100 beats·min⁻¹) that originate above the ventricles, including the sinus node, atria, and AV node. Paroxysmal supraventricular tachycardia (PSVT) encompasses several types of tachycardias that have sudden onset and termination. The three most common PSVT are AV nodal reentry tachycardia (AVNRT, 52%), AV reciprocating tachycardia (AVRT, 38%), and atrial tachycardia (10%).[10] The QRS complex is usually narrow in these arrhythmias but occasionally can show bundle branch block (BBB). The mean rates for AVNRT (181), AVRT (187), and atrial tachycardia (183) are very similar so the rate does not allow for differential diagnoses of these tachycardias.

According to the American College of Cardiology and American Heart Association (ACC/AHA) guideline,[11] the development of SVT is one of the relative indications for terminating exercise testing. The specific exercise-provoked SVTs include AVNRT, orthodromic AVRT, atrial tachycardia, atrial flutter-fibrillation, and junctional tachycardia.[12,13] Atrial fibrillation and flutter are induced by exertion only rarely and when they do occur may revert spontaneously.[13,14]

AV Nodal Reentrant Tachycardia

AV nodal reentrant tachycardia (AVNRT) is characterized by tachycardia with a QRS complex of supraventricular origin, with sudden onset and ter-

mination generally at regular rates between 150 and 250 beats·min⁻¹.[10] Usually AVNRT is initiated by a PAC that conducts down the slow AV nodal pathway and produces a prolonged P'R interval (figure 8.8). Once the impulse enters the AV node, it travels in two directions simultaneously, one down to the ventricles and one up to the atrium. The impulse that travels down to activate the ventricles produces a narrow QRS rhythm because the ventricles are activated through the normal His–Purkinje system. If bundle branch block or ventricular aberrancy is present, then the QRS complex is wide. The impulse that travels up to the atrium via the fast pathway produces a retrograde P' wave. Because the two impulses travel in two different directions simultaneously, the P' waves are generally buried in the QRS complex or just prior to or just after the end of the QRS, creating pseudo–s waves in the inferior leads (II, III, aVF) or pseudo–r' waves in lead V₁.[15]

Orthodromic AV Reciprocating Tachycardia

Orthodromic AV reciprocating tachycardia (AVRT) occurs in individuals who have an accessory pathway other than the normal AV conduction system that provides direct connection from the atria into the ventricles. A PAC usually initiates AVRT (figure 8.9). The early conducted PAC is unable to conduct down the accessory pathway because it is still refractory, so the impulse is conducted down the normal AV node pathway in an antegrade (orthodromic) direction from the atrium to ventricle. This results in a *narrow QRS* tachycardia that is identical to the sinus-initiated QRS complex because the ventricles are depolarized through the normal His–Purkinje system. If bundle branch block or ventricular aberrancy is present, then the QRS complex is wide. Once the ventricles are depolarized, the impulse conducts retrogradely from the ventricle to the atrium using the accessory pathway,[10] producing a P' wave in the ST segment or early in the T wave. The retrograde impulse depolarizes the atria and returns down the AV node, depolarizing the ventricles again and creating a circus movement tachycardia, referred to as orthodromic AVRT.

Atrial Tachycardia

Atrial tachycardia has a rapid atrial rate of 150 to 200 beats·min⁻¹ attributable to rapid firing of an ectopic atrial focus or to an atrial reentry circuit that allows an impulse to travel rapidly and repeatedly around a pathway in the atria. The P'-wave morphology in atrial tachycardia is different from that of the sinus P wave. As the atrial rate increases, the AV node begins to block some of the impulses to protect the ventricles from

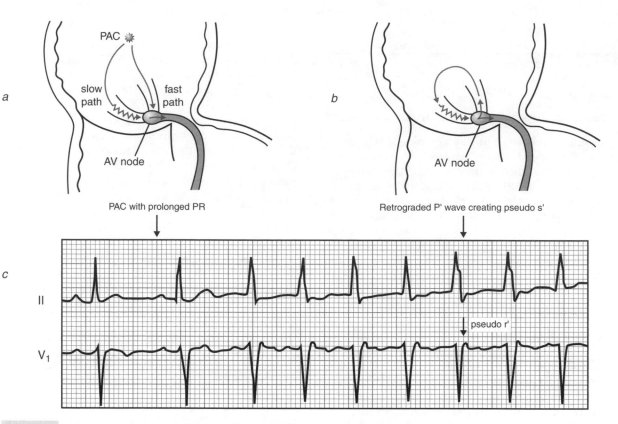

Figure 8.8 Atrioventricular nodal reentry tachycardia (AVNRT). *(a)* The onset of AVNRT is initiated by a premature atrial contraction (PAC). The premature P' wave can be seen at the tail end of the second T wave on the tracing below. The P'R interval is prolonged because the impulse is traveling through the slow rather the normal fast pathway. *(b)* Within the atrioventricular node, the impulse travels in two directions: down to activate the ventricles and up to the atrium via the fast pathway. During this tachycardia, the retrograde P' waves distort the QRS complexes creating pseudo–s waves in lead II and pseudo–r' waves in lead V_1. These are apparent when compared with the QRS complexes of the sinus rhythm (first and second beats).

Adapted from *Understanding Electrocardiography,* 8th ed., M.B. Conover, pgs. 121-122, Copyright 2003, with permission from Elsevier.

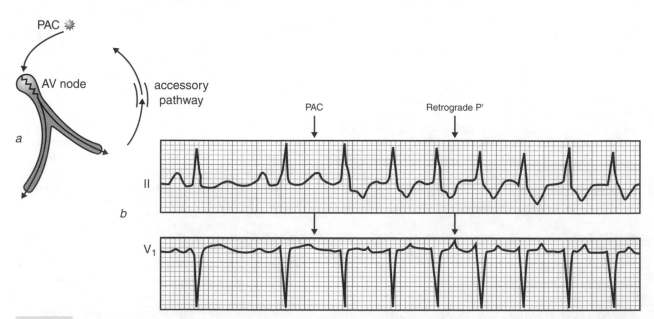

Figure 8.9 Orthodromic atrioventricular reciprocating tachycardia (AVRT). *(a)* The premature atrial contraction (PAC) is conducted down the atrioventricular (AV) node to produce a narrow QRS complex. Following ventricular depolarization, the impulse is able to conduct back to the atrium via the accessory pathway because it is no longer refractory. *(b)* The retrograde impulses to the atrium produce P' waves during the tachycardia that are seen immediately after and separate from the preceding QRS complexes.

Adapted from *Understanding Electrocardiography,* 8th ed., M.B. Conover, pgs. 124-125, Copyright 2003, with permission from Elsevier.

excessively rapid rates, and a Wenckebach (Mobitz type 1) second-degree AV block can occur (figure 8.10). When the arrhythmia has sudden onset and termination, the term *paroxysmal* is used.

Atrial Flutter

Atrial flutter is a rapid atrial rhythm sustained by a macro-reentrant circuit, which is a recycling of an impulse around a circuit that is large enough to be recorded on the surface ECG.[8] In typical atrial flutter, the reentry circuit is confined to the right atrium and usually travels in a counterclockwise direction up the septum and down the right atrial free wall.[16-18] Because of the circular conduction, the ECG typically reveals identically recurring regular sawtooth flutter (F) waves, best visualized in leads II, III, aVF, or V_1 (figure 8.11). The atrial rate during atrial flutter is typically 250 to 350 beats·min^{-1} with a mean of approximately 300 beats·min^{-1}. Because the AV node usually blocks

half of those atrial impulses, a ventricular rate of 150 beats·min^{-1} is common. When a ventricular rate of 150 beats·min^{-1} is seen, the diagnosis of atrial flutter with 2:1 conduction (atrial–ventricular rate of 300:150) should be suspected. The ratio of flutter waves to conducted ventricular complexes is usually an even number, such as 2:1 and 4:1. If the patient is treated with antiarrhythmic agents and the atrial rate is reduced to 200 beats·min^{-1} or less, the ventricles can respond to atrial impulse in a 1:1 fashion.[15]

Atrial Fibrillation

Atrial fibrillation is the most commonly sustained abnormal cardiac rhythm that is characterized by unorganized atrial depolarizations. These unorganized atrial depolarizations are detected on the ECG as f waves (irregular multiform atrial activity associated with fibrillation) that are variable in amplitude and morphology (figure 8.12). Atrial fibrillation can

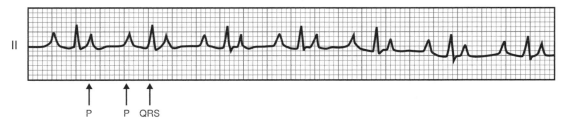

Figure 8.10   Atrial tachycardia with 2:1 conduction. The ectopic focus conducts 188 beats·min^{-1} in the atria. There are two P waves for every QRS complex. The atrioventricular node is unable to repolarize quickly enough to be ready for the next impulse, so it conducts only every other impulse.

Adapted, by permission, from H.J.L. Marriott, *Marriott's board review manual of electrocardiography,* 2nd ed. (Riverview, FL: American College of Cardiac Nurses), 23.

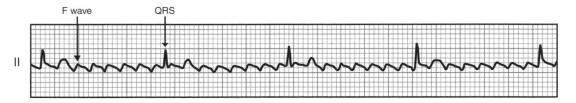

Figure 8.11   Atrial flutter with an 8:1 atrioventricular conduction. The flutter (F) wave rate is 250 beats·min^{-1} and the ventricular rate is 33 beats·min^{-1}. The regular sawtooth flutter waves are apparent in lead II.

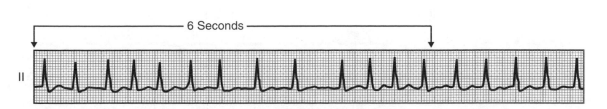

Figure 8.12   Atrial fibrillation with rapid ventricular response at a rate of 110 beats·min^{-1}. Absence of P waves and a fine fibrillatory line are noted. The ventricular response is rapid and grossly irregular.

be extremely rapid at a rate of 350 to 600 beats·min⁻¹. The small, fine, rapid f waves may not be visible on the standard 12-lead ECG. In atrial fibrillation, each f wave does not initiate QRS complexes. The ventricular response is irregular (irregularly irregular) at a rate of 100 to 160 beats·min⁻¹ in untreated patients with normal AV conduction. When the ventricular rate is very rapid or very slow, the rhythm may appear to be more regular.

Junctional Tachycardia

The rate in the AV junction is usually 40 to 60 beats·min⁻¹. Junctional tissue may exhibit an enhanced discharge rate and assume the role of the dominant pacemaker. Junctional tachycardia is recognized by narrow QRS morphology at a regular rate exceeding 100 beats·min⁻¹[15] (figure 8.13). During junctional rhythms, the possible relationships between the P' waves and QRS complexes include either (a) a constant P'R interval of less than 0.12 s (1:1 AV ratio), (b) an absent P wave (buried in the QRS complex), or (c) a retrograde P' following the QRS complex.[19]

Ventricular Arrhythmias

Ventricular arrhythmias originate in the ventricular muscles or Purkinje system and are considered to be more dangerous than other arrhythmias because of

their potential to severely limit cardiac output. According to the practice guidelines of the ACC/AHA,[11] sustained ventricular tachycardia is an absolute indication for terminating exercise testing, and polymorphic premature ventricular contractions (PVCs) and triplets of PVCs (three in succession) are relative indications for terminating exercise testing. R-on-T PVCs, frequent monomorphic or polymorphic PVCs (constituting ≥30% of the beats·min⁻¹), and coupling of PVCs (two in succession) are classified as "significant" or "complex" arrhythmias that may be a precursor to sudden cardiac death.[2] In addition, frequent ventricular ectopy, as defined by the presence of seven or more PVCs per minute, ventricular bigeminy or trigeminy, ventricular couplets or triplets, ventricular tachycardia (VT >100 beats·min⁻¹), torsade de pointes, ventricular flutter, or ventricular fibrillation, during recovery period after exercise has recently been found to be a better predictor of an increased risk of death than ectopy occurring during exercise only.[20]

PVC

PVCs are characterized by wide and premature QRS complexes that differ in morphology from the individual's normal beats (figure 8.14). Rhythm is irregular because of the early beats. They usually are not preceded by a P wave, although retrograde ventriculoatrial conduction may occur. Sinus rhythm is not usually interrupted, so frequently sinus P waves can be seen occurring regularly throughout the rhythm.

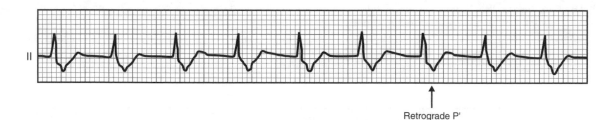

Figure 8.13   Junctional tachycardia at a rate of 110 beats·min⁻¹. Note that there are no P waves in front of QRS complexes. The retrograde P' waves are located immediately following the QRS complexes.

Adapted from *Understanding Electrocardiography,* 8th ed., M.B. Conover, pg. 117, Copyright 2003, with permission from Elsevier.

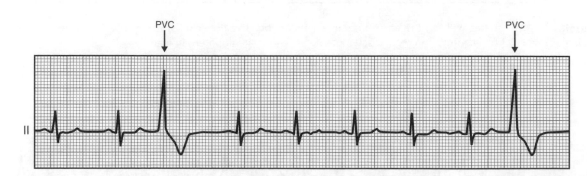

Figure 8.14   Monomorphic premature ventricular contractions (PVCs) with wide and premature QRS complexes. The rhythm is irregular because of the early beats. The sinus rhythm is not interrupted (the timing of the fourth beat is not altered by the preceding PVC). No premature P waves precede the PVCs. T waves are in the opposite direction from the QRS complexes in PVCs.

P' waves may follow PVCs because of retrograde conduction from the ventricle backward through the atria; these P' waves are inverted in the inferior leads II, III, and aVF. PR intervals are not usually present before most PVCs. If, by coincidence, a P' wave precedes a PVC, then the P'R interval is short. The QRS complex is wide and bizarre, usually of greater duration than 0.12 s. T waves are usually in the opposite direction from the QRS complex in PVCs. Bigeminy and trigeminy PVCs are arrhythmias in which every second or third beat, respectively, is premature. QRS complex may vary in morphology if PVCs originate from more than one focus in the ventricles, called *polymorphic* PVCs. PVCs may occur in groups of two or more in succession. Two PVCs in a row are called a *couplet* and a group of three is called a *triplet*. Three or more consecutive PVCs are known as *ventricular tachycardia* (VT).

Ventricular Tachycardia

VT is defined as a rapid ventricular rhythm that includes three or more consecutive PVCs. The usual rate of a VT is 100 to 240 per minute (figure 8.15). Although *AV dissociation* (atrial activity is independent of ventricular activity or the atria are depolarized in retrograde fashion by the ventricles) occurs in approximately 25% of VT,[3,21] it is considered to be a hallmark of VT. A *nonsustained* VT refers to a VT that

lasts less than 30 s. *Sustained* VT refers to VT that lasts longer than 30 s or that requires immediate termination because of hemodynamic compromise.

Monomorphic VT refers to VT with the same morphology in QRS complexes, and *polymorphic VT* refers to a VT with varied and random morphology in QRS complexes. A special type of VT is one in which the QRS complexes have continuously changing morphologies called *torsade de pointes (TdP)*, which means "twisting of the points." TdP is defined as a pause-dependent malignant polymorphic VT with a characteristic shifting morphology of the QRS complex that occurs in the setting of a prolonged QT interval and is extremely rapid, resembling VF.

Differentiating VT from SVT with wide QRS complex may be difficult; however, the distinction is important because of necessary differences in management strategies. Four criteria, including the presence of AV dissociation, QRS duration, QRS axis, and QRS morphology, can be used to differentiate VT from SVT.[21] First, the presence of AV disassociation indicates VT; however, absence of AV dissociation may suggest either SVT or VT. Second, extremely wide QRS complexes greater than or equal to 0.16 s indicate VT, and narrower QRS complexes (0.12-0.14 s) can either be SVT or VT. Third, a frontal QRS axis in the right superior quadrant (−90° to ±180°) strongly suggests VT; however, this abnormal QRS axis occurs only in approximately 20% of VT. Fourth, QRS morphology

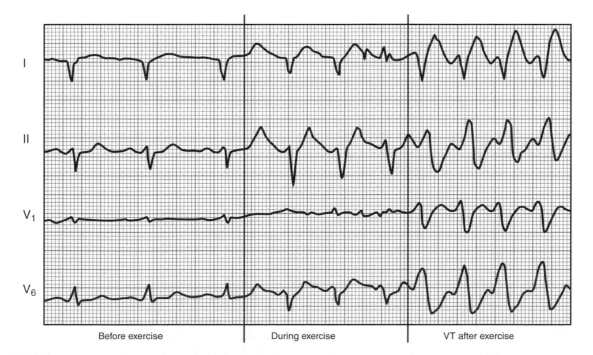

Before exercise   During exercise   VT after exercise

Figure 8.15 Ventricular tachycardia (VT) developed shortly after exercise. During VT, the ventricular rate is 136 beats·min⁻¹. The QRS duration is about 0.16 s. The QRS morphology (see figure 8.16) in lead V₁ showing an R duration of greater than 30 ms and the onset of QRS to S nadir greater than 60 ms indicates that this wide QRS tachycardia is VT. In lead V₆, the biphasic Rs complex with an R:S ratio of greater than one is unhelpful for diagnosing VT.

Adapted from Wellens and Conover 1992.

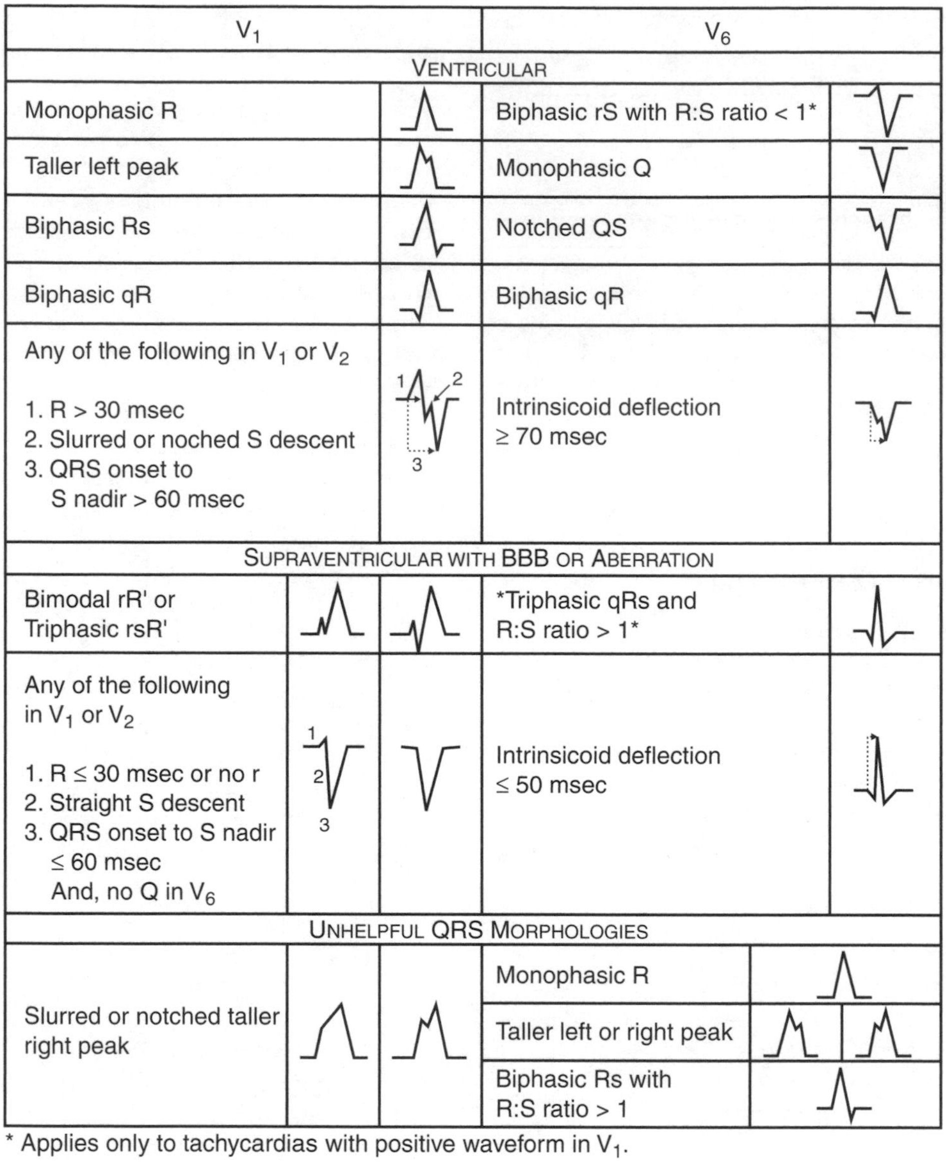

V₁		V₆	
VENTRICULAR			
Monophasic R		Biphasic rS with R:S ratio < 1*	
Taller left peak		Monophasic Q	
Biphasic Rs		Notched QS	
Biphasic qR		Biphasic qR	
Any of the following in V₁ or V₂ 1. R > 30 msec 2. Slurred or noched S descent 3. QRS onset to S nadir > 60 msec		Intrinsicoid deflection ≥ 70 msec	
SUPRAVENTRICULAR WITH BBB OR ABERRATION			
Bimodal rR' or Triphasic rsR'		*Triphasic qRs and R:S ratio > 1*	
Any of the following in V₁ or V₂ 1. R ≤ 30 msec or no r 2. Straight S descent 3. QRS onset to S nadir ≤ 60 msec And, no Q in V₆		Intrinsicoid deflection ≤ 50 msec	
UNHELPFUL QRS MORPHOLOGIES			
Slurred or notched taller right peak		Monophasic R	
		Taller left or right peak	
		Biphasic Rs with R:S ratio > 1	

* Applies only to tachycardias with positive waveform in V₁.

Figure 8.16 QRS morphology in leads V₁ or V₆, suggestive of VT.

Adapted from Drew BJ (1993). Wide QRS tachycardia: distinguishing SVT with bundle branch block or aberrant conduction from VT. Pamphlet from Hewlett-Packard.

in V₁, V₂, and V₆ can also be used to differentiate VT versus SVT (figure 8.16).[21] With VT, ventricular complexes are not initiated by atrial activity and have a morphology that is different from that of typical right bundle branch block (RBBB) or left bundle branch block (LBBB).

Ventricular Flutter

Ventricular flutter is similar to VT, but the rate is faster, usually 220 to 400 beats·min⁻¹. The rhythm is usually regular. P waves and PR interval are not measurable.

QRS complexes are wide, regular, and in a sine wave pattern (wide QRS complex that merges with the T wave).

Ventricular Fibrillation

Ventricular fibrillation is rapid, ineffective quivering of the ventricles and is a preterminal rhythm. P waves and PR intervals are not identifiable, and QRS complexes are not clear-cut. This erratic electrical activity may be coarse or fine.

Atrioventricular (AV) Blocks

The term *block* refers to a delay or failure of impulse propagation. Atrioventricular block occurs when the atrial impulse is conducted with delay or is not conducted at all. AV block can occur in the AV node, His bundle, bundle branches, fascicles, or any combination of these. AV block is traditionally categorized by severity: *first-degree* (PR interval >0.2 s with all atrial impulses conducted), *second-degree* (intermittent blocked beats), or *third-degree* (complete heart block, in which no supraventricular impulses are conducted to the ventricles). Although uncommon, first-degree, second-degree, and complete heart blocks during exercise have been observed.[22-25]

First-Degree AV Block

First-degree AV block is a delay or prolongation of impulse conduction in the AV node (PR >0.2 s), but all atrial impulses are conducted to the ventricles (figure 8.17). First-degree AV block with a narrow QRS is usually benign and does not require treatment. However, it should be observed for possible progression to more advanced blocks.

Second-Degree AV Block

Second-degree AV block is divided into Mobitz type I (Wenckebach) and Mobitz type II. Mobitz type I is characterized by progressive PR lengthening with a shortening of the RR interval ending in a nonconducted P wave, which produces a pause. In comparison with Mobitz type I block, Mobitz type II has intermittently nonconducted P waves but the PR interval remains constant without the progressive lengthening. Mobitz type I AV block with a normal QRS complex is generally more benign and does not progress to more advanced forms of AV conduction disturbances. Mobitz type II AV block is not as common as type I but is often associated with poor outcomes. Mobitz type II often occurs in a setting of an acute anterior myocardial infarction (MI), may require pacing, and is associated with more myocardial damage and a higher mortality rate.[26]

Third-Degree AV Block

Third-degree AV block or complete heart block occurs when no atrial impulse is conducted to the ventricles. Thus, the atria and ventricles are controlled by independent pacemakers and AV dissociation is observed. The atria rhythm may be sinus or ectopic (flutter or fibrillation) or from an AV junctional focus. The ventricular rhythm is usually regular and may be junctional or ventricular depending on the level of block.

Bundle Branch Blocks

The bundle branches are part of the specialized electrical conduction system of the heart located in the intraventricular septum. *Bundle branch block* (BBB) refers to a delay or failure of conduction within a bundle branch. BBB may be complete, incomplete, permanent, or intermittent. When one bundle branch is blocked, the atrial impulse is conducted through the normal bundle branch causing asynchronous depolarization of ventricles. Asynchronous ventricular depolarization takes longer than simultaneous depolarization of both ventricles, thus producing a widening of the QRS complex to 0.12 s or greater and best recognized in precordial leads V_1 and V_6. The wide QRS complex during BBB can produce a narrow, normal-looking QRS complex in lead II; therefore, lead II cannot be used to diagnose RBBB and LBBB.

The development of new RBBB, LBBB, left anterior fascicular block (LAFB), and left posterior fascicular block (LPFB) during exercise is infrequent.[27-29] Transient LBBB occurs in approximately 0.5% of all patients undergoing exercise testing.[29] A recent study showed that the risk of death and major cardiac events in patients with exercise-induced LBBB is increased approximately threefold compared with patients without LBBB.[29] Transient normalization of LBBB and RBBB patterns during exercise has also been reported.[30]

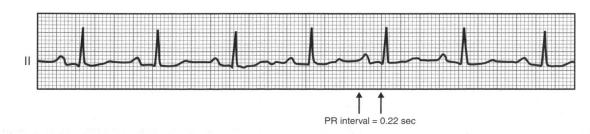

II

PR interval = 0.22 sec

Figure 8.17   First-degree atrioventricular (AV) block.

Left Bundle Branch Block

Left bundle branch block (LBBB) is recognized by a wide QS or rS complex in right precordial leads V_1 and V_2 and wide R waves without q waves in lateral leads V_5, V_6, I, or aVL. In LBBB, the septum does not depolarize in its normal left-to-right direction. This causes the loss of the normal small r wave in V_1 and loss of the q wave in lateral leads V_5, V_6, I, and aVL (figure 8.18). ST–T-wave changes are prominent in LBBB. In leads V_1 and V_2, the QRS complex is negative, the ST segment is elevated, and the T wave is upright. The ST segment is depressed and the T wave is inverted in leads with an upright QRS complex in leads V_5, V_6, I, or aVL.

Right Bundle Branch Block

Typical right bundle branch block (RBBB) may be recognized by a wide triphasic rsR' (rabbit ears) pattern that is best observed from a right precordial lead V_1 because the exploring electrode is located near the right ventricular free wall and there is a wide qRs pattern in leads V_5, V_6, I, and aVL (figure 8.19). If an individual with RBBB has a septal MI, the initial small r wave in lead V_1 (which represents septal depolarization) disappears and results in a qR pattern.

Myocardial Ischemia and Infarction

Myocardial ischemia occurs when myocardial oxygen demand is greater than the myocardial oxygen supply. Myocardial ischemia can produce changes in the QRS complex, the ST segment, and the T wave. Decreased R-wave amplitude or Q waves, ST-segment depression of at least 1 mm, an ST segment that forms a sharp angle with the upright T wave, and T-wave inversion are all indications of acute myocardial ischemia. Myocardial injury is most often indicated by ST-segment elevation of at least 1 mm from an individual's baseline. Other signs of acute injury include a straightening of the ST segment that slopes up to the peak of the T wave, tall peaked T waves, and symmetric T-wave inversion.

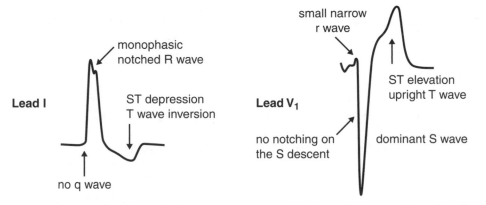

Figure 8.18   Left bundle branch block (LBBB): QRS characteristics in leads I and V_1. Approximately a third of individuals with LBBB have the QS complex (absence of the initial r wave) in lead V_1.

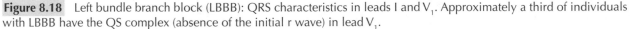
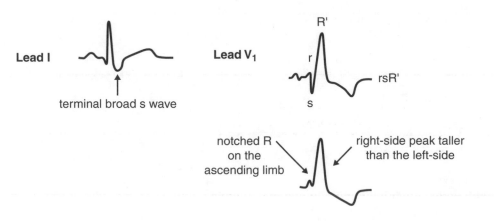

Figure 8.19   Right bundle branch block (RBBB): QRS characteristics in leads I and V_1. In lead V_1, the typical QRS is usually a triphasic rsR' (90%) and sometimes a notched monophasic R wave (10%).

Prolonged myocardial ischemia results in cellular necrosis or myocardial infarction (MI). Necrosis of the myocardium produces depolarization abnormalities affecting the QRS complex (development of new Q waves or loss of R waves). Pathologic Q-wave and R-wave durations are summarized in table 8.1.[31] Traditional thought was that the presence of Q waves indicated transmural MI extending through the entire thickness of the myocardium and that subendocardial infarction did not produce Q waves because it involves less than the entire thickness of the muscle. However, current thinking is that the Q waves can develop transiently with severe ischemia and that MI can occur without any development of Q waves. The newer terms *ST-elevation MI (STEMI)* and *non-ST-elevation MI (NSTEMI)* replace the older terms *transmural–Q wave* and *subendocardial–non-Q-wave* infarction.[32]

Evolution of ECG Changes With MI

The progression of the infarction from the acute phase through the fully evolved phase can be reflected on the ECG. Ischemic ST-segment deviation and tall, positive (hyperacute) T waves are the earliest sign of an acute MI. ST-segment elevation can persist for hours to several days but resolves quickly with successful reperfusion. Once the ST segment has returned to baseline, ECG evidence of the acute stage is lost. Q waves appear within hours of symptom onset and usually remain indefinitely, although they may disappear over the years following an MI. T-wave inversion occurs within hours of an MI and may last for days or weeks or persist indefinitely.

Localization of MI

The ECG leads are helpful in localizing MI. ST-segment elevations, Q waves, and T-wave inversions are recorded in the leads facing the damaged myocardium and are referred as indicative changes of MI. The ECG leads opposite the damaged myocardium record mirror images known as reciprocal changes.

Anterior wall MI may be caused by occlusion of the left anterior descending (LAD) coronary artery circulation and is recognized by indicative ST-segment elevations in leads facing the anterior wall (V_1-V_4; figure 8.20). If only the septum is infarcted, ECG changes occur in leads V_1 through V_2. An anterior

Table 8.1		Quick and Simple Method for Diagnosing Pathologic Q- or R-Wave Duration					
I	Q ≥ 30 ms	aVR		V_1	Any Q wave R ≥ 40 ms	V_4	Q ≥ 30 ms
II	Q ≥ 30 ms	aVL	Q ≥ 30 ms	V_2	Any Q wave R ≥ 50 ms	V_5	Q ≥ 30 ms
III		aVF	Q ≥ 30 ms	V_3	Any Q wave	V_6	Q ≥ 30 ms

The numbers next to each of the 12 leads correspond to pathologic widths for Q waves and R waves.
Adapted from Evans 1996.

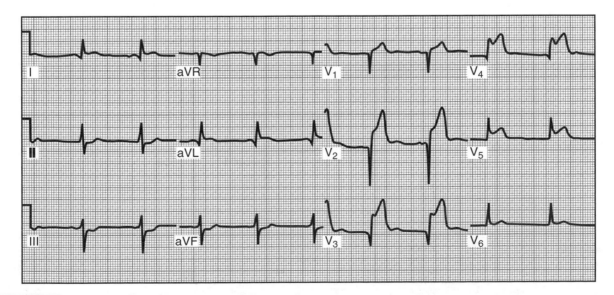

Figure 8.20   Acute anteroseptal wall myocardial infarction with lateral and apical involvement. ST-segment elevations are noted in lead V_1 through V_6 as well as leads I and aVL. Reciprocal ST-segment depression are seen in leads II, III, and aVF.

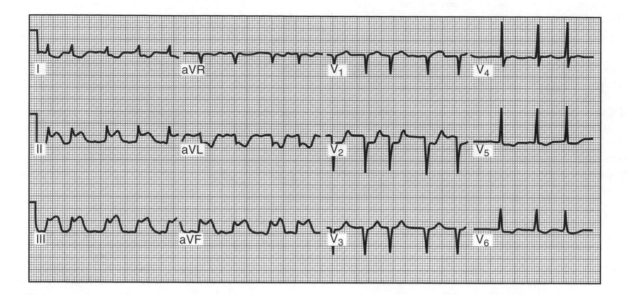

Figure 8.21 Atrial fibrillation with rapid ventricular response (120 beats·min⁻¹) with acute inferoposterior myocardial infarction (MI) and right ventricular involvement. Acute inferior wall MI is evidenced by ST-segment elevations in the inferior leads II, III, and aVF and reciprocal ST-segment depression in leads I and aVL. Acute posterior injury is evident from the reciprocal ST-segment depression in leads V_2 and V_3. Right ventricular involvement is shown by ST-segment elevation in lead V_1 and ST-segment depression in lead V_2, ST-segment depression in lead aVL greater than in lead I, and ST-segment elevation in leads III greater than in lead II.

wall MI that extends laterally and involves leads I and aVL is referred to as *anterolateral MI*. Anterior wall MI that extends to the apex and involves leads V_5 and V_6 is referred to as *anteroapical MI*. In anterior MI, the reciprocal ST-segment depressions are seen in inferior leads II, III, and aVF.

Lateral wall infarction usually is caused by occlusion of the circumflex coronary artery and results in indicative changes in leads I, aVL, V_5, and V_6 with reciprocal changes in inferior leads II, III, and aVF.

Inferior MI is usually the result of occlusion of the right coronary artery (RCA) circulation and is diagnosed by indicative ST-segment elevations in leads II, III, aVF and reciprocal ST-segment depression in leads I and aVL (figure 8.21). ST-segment depressions in the precordial leads may indicate reciprocal changes of an acute inferior or posterior wall MI.

Right ventricular (RV) involvement is not common and usually is caused by proximal occlusion of the RCA proximal to the right ventricular branch. Several changes on the 12-lead ECG suggest RV involvement: ST-segment elevation in lead III greater than in lead II, ST-segment elevation in lead V_1 accompanying ST depression in V_2, and ST depression in lead aVL greater than in lead I (figure 8.21). Right-sided leads may be obtained to confirm right ventricular myocar-

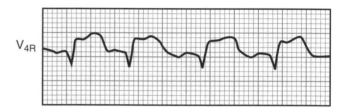

Figure 8.22 Acute right ventricular involvement. ST-segment elevation of at least 1 mm in the right ventricular lead V_{4R} confirms right ventricular involvement in the individual presented in figure 8.21.

dial infarction (RVMI), and ST-segment elevation of at least 1 mm in lead V_{4R} has been suggested to diagnose RVMI (figure 8.22).[33]

Posterior wall MI is caused by occlusion of left circumflex (LC) artery or the RCA. The reported incidence of acute posterior wall MI is approximately 15% to 20% of all acute MIs, and the incidence of isolated posterior MI is approximately 3% to 4%. Because none of the 12 standard leads are placed over the posterior chest to record indicative changes, the diagnosis of acute posterior MI has traditionally been based on the presence of reciprocal changes in precordial leads V_1 through V_3. These reciprocal changes include

ST-segment depression (a mirror image of ST elevation in posterior leads), wider and taller R waves (a mirror image of Q waves in posterior leads), and tall, upright T waves (a mirror image of T-wave inversion in posterior leads). Posterior ECG leads V_7 through V_9 have been found to be more efficacious in detecting LC-related changes than reciprocal ST-segment depression in precordial leads V_1 through V_3.[34] Because the ECG amplitudes in the posterior leads are small, ST elevation of 0.5 mm in posterior leads V_7 through V_9 is significant for detecting an acute myocardial ischemia in the posterior wall of the left ventricle (figure 8.23).[34] Electrode locations for recording posterior ECGs are shown in figure 8.24.

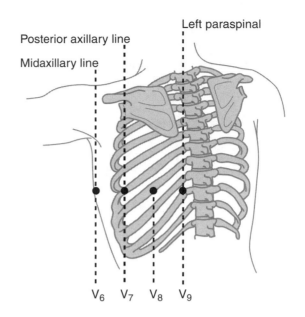

Figure 8.24   Electrode locations for recording posterior electrocardiogram leads. Posterior leads V_7 through V_9 are located at the same horizontal level as leads V_4 through V_6. Lead V_7 is at the posterior axillary line, V_9 is at the left paraspinal line, and V_8 is halfway between V_7 and V_9.

Reprinted from *AACN procedure manual for critical care*, 4th ed., S.F. Wung and B.J. Drew, pg. 343, Copyright 2001, with permission from Elsevier.

ST-Segment Deviations During Exercise

When a clinician interprets exercise-induced ECG changes, the ST-segment level is measured relative to the PR segment or the PQ junction because the TP segment can be difficult to determine at a rapid heart rate. Exercise-induced myocardial ischemia may manifest as either ST-segment depression or elevation. The presence of LBBB, left ventricular hypertrophy with repolarization abnormalities, and resting ST-segment depression 1 mm or more and the use of digoxin confound the interpretation of the ST segment for ischemia.

ST-Segment Depression

The most common manifestation of exercise-induced myocardial ischemia is ST-segment depression. Although many criteria can be used to determine abnormal exercise response, the standard criterion is defined as horizontal or downward-sloping

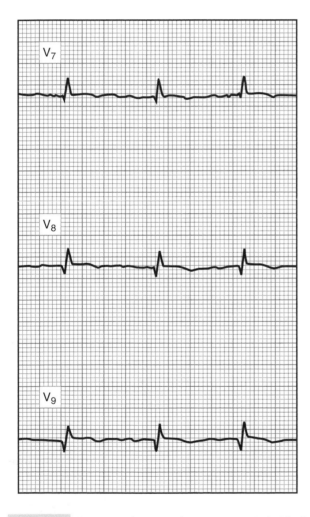

Figure 8.23   Posterior electrocardiograms in an individual with an acute posterior wall myocardial infarction (MI). Acute posterior wall MI is evident by ST-segment elevations of 0.5 mm and pathological Q waves in the posterior leads V_8 and V_9 in this individual.

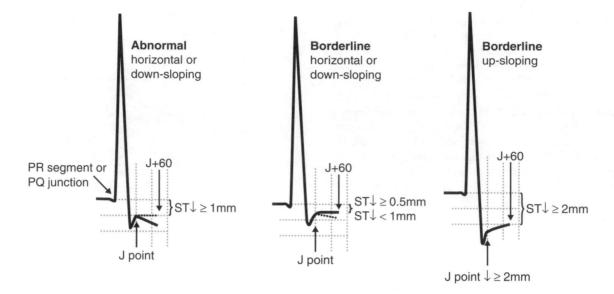

Figure 8.25   Abnormal and borderline ST-segment depression during exercise. The standard criterion for an abnormal ST-segment depression response during exercise is horizontal or down-sloping ST-segment depression greater than or equal to 1 mm at J+60 ms (1.5 boxes following the J point) in relation to the isoelectric PR segment or the PQ junction. Down-sloping ST-segment depression is worse than horizontal ST-segment depression. Borderline ST-segment depression is defined as horizontal or down-sloping ST-segment depression greater than or equal to 0.5 mm but less than 1 mm at J+60 ms. To be considered a borderline ST-segment depression response, the up-sloping ST-segment depression as well as J-point depression should be at least 2 mm in amplitude.

Adapted from Fletcher et al. 2001.

ST-segment depression of more than 1 mm at J+60 ms or J+80 ms in three consecutive beats with a stable baseline (figure 8.25).[3] Exercise-induced ST-segment depression does not localize the site of myocardial ischemia, nor does it suggest that the coronary artery involved. For example, patients with isolated RCA disease may exhibit exercise-induced ST-segment depression only in leads V_4 through V_6. Patients with LAD coronary artery disease may exhibit exercise-induced ST-segment deviation in leads II, III, and aVF.

The slope of the ST-segment depression is used as a predictor of coronary heart disease (CHD). Down-sloping and horizontal ST-segment depressions are more predictive of CAD than up-sloping ST-segment depression. Up-sloping ST-segment depression is considered to be "borderline" or negative (figure 8.25).

ST-Segment Elevation

Prior MI (with pathologic Q waves on the resting ECG) is the most frequent cause of ST-segment elevation during exercise. Approximately 30% and 15% of subjects with anterior wall MI and inferior wall MI, respectively, who exercise within 2 weeks of MI demonstrate exercise-induced-ST-segment elevation in Q-wave leads.[3] The importance of this finding remains controversial.[3] ST-segment elevation in an infarcted area usually indicates a wall motion abnormality and is not considered an ischemic response (figure 8.26).[3]

In subjects without previous MI, ST-segment elevation during exercise localizes the site of severe transient ischemia resulting from significant proximal

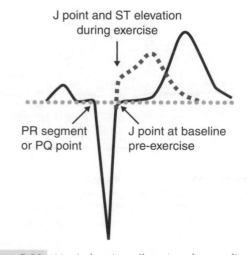

Figure 8.26   Nonischemic wall motion abnormality during exercise exhibited as J-point and ST-segment elevation over Q wave leads.

coronary artery disease or spasm.[3,35] Exercise-induced ST-segment elevation corresponds to the territory of myocardial ischemia and the coronary artery involved. For example, ST-segment elevation in leads V_2 through V_4 indicates LAD involvement, and ST-segment elevation in leads II, III, and aVF indicates RCA involvement. Concomitant ST elevation and depression in the same exercise test may indicate multivessel CAD.[3] Ventricular arrhythmias during exercise are more frequent in patients who demonstrate exercise-induced ST elevation.[3]

ECG Monitoring During Exercise Testing

Exercise testing typically includes a 12-lead ECG and should be recorded at standardized intervals throughout exercise and recovery. However, most computer-based exercise testing systems allow for the continuous monitoring of only three leads during exercise. The choice of which three leads to monitor is important for detecting significant myocardial ischemia. ECG monitoring during supervised exercise training sessions is usually limited to one ECG lead, and again the choice of which lead to monitor affects the ability to detect myocardial ischemia.

- Mason–Likar Lead System

  Electrode placement affects the slope and amplitude of the ST segment. Standard resting 12-lead ECGs are recorded with arm and leg electrodes on the wrists and ankles. However, recording exercise ECGs with electrodes placed on the distal end of extremities is impractical. The Mason–Likar modification is used to record 12-lead exercise ECGs by placing the arm electrodes immediately below the distal end of the clavicles and the leg electrodes immediately above the iliac crest and on the midclavicular line. Although the Mason–Likar modification minimizes motion artifacts, it results in a right-axis shift and increased voltage in the inferior leads, which may produce a loss of inferior Q waves and the development of new Q waves in lead aVL.[3]

- Lead Selection

  Most ST-segment changes during exercise occur in the lateral precordial leads V_4 through V_6.[3] The lateral precordial leads V_4 through V_6 are capable of detecting approximately 90% of ST-segment depression observed in multiple-lead ECG systems. ST-segment elevation is rare but occurs with equal frequency in leads V_2, aVF, and V_5. During ECG-monitored exercise training, only one lead is monitored at a time on the typical telemetry system. The lead that is most sensitive to ST-segment depression and is also stable during exercise is modified chest lead V_5 (MCL_5). This involves having the positive electrode in the standard V_5 position and the negative electrode on the right arm (RA) position. Although detecting ischemia during monitored exercise may be important in an individual patient, detecting and documenting significant arrhythmias may be equally important in certain patients.

- Additional ECG Leads

  The sensitivity of exercise 12-lead ECG for the detection of single-vessel CAD is low, ranging from 35% to 61%,[36,37] and even lower in RCA disease.[38] Although not common in clinical practice, there has been increased interest in using additional ECG leads during exercise testing to improve sensitivity. Several studies have found that using an additional single lead V_{4R} during exercise results in a small improvement in the detection of RCA disease.[39,40] Recently, researchers reported a significant improvement in sensitivity for detecting single-, two-, and three-vessel disease by using three additional right precordial leads V_{3R} to V_{5R}.[38] In addition, the use of extra leads may help to differentiate stenosis in the right versus left circumflex coronary artery. For example, exercise-induced ST-segment changes in leads V_{3R}, V_{4R}, or both but not in V_{5R} may identify RCA stenosis, whereas ST-segment changes in leads V_{4R}, V_{5R}, or both but not in V_{3R} may identify disease of the LC coronary artery. However, two recent studies reported that the use of additional right-side and posterior leads V_7 through V_9 did not increase detection of myocardial ischemia during exercise stress testing.[41,42]

- Pseudonormalization

  Pseudonormalization is defined as a normal-looking isoelectric ST segment during acute myocardial ischemia. Patients with chronic ST-segment deviations on the resting ECG attributable to conditions other than acute myocardial ischemia, such as BBBs and early repolarization, can produce a deceptively normal-looking isoelectric ST segment during acute myocardial ischemia while exercising. Thus, when the resting baseline ST-segment depression is 1 mm or greater, the exercise ECG changes become less specific for myocardial ischemia,[3] and an exercise or pharmacological imaging study should be considered.[11] Exercise-induced ST-segment depression is found in most patients with LBBB and cannot be used as a diagnostic or prognostic indicator regardless of the degree of ST-segment abnormality.

ECG Monitoring During Exercise Training

The ACC/AHA exercise standards for testing and training[3] suggest that patients with known, stable cardiovascular disease with low risk for complications with vigorous exercise (*Guidelines,* figure 5.1) should be monitored by ECG for 6 to 12 sessions during the early prescription phase. In addition, continuous ECG monitoring should be performed during exercise sessions until safety is established (usually ≥12 sessions) for those who have a moderate to high risk for complications during exercise or are unable to self-regulate activity or understand recommended activity level.[3] In addition, the working group suggests that ECG monitoring sessions should be conducted by personnel who have a working knowledge of electrocardiography and arrhythmia detection.

Summary

Cardiac rehabilitation professionals must understand basic electrocardiography and exercise-related arrhythmias. These professionals must also

- fully understand medical reports that contain ECG recordings or ECG interpretation information,
- be able to compare current with previous ECG recordings, and
- recognize serious ECG abnormalities (e.g., VT, high-degree AV blocks, significant ischemic ST-segment changes) so that appropriate action may be taken.

PART III

Special Considerations

Women

Lauralyn B. Cannistra, MD

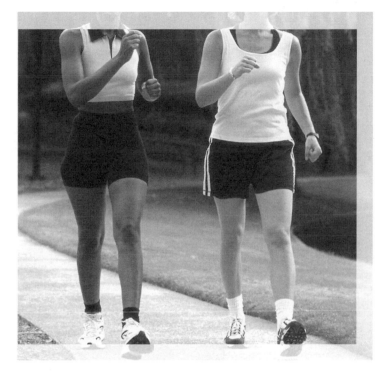

Cardiovascular disease (CVD) is the leading cause of death in women, and the majority of these deaths are attributable to coronary heart disease (CHD).[1] Nearly one of every two women will die of CVD, and since 1984, the number of CVD deaths in women has exceeded that of men. Although CVD mortality rates have been decreasing for men and women, they have been decreasing less for women, and the absolute number of women dying from CVD is actually increasing because of the aging of the population. African American women have experienced less of a decline in their mortality rate from CVD, and their death rate from CHD is significantly higher than that of white women. Despite these overwhelming statistics, according to a recent American Heart Association (AHA) survey, most women (51%) still believe that cancer is their greatest health threat, whereas only 13% of them correctly perceive heart disease or a heart attack as their greatest health problem.[2]

There is, unfortunately, more bad news. Once a woman develops coronary artery disease, her prognosis is worse than that of a man. The Multicenter Investigation of the Limitation of Infarct Size (MILIS) study documented a higher in-hospital (13% vs. 7%) and 48-month (36% vs. 21%) mortality rate for women compared with men.[3] Black women had an especially high mortality rate at 48 months (48%). At the 6-month follow-up visit, women were also more likely to have angina, congestive heart failure, and reinfarction compared with men. A meta-analysis of fibrinolytic trials[4] and a national myocardial infarction registry database[5] confirmed higher in-hospital and short-term mortality rates for women after myocardial infarction.

GUIDELINES, 4TH EDITION

- Chapter 9, pages 140-142

Treatment Issues

Possible reasons for the poorer prognosis for women include their increased age and more advanced disease at presentation and increased comorbidity.[6] In patients with established CHD, women are more likely to have hypertension and diabetes and to have higher cholesterol levels than men.[7,8,9] Other possible explanations may be related to differences in the use or effectiveness of established medical therapies, noninvasive and invasive diagnostic procedures, and interventional or surgical revascularization in women compared with men. For patients presenting with acute or suspected myocardial infarctions and eligible to receive these medical therapies according to American Heart Association guidelines, several studies have shown less utilization of aspirin, β-blockers, and thrombolytic therapy for women compared with men.[4,10,11,12] Among women and men with CHD and elevated low-density lipoprotein (LDL) cholesterol levels, lipid-lowering drugs are prescribed less often for women.[13] It is reasonable to believe that greater use of these therapies would have improved women's outcomes because they have been proven effective in women as well as men.[14-17]

Women are less likely to undergo cardiac catheterization procedures for suspected coronary disease after an abnormal stress test[18] or in the setting of a myocardial infarction.[19] They are also less likely to be referred for coronary angioplasty and coronary bypass surgery when hospitalized for a myocardial infarction.[19] These procedures do impose a higher risk on women, with three times the periprocedural morbidity and mortality rates for angioplasty in women and a higher operative mortality rate for bypass surgery.[6] Possible reasons for these increased procedural risks

include a woman's older age, presentation at a later stage of disease, comorbidities, and smaller vessel size. If women survive the procedure, they experience a long-term benefit similar to that of men.

After a myocardial infarction or revascularization procedure, women in cardiac rehabilitation programs have similar improvements in functional capacity, risk factor modification, and psychosocial functioning compared with men.[9,20] Unfortunately, this is another area in which women are underrepresented compared with men. In a national survey of participation rates in cardiac rehabilitation after myocardial infarction and coronary bypass surgery, only a minority of patients enrolled in these programs. The rates were particularly low for women, with only 6.9% of women enrolling after myocardial infarction and 20.2% participating after bypass surgery.[21]

There is, however, reason for hope. The information discussed here highlights the recent literature concerning the problems of diagnosis, treatment, and worse outcomes for women with CHD. This awareness is the first critical step. More attention is now being given to including women in clinical trials of coronary heart disease. Recent articles, consensus statements, and guidelines have been published to enhance clinician awareness and implementation of primary and secondary prevention strategies for women (see sidebar).

Evaluation of Chest Pain

The diagnosis of CHD presents a greater challenge in women than men because of differences in clinical presentation and the lower accuracy of noninvasive diagnostic tests for women. Part of this decreased

Important Publications for Health Care Professionals About Women and Cardiovascular Disease

- Cardiovascular disease in women: A statement for health care professionals from the AHA[7]
- AHA guidelines: Evidence-based guidelines for cardiovascular disease prevention in women[22]
- Guide to preventive cardiology for women: AHA/American College of Cardiology (ACC) scientific statement consensus panel statement[22]
- AHA scientific statement: Role of noninvasive testing in the clinical evaluation of women with suspected coronary artery disease[22]
- Hormone replacement therapy and cardiovascular disease: A statement for health care professionals from the AHA[24]
- Women and cardiovascular disease: The risks of misperception and the need for action[25a]
- Percutaneous coronary intervention and adjunctive pharmacotherapy in women: A statement for health care professional from the AHA[25b]

accuracy is the result of the lower age-specific prevalence of CHD in women. Longitudinal studies such as the Framingham Heart Study, which was initiated in 1948, concluded that women with angina had a more benign course and a much more favorable outcome.[23] This has possibly led to a misperception that chest pain in women does not have to be evaluated with such an intense search for CHD. In that study, however, the presence of angina was a clinical diagnosis without documentation by coronary angiography. The Coronary Artery Surgery Study (CASS) documented that for men and women presenting with chest pain, only 50% of women versus 83% of men had significant CHD at catheterization.[24] Many of the women with "angina" in the Framingham study cohort, then, had a better prognosis because they did not actually have significant CHD. Further analysis of the Framingham data reveals that the more favorable prognosis was limited to the younger women. The prognosis for women 60 years old or older was nearly identical to that of men.

The predictive value of chest pain in women may be further improved by defining the chest pain as typical angina, probable angina, or nonspecific chest pain. The CASS trial provides the data shown in table 9.1.[24] All forms of chest pain are associated with a lower prevalence of CHD documented by cardiac catheterization in women than in men. Women are also more likely than men to present with atypical symptoms such as upper-abdominal pain, nausea, and fatigue.[26] However, although chest pain is a less sensitive and specific predictor of CHD in women, it is still their most common presenting symptom of CHD, and the majority of women with an acute myocardial infarction experience chest pain similar to that of men.[23,26] We therefore need better ways to evaluate this symptom in women. The Women's Ischemia Syndrome Evaluation (WISE) study[27] evaluated several aspects of chest pain and diagnostic testing in women. Results of this study indicated that only 39% of women referred for coronary angiography had CHD, which was defined as a stenosis greater than 50% in more than one coronary artery. In addition, the classification of women experiencing "typical" symptoms of angina did not correctly identify 65% of women who actually had CAD.[28] It is speculated that symptoms experienced by women in the absence of CAD may be symptoms that are related to microvascular ischemia or ischemia related to coronary constriction.[29]

Douglas and Ginsburg published a specific approach to the evaluation of chest pain in women that characterizes various clinical determinants of CHD into major, intermediate, or minor based on the strength of their association with the disease[55] (table 9.2). This approach is an attempt to optimize the use of diagnostic testing in women in a cost-efficient and

Table 9.1   Predictive Value of Chest Pain in Women

Number of positive responses	Classification	PRETEST PROBABILITY OF DISEASE (%)	
		Women	Men
3	Definite angina	72	93
1-2	Probable angina	36	66
0	Nonspecific chest pain	6	14

Note. Determine whether pain or discomfort is substernal, brought on by exertion, or relieved within 10 min by cessation of exercise or sublingual nitroglycerin.

Adapted from Pepine 2004.

Table 9.2   Determinants of Coronary Heart Disease in Women With Chest Pain

Minor	Intermediate	Major
Age >65 years	Hypertension	Typical angina pectoris
Obesity, especially central obesity	Smoking	Postmenopausal status
Sedentary lifestyle	Lipoprotein abnormalities, especially low HDL cholesterol levels	Diabetes mellitus
Family history of coronary artery disease		Peripheral vascular disease

Note. HDL = high-density lipoprotein.

most informative manner. If a woman with chest pain has a low risk of having CHD after this analysis, reassurance without further testing and careful clinical observation are recommended. For women with a high likelihood of CHD by this analysis, stress testing is recommended for prognostic information. The vast majority of women will fall into a category of intermediate likelihood of disease, and diagnostic stress testing is recommended for these women. For all women, this evaluation should result in a discussion of their cardiac risk factors and either primary or secondary prevention of CHD.

Cardiac Risk Factors

When evaluating chest pain in women, identification of other clinical variables and their cardiac risk factors can improve the clinician's ability to estimate the likelihood of CHD and decide on the need for further testing. Stratification by the presence of risk factors has been shown to help predict the presence of significant CHD at catheterization. The predictive value of coronary risk factors is better for women than men and is particularly strong in young women.[31,32] Identification of risk factors is not only helpful in assessing chest pain in women but is very important in preventing death from CHD in women. This is highlighted by data from the Framingham study, in which nearly two-thirds of sudden cardiac deaths in women occurred in women without prior cardiac symptoms.[6] Identification and treatment of cardiac risk factors are therefore essential in women's health and are the subject of two recent ACC/AHA guidelines.[6,33,34] Chapter 3 illustrates the major established risk factors for CHD in both women and men. There are some important differences, however, in cardiac risk factors for women.

Smoking

Smoking is the leading preventable cause of CHD in women, with more than 50% of myocardial infarctions in middle-aged women occurring among women who smoke.[35] Although overall smoking prevalence is declining for men and women, it is declining more slowly in women and their smoking prevalence rates are soon expected to exceed those in men. Especially concerning is the increase in cigarette use among young women.[6] Smoking may be more hazardous to a woman's health than to a man's because it lowers the age at first myocardial infarction more for a woman than for a man.[36] Smoking is, therefore, another risk factor that appears to negate the age advantage in women.

Dyslipidemia

Elevated total cholesterol and LDL levels are coronary risk factors in both men and women. A low level of high-density lipoprotein (HDL) cholesterol, however, is a better predictor than elevated LDL cholesterol in women, but not in men.[37] In addition, elevated triglyceride levels appear to be an important risk factor for CHD in older women.[38] The recent ACC/AHA scientific guidelines for preventive cardiology in women acknowledge these differences and suggest that the optimal triglyceride level may be lower and the HDL level higher for women than the current National Cholesterol Education Program (NCEP) guidelines.[33,39]

Diabetes Mellitus

Diabetes appears to be a more powerful risk factor for women than men. Women without diabetes generally present 10 years later than men with CHD. The presence of diabetes negates this age advantage in women.[40] It is associated with a three- to sevenfold increase in CHD risk in women compared with a two- to threefold increase in men.[41] The increased risk may be attributable to the worse effects of diabetes on lipids and blood pressure in women.

Estrogen Deficiency and Hormone Replacement Therapy

A cardiac risk factor that is certainly unique to women is the relative estrogen deficiency of the postmenopausal state. A natural protective effect of estrogen in premenopausal women is postulated to account for the age advantage for women before the onset of cardiovascular disease.[42] Estrogen deficiency is associated with increases in total and LDL cholesterol, decreases in HDL cholesterol, and adverse effects on coagulation parameters and endothelial function.[43] Theoretical benefits of estrogen replacement therapy seemed to be verified by observational studies that suggested a 35% to 50% reduction in cardiovascular risk associated with hormone replacement therapy.[44-46] Unfortunately, in the last few years, randomized, controlled trials have not supported the observational data. Recently, the data and safety monitoring board for the primary prevention Women's Health Initiative trial recommended stopping the combined estrogen–progestin arm of the trial because the health risks exceeded the benefits after 5.2 years of follow-up.[47] One explanation for this discrepancy in results is that observational studies are limited by potential biases. One such bias is the "healthy women bias," which explains the more favorable outcome for women taking hormone therapy with their healthier behaviors. This bias has been demonstrated in a group of women followed from their premenopausal years through menopause.[48] Women who decided to take hormone replacement therapy were less obese, were more educated, had higher HDL levels, had lower blood pressure and fasting insulin levels, and engaged in more physical activity when they were premenopausal compared with women who did not take hormone replacement therapy. It may be these or other factors instead of the hormone replacement therapy that caused the favorable results in the observational studies.

The first of the recent randomized, controlled trials to challenge the benefit of hormone replacement therapy for the prevention of cardiovascular disease was the Heart and Estrogen/Progestin Replacement Study (HERS).[49] This was a secondary prevention trial in women with known CHD who were randomized to conjugated equine estrogen (0.625 mg) plus 2.5 mg of medroxyprogesterone or placebo. After 4 years, there were no overall differences between the two groups in nonfatal myocardial infarction or death from CHD. Further evaluation of these results, however, revealed a 50% higher risk of cardiovascular events in the hormone treatment group during the first year with fewer events in this group after 2 years. The hormone treatment group also had a higher incidence of thromboembolic and gallbladder disease.

It is postulated that the "early hazard" of hormone replacement therapy may be related to procoagulant or proinflammatory effects, but this is not clear. The possibility of an early hazard is further suggested by more recent observational data. In a retrospective analysis of women with a recent myocardial infarction, initiation of hormone replacement therapy after their infarction was associated with a higher incidence of the composite end point of death, myocardial infarction, and unstable angina compared with women who had never used hormone replacement therapy. Women who were on hormone replacement therapy at the time of their infarction did not have any increased risk of this composite end point during follow-up.[50] Data from women in the Nurses' Health Study also reveal a similar trend. In women with a prior myocardial infarction or atherosclerotic disease, use of hormone replacement therapy for less than 1 year was associated with an increased risk of recurrent coronary events. Increasing duration of use was associated with a trend of decreasing risk.[51] A second, randomized, controlled trial of hormone replacement therapy added to the negative information about this treatment for secondary prevention of cardiovascular disease. The Estrogen Replacement and Atherosclerosis (ERA) study showed the same progression of atherosclerosis as assessed by repeat coronary angiography whether women were taking hormone replacement therapy or placebo.[52]

For primary prevention of CHD, two large-scale controlled trials of hormone replacement therapy have been initiated, but as noted previously, the combined hormone replacement versus placebo arm of the Women's Health Initiative was terminated because of increased health risks found in the hormone replacement group. Preliminary data from the Women's Health Initiative had revealed a nonsignificant increased risk of blood clots, myocardial infarction, and stroke in women during the first 2 years of treatment with hormone replacement therapy compared with women randomized to placebo.[53] The health risks that prompted termination of the study suggest that for 10,000 women treated with a daily regimen of combined estrogen and progestin for 1 year, there would be seven more CHD events, eight more invasive breast cancers, eight more strokes, and eight more pulmonary emboli compared with women not receiving hormone replacement therapy. Health benefits of a lower risk of colorectal cancer and hip fractures were also found, but overall the harm outweighed the benefit. Even before publication of the Women's Health Initiative data, the AHA in a scientific advisory about hormone replacement therapy and cardiovascular disease recommended that hormone replacement therapy should not be initiated for primary or secondary prevention of CHD because of the randomized, controlled study data that were becoming available. Prevention of osteoporosis can be accomplished with other treatments,[54] and therefore in light of the Women's Health Initiative data, it seems prudent not to initiate combined hormone replacement therapy for this reason. The decision to use this therapy short-term for its known benefit of menopausal symptom management must be carefully weighed against the increased CHD and thromboembolic risks during the first year of therapy. These data do not apply to treatment with estrogen alone in women without a uterus, and we await the final results of this arm of the Women's Health Initiative study for more information about this form of hormone replacement therapy.

Noninvasive Stress Testing

For the women in whom a diagnostic stress is indicated, there are further challenges in the selection and interpretation of these tests. Exercise stress testing without imaging is the most frequently used noninvasive test for the diagnosis of CHD. For women, it is unfortunately not as sensitive or specific a test as for men and carries a high incidence of false positive results in women.[55-57] Some potential reasons for this decreased diagnostic accuracy in women are shown in the sidebar.

The addition of radionuclide imaging with thallium 201 improves the sensitivity of the test but in women is limited by false-positive results caused by breast tissue artifacts.[58] Technetium-99m sestamibi is a newer, higher-energy radionuclide agent that decreases the breast tissue artifact. In addition, with sestamibi imaging it is also possible to obtain gated images that are synchronized to the patient's electrocardiogram (ECG) and allow visualization of wall motion. This modality aids the interpretation of any perfusion abnormalities and improves the specificity of the test. Information on the use of sestamibi stress testing in women is becoming available.[58,59] The role of computed tomography,

Factors That Reduce Diagnostic Accuracy of Exercise Electrocardiogram in Women[49-51]

Reduced specificity

- Lower incidence of coronary heart disease in premenopausal women
- Higher incidence of mitral valve prolapse
- Premenopausal estrogen or hormone replacement therapy

Reduced sensitivity

- Higher incidence of single-vessel disease
- Lower peak exercise workload

magnetic resonance imaging, and carotid intima media thickness in the evaluation of women with suspected CHD is not clear at this time.[60] More data are necessary before any recommendations can be made as to the usefulness of these technologies in women. Another alternative noninvasive test is a stress testing with echocardiographic imaging. This modality has the advantages of being less expensive and faster than nuclear imaging without breast tissue artifacts. Stress echocardiography has been shown to be accurate in the detection of CHD in women[61] and to provide prognostic information for the prediction of their future cardiac events (see figure 9.1).[62] The technique can be limited by echocardiographic image quality, but use of harmonic imaging and intravenous contrast agents will likely minimize this limitation.

For the initial noninvasive diagnostic test in women with a moderate risk of having CHD, an exercise stress test is recommended in women with a normal baseline ECG who can exercise. Some advocate stress testing with imaging as the most cost-effective initial approach because of the higher costs of repeat testing or angiography with false-positive ECG responses.[59,62] As for the choice of imaging modalities, stress echocardiograpy and stress technetium-99m sestamibi imaging have similar sensitivity and specificity for the diagnosis of CHD in women and are better than exercise ECG alone (figure 9.1). For a particular facility, the choice of imaging modality will depend on local expertise and preference.

Exercise Benefits

When cardiac risk factors or CHD is identified in women, primary or secondary prevention strategies should be implemented. Exercise has beneficial effects on cardiovascular morbidity and mortality rates and several cardiac risk factors. It should, therefore, be an integral part of any risk factor modification program.

Reduced Cardiovascular Mortality and Morbidity Rates

Several population-based studies show that incremental levels of regular physical activity are inversely proportional to long-term cardiovascular mortality rates when controlled for the presence of other risk factors in both men and women.[63-65] Specifically in older women, a study of more than 32,000 postmenopausal women found a graded inverse relationship between leisure-time physical activity and cardiovascular mortality over 7 years of follow-up.[66] As for exercise as secondary prevention in women, the data are very limited. In a meta-analysis of the 4,500 patients enrolled in the randomized trials of cardiac rehabilitation after myocardial infarction, only 3% were women.[67] This meta-analysis showed a 20% reduction in overall mortality rate, but the small number of women precludes generalizing these results. As for the benefit of exercise on cardiovascular morbidity in women, a case-control study showed that leisure-time activity equivalent to walking for 30 to 45 min, three times a week, decreased the risk of nonfatal myocardial infarction in postmenopausal women by 50%.[68]

Exercise Training

Women demonstrate a 15% to 30% improvement in $\dot{V}O_2$peak in response to the type of aerobic exercise training used in cardiac rehabilitation, and this response is similar to that of men. In women with established CHD, a limited number of studies with small numbers of women show similar results to exercise training.[9,69-72] A study by Ades and colleagues[69] is the only one that measured peak $\dot{V}O_2$ before and after exercise training and included only women 62 years old or older. All of

Intermediate to High Likelihood Women with Atypical or Typical Chest Pain Symptoms

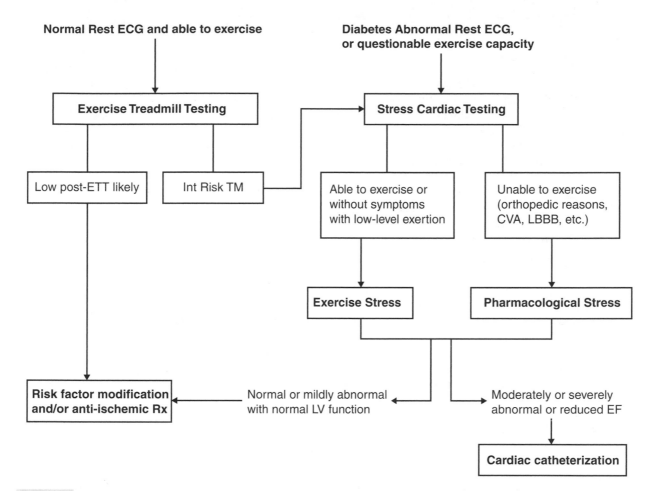

Figure 9.1   Algorithm for evaluation of symptomatic women using exercise electrocardiogram (ECG) or cardiac imaging. ETT = exercise tolerance test; Int = intermediate; TM = treadmill; Rx = prescription; CVA = cerebrovascular accident; LBBB = left bundle branch block; LV = left ventricular; EF = ejection fraction.

these studies found that women had a lower exercise capacity than men at baseline but showed similar improvements after exercise training. These results suggest that women with CHD may even derive a greater benefit from exercise training than men. Ades and colleagues also showed a more efficient response to submaximal exercise in older women with a lower rate–pressure product (heart rate × blood pressure) at an exercise intensity of 3 metabolic equivalents (METs) after exercise training. Kavanagh and colleagues[71] compared work rates on a cycle ergometer and measured $\dot{V}O_2$peak values in women and men during exercise testing at the beginning and after the completion of a 12-month outpatient cardiac rehabilitation program. The sample included 547 women and 547 men matched for age and was divided into four age-decade groups from 40 to 79 years of age. Peak work rate increased significantly on the final exercise test in both men and women in all four age decades with the increase being less in women than men. There were similar results for $\dot{V}O_2$peak with mean values for the women ranging from 17.3 to 13.4 ml·kg^{-1}·min^{-1} in the in the youngest and oldest age-decade groups, respectively.

Improved Coronary Risk Factors

One study of 500 healthy, middle-aged women[73] found an association between aging and increases in weight, diastolic blood pressure, and LDL cholesterol levels over 3 years, whereas HDL cholesterol levels declined. However, women who reported an increase in their physical activity of at least 300 kcal·week^{-1} (equivalent to walking an additional 3 miles a week) over the 3 years experienced less weight gain and less decline in HDL cholesterol. Physical activity has been associated with favorable effects on obesity, body composition, insulin sensitivity, and blood pressure, along with modest effects on lipoprotein profiles. In addition, regular exercise also seems to encourage beneficial lifestyle changes such as smoking cessation and stress reduction.

Decreased Body Weight

Exercise training appears to be an important component for weight loss and the development of a more favorable body composition and fat distribution with regard to CHD risk. The best results occur when diet modification is added to an exercise program. Although data for women are limited, a well-controlled, 1-year randomized trial[74] that included 112 women demonstrated a significant 5.1-kg weight loss, most of which was body fat, in women in the exercise and diet intervention. Those in the control group increased their weight by an average of 1.3 kg. Physically active women have a more favorable waist-to-hip ratio than do sedentary individuals.[75]

Reduced Risk of Developing Type 2 Diabetes Mellitus

The beneficial effects of exercise on glucose metabolism include increased sensitivity to insulin, decreased production of glucose by the liver, and reduction of obesity.[76] Although a study in men documented a decreased risk of the development of type 2 diabetes in a high-fitness group of men compared with men in the low-fitness group over 6 years of follow-up,[77] similar data for women were lacking until recently. Recent observational data from the Nurses' Health Study revealed the lowest risk of the development of type 2 diabetes in women who were consistently active compared with women who remained sedentary. Women who increased their physical activity level during the study period had an intermediate risk of developing diabetes over the 8 years of follow-up compared with women in the two other groups with lower levels of physical activity.[78] More data are clearly needed for women in this area.

Reduced Blood Pressure

Observational data have also suggested an inverse relationship between physical activity and blood pressure in women.[79] A study of 8 weeks of exercise training in women and men demonstrated systolic blood pressure reductions of 10 to 16 mmHg and diastolic blood pressure reductions of 5 to 14 mmHg. The benefit of exercise was similar for women and men.[80] A recent randomized controlled trial that included women demonstrated significant reductions in blood pressure with aerobic exercise alone or in combination with a behavioral weight management program compared with controls.[81] The combination of exercise and weight management had the greatest impact on blood pressure and supports the multidisciplinary approach to risk factor reduction.

Improved Lipoprotein Profiles

Beneficial effects of exercise on blood lipids have been suggested in studies of both men and women,[82] but few investigations of the effect of exercise on lipid and lipoproteins have been performed in women. A cross-sectional study examined the effects of vigorous exercise on HDL cholesterol in women runners. HDL cholesterol levels were higher with increasing amounts of exercise and continued to increase further in women who ran more than 64 km·week^{-1}.[83] A study was performed of postmenopausal women randomized to moderate-intensity exercise (equivalent to 10 miles of brisk walking per week), Step 2 American Heart Association diet, and the combination of diet plus exercise.[84] Decreases in LDL cholesterol were greatest in the diet-plus-exercise group, which experienced an 8% reduction in LDL cholesterol after 1 year. The effects of exercise on lipoprotein profiles are certainly modest, and other studies have had conflicting results. Because estrogen is associated with increases in HDL and triglyceride levels and a decrease in LDL cholesterol, the variable results may arise, in part, from the lack of control in these studies for menopausal status and estrogen use.

For women with CHD, data examining the effect of multidisciplinary cardiac rehabilitation programs on their lipid profiles are very limited. The two studies of 12 weeks of cardiac rehabilitation showed no significant improvements in lipid profiles among women.[9,20] This finding was also seen in the men in the programs. One potential reason for the negative results is the short duration of the intervention. In support of this explanation is a study by Warner and colleagues[85] showing a 20% increase in HDL cholesterol levels among women after 5 years of cardiac rehabilitation. This result was significantly better than that seen in the men in the group, who increased their HDL levels after the first year but then showed no further increase, resulting in a 5-year increase of only 5%.[85]

Enrollment and Adherence in Cardiac Rehabilitation Programs

The long-term success of any prevention program is directly related to patient compliance. For women with CHD, enrollment in cardiac rehabilitation programs is much less than expected based on their prevalence of coronary events, as mentioned earlier.[21] The reasons for this gender difference in participation rates are not clear. Recent studies have begun to investigate the potential barriers to women's participation in cardiac rehabilitation. Women candidates for cardiac rehabilitation are more often unmarried, may have less social support, are more likely to have a dependent spouse at home, and are less likely to own and drive a car.[9,69] In addition, women have more noncardiac morbidity such as arthritis and low back pain.[69,86] These patient-related factors certainly may play a role in the low participation rates. In addition, Ades and colleagues[70] found that the strength of the physicians' referral to cardiac rehabilitation was the most powerful predictor of participation among older coronary patients, and in this study, physicians did not recommend cardiac rehabilitation as strongly to their women patients.[69]

Once women enroll in cardiac rehabilitation, it is not clear if their compliance and attendance rates differ from those of the men, because the results are conflicting.[9,69,85] Cannistra and colleagues[9] demonstrated no significant difference in compliance rates between women and men and no difference with respect to the reasons given for lack of program completion. By univariate analysis, younger women and those who smoked were less likely to be compliant. Other patient-related factors associated with noncompliance included physically inactive leisure time, blue-collar employment, and sedentary occupations.[87] Preferences for program features may differ between women and men as well.[88]

Summary

CHD is clearly the major cause of morbidity and mortality in women, and, fortunately, many of the factors that place women at risk from this disease are modifiable. It is crucial, therefore, to educate women and their health care providers about the diagnosis, evaluation, and treatment of this disease in women. Fortunately, more cardiovascular research is being conducted in women that has helped to identify some treatment differences and to provide information about the effectiveness of standard therapies in women. It is also encouraging that articles, consensus statements, and guidelines about women's cardiovascular health have recently been published to help disseminate this information[22,89] (see table 9.3). There are some differences in presentation, diagnosis, and risk factors for CHD in women, but risk factor modification through an exercise-based multidisciplinary approach is as effective for women as for men. An excellent summary intended for patient education use of important issues related to women and heart disease is provided by the AHA.[22] The challenge, then, is to encourage more women to identify their cardiac risk factors and engage in primary or secondary prevention programs.

Table 9.3	Clinical Recommendations for Cardiovascular Disease (CVD) Prevention in Women
Lifestyle interventions	
Cigarette smoking	Consistently encourage women not to smoke and to avoid environmental tobacco.
Physical activity	Consistently encourage women to accumulate a minimum of 30 min of moderate-intensity physical activity (e.g., brisk walking) on most, and preferably all, days of the week.
Cardiac rehabilitation	Women with a recent acute coronary syndrome or coronary intervention or new-onset or chronic angina should participate in a comprehensive risk-reduction regimen, such as cardiac rehabilitation or a physician-guided home- or community-based program.
Heart-healthy diet	Consistently encourage an overall healthy eating pattern that includes intake of a variety of fruits, vegetables, grains, low-fat or nonfat dairy products, fish, legumes, and sources of protein low in saturated fat (e.g., poultry, lean meats, plant sources). Limit saturated fat intake to <10% of calories, limit cholesterol intake to <300 mg per day, and limit intake of *trans* fatty acids.
Weight maintenance or reduction	Consistently encourage weight maintenance or reduction through an appropriate balance of physical activity, caloric intake, and formal behavioral programs when indicated to maintain or achieve a BMI between 18.5 and 24.9 $kg \cdot m^{-2}$ and a waist circumference <35 in.
Psychosocial factors	Women with CVD should be evaluated for depression and referred and treated when indicated.
Omega 3 fatty acids	As an adjunct to diet, omega-3 fatty acid supplementation may be considered in high-risk[a] women.
Folic acid	As an adjunct to diet, folic acid supplementation may be considered in high-risk[a] women (except after revascularization procedure) if a higher than normal level of homocysteine has been detected.

(continued)

Table 9.3 *(continued)*

	Major risk factor interventions
Blood pressure—lifestyle	Encourage an optimal blood pressure of <120/80 mm Hg through lifestyle approaches.
Blood pressure—drugs	Pharmacotherapy is indicated when blood pressure is ≥140/90 mm Hg or even lower in the setting of blood pressure-related target-organ damage or diabetes. Thiazide diuretics should be part of the drug regimen for most patients unless contraindicated.
Lipid, lipoproteins	Optimal levels of lipids and lipoproteins in women are LDL-C <100 mg·dl^{-1}, HDL-C >50 mg·dl^{-1}, triglycerides <150 mg·dl^{-1}, and non-HDL-C (total cholesterol minus HDL-C) <130 mg·dl^{-1} and should be encouraged through lifestyle approaches.
Lipids—diet therapy	In high-risk women or when LDL-C is elevated, saturated fat intake should be reduced to <7% of calories, cholesterol should be reduced to <200 mg·day^{-1}, and *trans* fatty acid intake should be reduced.
Lipids—pharmacotherapy, high risk[a]	Initiate LDL-C-lowering therapy (preferably a statin) simultaneously with lifestyle therapy in high-risk women with LDL-C ≥100 mg·dl^{-1} and initiate statin therapy in high-risk women with an LDL-C <100 mg·dl^{-1} unless contraindicated. Initiate niacin[b] or fibrate therapy when HDL-C is low or non-HDL-C is elevated in high-risk women.
Lipids—pharmacotherapy, intermediate risk[c]	Initiate LDL-C-lowering therapy (preferably a statin) if LDL-C level is ≥130 mg·dl^{-1} on lifestyle therapy or niacin[b] or fibrate therapy when HDL-C is low or non-HDL-C is elevated after LDL-C goal is reached.
Lipids—pharmacotherapy, lower risk[d]	Consider LDL-C-lowering therapy in low-risk women with 0 or 1 risk factor when LDL-C level is ≥190 mg·dL^{-1} or if multiple risk factors are present when LDL-C is ≥160 mg·dL^{-1} or niacin[b] or fibrate therapy when HDL-C is low or non-HDL-C is elevated after LDL-C goal is reached.
Diabetes	Lifestyle and pharmacotherapy should be used to achieve near-normal HbA1c (<7%) in women with diabetes.
	Preventive drug interventions
Aspirin—high risk*	Aspirin therapy (75-162 mg), or clopidogrel if patient is intolerant to aspirin, should be used in high-risk women unless contraindicated.
Aspirin—intermediate risk[c]	Consider aspirin therapy (75-162 mg) in intermediate-risk women as long as blood pressure is controlled and benefit is likely to outweigh risk of gastrointestinal side effects.
β-blockers	β-blockers should be used indefinitely in all women who have had a myocardial infarction or who have chronic ischemic syndromes unless contraindicated.
ACE inhibitors	ACE inhibitors should be used (unless contraindicated) in high-risk[a] women.
ARBs	ARBs should be used in high-risk[a] women with clinical evidence of heart failure or an ejection fraction <40% who are intolerant to ACE inhibitors.
	Atrial fibrillation/stroke prevention
Warfarin—atrial fibrillation	Among women with chronic or paroxysmal atrial fibrillation, warfarin should be used to maintain the INR at 2.0 to 3.0 unless they are considered to be at low risk for stroke (<1% per year) or high risk of bleeding.
Aspirin—atrial fibrillation	Aspirin (325 mg) should be used in women with chronic or paroxysmal atrial fibrillation with a contraindication to warfarin or at low risk for stroke (<1% per year).

(continued)

	Class III interventions
Hormone therapy	Combined estrogen plus progestin hormone therapy should not be initiated to prevent CVD in postmenopausal women.
	Combined estrogen plus progestin hormone therapy should not be continued to prevent CVD in postmenopausal women.
	Other forms of menopausal hormone therapy (e.g., unopposed estrogen) should not be initiated or continued to prevent CVD in postmenopausal women pending the results of ongoing trials.
Antioxidant supplements	Antioxidant vitamin supplements should not be used to prevent CVD pending the results of ongoing trials.
Aspirin—lower risk[d]	Routine use of aspirin in lower-risk women is not recommended pending the results of ongoing trials.

BMI = body mass index; HDL-C = high-density lipoprotein cholesterol; LDL-C = low-density lipoprotein cholesterol; HbA1c = hemoglobin A1c; ACE = angiotensin-converting enzyme; ARB = angiotensin receptor blocker; INR = International Normalized Ratio.

[a]High risk is defined as coronary heart disease (CHD) or risk equivalent, or 10-year absolute CHD risk >20%; [b]dietary supplementation of niacin must not be used as a substitute for prescription niacin, and over-the-counter niacin should only be used if approved and monitored by a physician; [c]intermediate risk is defined as 10-year absolute CHD risk 10% to 20%; [d]lower risk is defined as 10-year absolute CHD risk <10%.

Adapted, by permission, from L. Mosca et al., 2004, "Evidence-based guidelines for the prevention of cardiovascular disease in women," *Circulation* 109: 372-693.

10

Older Patients

Nanette K. Wenger, MD

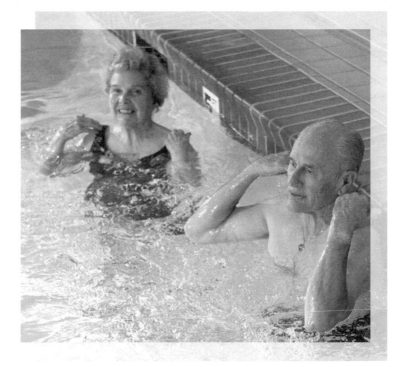

About half of the 25 million people in the U.S. older than 65 years have cardiovascular disease, which is the major cause of death and disability in elderly persons. Coronary heart disease (CHD) is the predominant cardiac problem, followed by hypertensive cardiovascular disease; valvular and pulmonary heart diseases are other important causes.[1] CHD prevalence per 1,000 men and women aged 65 years and older is 83 and 90, respectively, increasing to 217 and 129, respectively, at age 75 years and older.[2]

An overall decline in functional status was documented in the Cardiovascular Health Study between individuals aged 75 to 84 years and those 85 years of age and older.[3] The goal of clinical care is to return elderly patients to independent living for as long as reasonable.[4]

GUIDELINES, 4TH EDITION

- Chapter 9, pages 137-138

Cardiovascular Physiological Changes of Aging

Both functional and structural changes of aging in the cardiovascular system decrease the cardiac functional reserve capacity, limit the performance of physical activity, and lessen the ability to tolerate a variety of stresses and illnesses.[5]

Maximal heart rate and maximal aerobic capacity both decrease progressively with aging, independent of habitual physical activity.[6] However, the maximal oxygen uptake and maximal work capacity of sedentary elderly individuals are 10% to 20% less than in their physically active counterparts. Peak exercise cardiac output and exercise ejection fraction also decrease in elderly individuals. An increase in stroke volume, mediated by cardiac dilation, compensates for the diminished heart rate response to maintain the increased cardiac output required for exercise.

The increased aortic and large artery thickness and vascular stiffness of aging increase arterial systolic pressure and the impedance to left ventricular ejection. Both systolic blood pressure and mean blood pressure increase with aging, with widening of the pulse pressure.

The diastolic dysfunction of aging, that is, decreased ventricular compliance with substantial reduction in the early diastolic filling rate, increases the dependence on the contribution of atrial contraction to late left ventricular filling to maintain cardiac output. Both myocardial contraction and relaxation times are prolonged, and there is a lessened chronotropic and inotropic response to sympathetic stimulation.[7]

Baroreceptor responsiveness decreases with aging, caused in part by loss of vascular distensibility. More than 18% of community-dwelling individuals in the Cardiovascular Health Study[8] had orthostatic hypotension, with the prevalence increasing with age. Pacemaker cells and the number of bundle branch fibers decrease with age,[9] resulting in the sick sinus syndrome, atrioventricular block, atrioventricular conduction delay, and bundle branch block, which are accentuated by fibrosis and calcium deposition in the cardiac skeleton. The combination of atrial dilation and fibrosis likely underlies the increased prevalence of atrial arrhythmias at elderly age.

Collagen degeneration and calcium deposition in the cardiac valves are common in elderly individuals; one-third of patients aged 70 and over have calcium deposition in either the aortic or mitral valve.[10]

Coronary Heart Disease

Most patients in the United States with new episodes of myocardial infarction (MI) and with heart failure secondary to CHD are older than 65 years.[11] Sixty percent of patients hospitalized for acute MI are older than 65.[12] Eighty-five and 55% of men and women, respectively, aged 75 years and older have activity limitation attributable to CHD, compared with 50% and 20% of men and women, respectively, aged 55 to 64 years. Although octogenarians represent 5% of the U.S. population, they contribute to 20% of all hospital admissions for MI and 30% of all hospital deaths from MI.[4]

Patients with angina in a recent study[13] had a mean age of 69 years, and 75% of the population were women. Although typical angina pectoris remains common in elderly patients, angina at elderly age is less likely to be activity induced, in that arthritis, claudication, chronic pulmonary disease, musculoskeletal problems, or neurologic disorders limit activity before angina occurs. Alternatively, this may reflect habitual physical inactivity. More older than younger patients have atypical manifestations of myocardial ischemia including dyspnea and worsening heart failure, likely mediated by an ischemia-related increase in left ventricular end-diastolic pressure superimposed on the ventricular diastolic dysfunction of aging. Also, angina is more likely to be precipitated by an intercurrent medical or surgical problem. Therapy for angina is as for younger patients. Unstable angina and non-Q-wave MI are more common in elderly than younger patients.[14]

Eighty percent of all MI deaths occur after age 65,[15] with functional disability before MI predicting both the severity of infarction and postinfarction survival.[16] Chest pain is less frequent as the presenting manifestation of MI in elderly individuals[17,18]; common presentations include dyspnea, exacerbation of heart failure, and pulmonary edema. Atypical symptoms may in part explain the delayed presentation to hospital at elderly age,[19] with delayed presentation often limiting optimal therapy. Atypical symptoms may partially explain the high rates of unrecognized MI at elderly age, particularly in elderly women.

In large, randomized, placebo-controlled trials of thrombolytic therapy for acute MI, there is comparable benefit at younger and older ages up to age 75 years,[20] but for patients older than 75 years, caution is warranted in that observational data from a Medicare database suggest less favorable survival with coronary thrombolysis.[21] Primary percutaneous transluminal coronary angioplasty appears associated with more favorable outcomes than coronary thrombolysis in very elderly persons.[22]

Complications of MI are more frequent in elderly patients. These, plus an increased prevalence of comorbid illnesses, contribute to the increased mortality rate from MI at elderly age. Although significant underuse of beneficial therapies at elderly age persists,[23,24] increased use of pharmacological and invasive interventions at elderly age has substantially improved the survival of elderly patients with MI, particularly those younger than 85 years.[25-27] Pharmacologic management is comparable to that for a younger population, with recommendations that initial drug dosage be lower and the drug doses be gradually increased as tolerated.[28] Emphasis should be on use of aspirin, β-blocker, angiotensin-converting enzyme (ACE) inhibitor, and statin therapy in the absence of contraindications.

A substantial number of elderly patients have an uncomplicated clinical course with MI. These patients are ideal candidates for early ambulation and subsequent rehabilitation. Predischarge exercise testing to define risk status and suggest the need for invasive intervention is safe for appropriately selected elderly patients.[29] Exercise test data can also guide the recommended intensity of physical activity following hospital discharge.

Often, the habitual activity level of older cardiac patients is underestimated,[30] and excessive immobilization is prescribed. Rehabilitative exercise training can limit the high risk of disability in elderly patients after a coronary event, and rehabilitative education can encourage coronary risk reduction.[30,31] Comparable improvements in physical work capacity and endurance occur in elderly persons as in younger men and women, and appropriate exercise entails no greater risk.[32-34] The ideal exercise regimen after hospital discharge is walking, with gradual increases in pace and distance. Additional benefits of exercise include improved neuromuscular coordination, joint mobility, coordination, and flexibility and the potential to limit bone demineralization. High-impact aerobic activities are inappropriate, because they are associated with an increase in musculoskeletal complications.[35] Lack of emotional or social support independently predicts mortality risk following MI.[36]

Older patients now constitute more than half of the population undergoing cardiac catheterization with coronary angiography, percutaneous coronary interventions (PCIs), and coronary artery bypass graft (CABG) surgery.[12] At coronary arteriography, coronary disease is more extensive at elderly age, with more prevalent multivessel disease, coronary artery calcification, and evidence for prior MI. The elderly patient presenting for myocardial revascularization is more likely to have severe and unstable angina, to be female, and to have hypertension, peripheral vascular disease, and heart failure. Because octogenarian patients with unstable angina treated medically have an event-free survival of about 55% and often tolerate antianginal therapy poorly, revascularization is increasingly undertaken to reduce symptoms and limit recurrent hospitalizations.[27] However, older age is an independent risk factor for morbidity and mortality from CABG surgery, with elderly women and patients undergoing reoperation at highest risk.[37] Octogenarian patients in the Society of Thoracic Surgeons database had an operative mortality rate of 4% to 7% for isolated CABG surgery.[38] However, octogenarian survivors are pain free, often with restored performance status, and with a 5-year survival rate comparable to that of the general U.S. octogenarian population.[39] Elderly patients can be anticipated to have a longer hospital stay following CABG, with more time in an intensive care setting.[40] This reflects higher rates of postoperative cardiac complications, which occur in as many as 30% to 50% of patients. Prominent among these are atrial fibrillation and stroke. Early ambulation and progressive physical activity after CABG surgery can help limit complications and improve functional status. Nonrandomized comparisons show a 3-year survival for elderly patients who undergo elective CABG surgery of 77% compared with 54% with medical therapy.[41]

Recent reports of PCI at elderly age document angiographic success rates of 80% to 90%, even with multivessel PCI, without excess occurrence of procedural complications and with functional improvement and patency rates comparable to those at younger age.[42-44] Nonetheless, older age continues to predict procedural mortality and decreased survival rates, particularly for patients older than 80 years.[43,45] Newer transcatheter procedures including stenting have shown improved outcomes,[46] with similar success rates at age 70 and older as in younger patients in the Newer Approaches to Coronary Interventions (NACI) Registry. However, an excess of both non-Q-wave MI and vascular complications is reported in other studies.

Systemic Arterial Hypertension

Hypertension is present in half of the U.S. population older than 65 years.[47] Whereas diastolic blood pressures level off in the 50- and 60-year-old age group, systolic blood pressure increases into the eighth and ninth decade, rendering isolated systolic hypertension prominent at elderly age.[48] Isolated systolic hypertension accounts for about two-thirds of the hypertension after age 65.

Hypertension is a powerful predictor of cardiovascular events even at elderly age, with systolic hypertension more closely correlated with cardiovascular and cerebrovascular morbidity and mortality in the elderly population[49,50] and with a widened pulse pressure ($\geq$50 mmHg), highly predictive of risk for cardiovascular disease and heart failure.[51]

Hypertension contributes to accelerated CHD, heart failure, cerebrovascular accident, peripheral vascular disease, renal failure, aortic dissection, and aortic aneurysm rupture in both younger and elderly populations. Control of isolated systolic hypertension in the Systolic Hypertension in the Elderly Program (SHEP)[52] using diuretics and low-dose β-blockade as needed reduced stroke by 36% and fatal and nonfatal cardiovascular events by 32% in an elderly population, with heart failure reduced about 50%. Although data from large hypertension treatment trials are limited for patients older than 80 years, therapy appeared beneficial in the Systolic Hypertension Europe (SYST-EUR) trial and in subgroup meta-analysis from other trials[53,54] for reduction of stroke, heart failure, and major cardiovascular events; no reduction in cardiovascular mortality or total mortality was evident.

Nonpharmacologic interventions for control of hypertension in elderly patients with mild elevation of blood pressure include reduction of sodium intake, weight reduction, moderation of alcohol consumption, and regular moderate-intensity physical activity.[55] In the randomized Trial of Nonpharmacologic Intervention in the Elderly (TONE), sodium restriction combined with weight loss effected the best result.[56] Major randomized clinical trials show comparable or greater benefit of pharmacotherapy at least to age 80 in elderly compared with younger patients.[48,57]

Goal blood pressure is less than 140/90 mmHg, with avoidance of postural hypotension and maintenance of renal function. A target blood pressure of less than 130/80 mmHg is recommended for patients with heart failure, renal insufficiency, and type 2 diabetes.[55] Goal blood pressure of less than 130/85 mmHg is a cost-effective intervention in elderly hypertensive diabetic patients.[58] Drug dosage should be initiated at half the usual adult dose, with gradual increments in drug dosage. Selection of pharmacotherapy should reflect the presence of comorbidities and risk factors, the severity of the hypertension, and target organ damage. Blood pressure should be checked in the sitting and standing positions because of impaired baroreflex control of blood pressure at elderly age.

Heart Failure

Heart failure is the most frequent hospital discharge diagnosis for patients older than 65 years[59] and is more common in men than women until about age 80 (see chapter 12 for a general discussion of chronic heart failure). The prevalence of heart failure increases with increasing age and involves about 5% of individuals aged 65 to 75 years and 10% of those older than 75 years.

CHD and calcific aortic stenosis are the most prevalent causes of heart failure, and heart failure is more frequently precipitated or exacerbated by associated medical problems at elderly age.

Echocardiography has substantially improved the recognition of heart failure in elderly patients and is the best test to differentiate systolic from diastolic ventricular dysfunction.[60] More than half of octogenarians with heart failure have diastolic dysfunction with intact ventricular systolic function.[61] Therapy for the patient with ventricular systolic dysfunction includes dietary sodium restriction, activity limitation until compensation is achieved, digitalis, diuretic drugs, vasodilator drugs, β-blocking drugs, and spironolactone.[62-65] ACE inhibitor benefit has been demonstrated at very old age.[66] Limited experience shows benefit of β-blocking drugs in patients up to 75 years of age,[67-69] and spironolactone has been shown effective up to age 80.[70]

Deconditioning of skeletal muscles and impaired skeletal muscle vasodilator response to exercise more frequently impair functional capacity at elderly age. Resumption of a regular physical activity regimen is recommended once compensation is achieved[60] because improvement in functional capacity decreases dependency and disability.[32]

Particularly at elderly age, an intensive multidisciplinary treatment strategy for heart failure involving education, assessment, and management has proved cost-effective because it limits subsequent hospitalizations.[71,72]

Arrhythmias and Conduction Abnormalities

Arrhythmias and conduction abnormalities are more prevalent at elderly age,[73-75] owing to age-related changes in conduction tissue and atrioventricular myocardium.[9]

Atrial fibrillation is present in almost 10% of the population older than 80 years[76] and is the major contributor to stroke.[77] CHD, hypertension, and valvular disease are the most common etiologies, with heart failure a concomitant problem. Anticoagulation can reduce stroke risk by almost 70%,[78] even in patients older than 75 years.

Asymptomatic ventricular arrhythmias in healthy elderly patients in the absence of myocardial ischemia or ventricular dysfunction do not impart excess risk and rarely require treatment. Ventricular arrhythmias, including premature ventricular contractions and nonsustained ventricular tachycardia, are common at elderly age,[75,79] even in the absence of cardiac disease. Both sick sinus syndrome and complete atrioventricular block are frequent in an elderly population and are the major indications for pacemaker implantation. Pacemaker implantation can improve symptoms and the quantity and quality of life even at elderly age.[80] The median age of pacemaker recipients in the United States is 70 years.

Valvular Heart Disease

Hemodynamically significant symptomatic calcific aortic stenosis is the major valvular disease requiring surgical intervention at elderly age.[81] Atrial fibrillation is present in up to one-fourth of patients with severe aortic stenosis and often precipitates heart failure. Symptomatic severe aortic stenosis requires aortic valve replacement[82] because of the excessive mortality once angina, heart failure, or syncope occurs. Mortality rates as high as 50% have been described in the first year.[83] Perioperative mortality rates as low as 4% to 5% have been described with aortic valve replacement,[84] with increased mortality rates when concomitant CABG surgery is required.

Risk Factor Management

As increased numbers of reasonably healthy and active individuals enter elderly age, there will be greater interest in and requirements for cardiovascular preventive care. As well, more precise assessment of their functional capabilities will be requisite to recommend levels of recreational and leisure activities.

Modifiable coronary risk factors are highly prevalent and continue to predict coronary events and mortality in old age.[85,86] Because estimated life expectancy at age 65 is 16.9 years and at age 75 is 10.7 years, coronary risk reduction strategies are appropriate. Although the relative risk of coronary risk factors decreases somewhat at elderly age, the absolute or attributable risk is greater because of excess coronary morbidity and mortality in an elderly population.[87] Preventive approaches should address hypertension control, weight reduction and control, dietary sodium and fat restriction, control of hyperlipidemia, regular modest-intensity physical activity, and smoking cessation.

The Adult Treatment Panel of the National Cholesterol Education Program (NCEP) recommends that all adults with total blood cholesterol levels greater than 200 mg·dl^{-1} be evaluated and that those with elevated low-density lipoprotein cholesterol levels be treated.[88] Based on NCEP guidelines, about one-third of elderly men and one-half of elderly women have elevated cholesterol levels warranting intervention.[89] Most recommendations for cholesterol lowering at elderly age are based on extrapolation of data derived from younger populations, although subanalyses of older subjects in reported studies have demonstrated a comparable value of lipid lowering in those older and younger than 65 years. The Prospective Pravastatin Pooling Project analyzed the effects of this statin in older (≥65 years of age) versus younger patients with CHD.[90] The relative risk for CHD death or nonfatal MI was 32% in persons less than 55 years of age, 21% in those 55 to 64 years old, and 26% in the patients 65 to 75 years old.

Because mortality rates are greater at older age, absolute risk reduction for all-cause and CHD mortality is almost twice as great in older individuals. Analysis from the Cholesterol and Recurrent Events (CARE) trial regarding prevention of coronary events with lipid lowering[90] identified that, for every 1,000 patients treated, 225 cardiovascular hospitalizations would be prevented in elderly patients versus 121 hospitalizations at younger age.

One study of postinfarction patients that included a sizeable elderly cohort[92] reported a 28% reduction in total mortality rate in patients treated with lipid-lowering agents. In the recently reported British Heart Protection Study,[93] patients older and younger than age 65 derived comparable benefit from statin therapy, without evidence of excess risk at elderly age.

Recommended dietary therapy at elderly age includes a regimen restricted in saturated fat and cholesterol and high in fruits, vegetables, and grains. Additional dietary components include lean meats, fish, and low-fat diary products. This diet may confer other health benefits as well.

Smoking cessation decreases cardiovascular risk, independent of the age at smoking cessation[94]; benefit is often evident within the first year of smoking cessation. Even in older men and women (>70) with angiographically documented coronary disease in the Coronary Artery Surgery Study (CASS) Registry,[95] smoking cessation decreased the risk of MI or mortality. Repeated interventions may be required to effect smoking cessation, but strategies effective at younger age are equally applicable to elderly patients with cardiovascular disease.[96,97]

A physically active lifestyle should be encouraged at elderly age, because deconditioning attributable to physical inactivity occurs more rapidly in elderly individuals. Even in previously sedentary individuals, physical activity can enhance endurance and functional capacity. In one study, resistance training improved walking endurance in healthy individuals.[98] Although there has not been a systematic evaluation of the effect of exercise on coronary risk at elderly age, high-level physical activity (>2,000 kcal weekly) in individuals 65 to 79 years of age in one study was associated with improved survival compared with individuals with lower physical activity levels.[99] As well, moderate- and high-intensity walking lowered blood pressure in normotensive elderly subjects,[100] with lower rates of hypertension described in physically active elderly women.[101]

Regular walking in men with a mean age of 69 years in the Honolulu Heart Program was associated with decreased mortality rate at 12-year follow-up.[102] There was comparable inverse association between physical activity and all-cause mortality in menopausal women (mean age 62 years) in the Iowa Women's Health Study.[103] Physical activity level independently predicted 5-year mortality in community-dwelling elderly individuals (mean age 73 years) in the Cardiovascular Health Study.[104]

Hypertension is the dominant risk factor at elderly age; it is present in more than half of U.S. individuals older than 60 years, and its incidence increases with advancing age. Nearly two-thirds of persons older than 75 have uncontrolled hypertension, that is, 140/90 mmHg or more. Isolated systolic hypertension is the most prevalent problem. Meta-analysis has shown prominent benefit of antihypertensive therapy at ages 60 to 80 years.[105] Control of blood pressure limits cerebrovascular complications and facilitates the management of angina and heart failure. Dietary sodium restriction is important in blood pressure control.

Control of obesity decreases cardiac work and cardiovascular risk and favorably affects glucose tolerance, blood pressure, and serum lipid levels. Framingham Heart Study data confirm obesity as a risk factor for recurrent coronary events at older age, likely reflecting the prominent clustering of obesity, dyslipidemia, and insulin resistance at elderly age.[106,107] A combination of diet and exercise is likely to be beneficial, but few intervention data are available for older populations. Exercise training, in the absence of dietary intervention, has shown little benefit in older patients,[31] although more frequent and prolonged walking training appears favorable.[108]

Diabetes mellitus and glucose intolerance remain independent predictors of cardiovascular risk in old age and are powerful predictors of recurrent coronary events.[109] Exercise training can improve insulin resistance and diabetic control at older age,[110] and control of obesity can improve glucose and insulin levels.

Although postmenopausal estrogen use by women in the Cardiovascular Health Study was associated with a more favorable cardiovascular risk profile well into the eighth decade, it is controversial whether this reflects hormone effect, the baseline characteristics of women who continue hormone therapy, or both.

The role of dietary and pharmacologic antioxidants remains uncertain,[111] but recent studies of antioxidant vitamins have not shown benefit.[92]

Further validation of risk intervention at elderly age is provided by Framingham data[11] showing that the 10% of individuals aged 65 to 74 years with the highest multivariate coronary risk scores had a doubled occurrence of coronary events among men and a fourfold greater occurrence among women. Elevated risk levels for cardiovascular disease in the elderly Framingham cohort were associated with increased Medicare costs.[112]

Exercise Training

Exercise training comparably improves functional capacity at younger and elderly age, although absolute levels are lower in an aged population.[113-115] This occurs both in healthy individuals and in patients following MI and myocardial revascularization.

Lavie and Milani[115] compared the effects of exercise-based cardiac rehabilitation in older (>70 years) and younger (<55 years) patients with CHD. Younger patients had greater improvement in estimated aerobic capacity, $\dot{V}O_2$peak, and total quality of life scores; the elderly patients showed highly significant ($p < .0001$) improvements in estimated aerobic capacity, measured $\dot{V}O_2$peak, total function scores, and total quality of life scores compared with baseline values at the start of exercise training.

In a randomized, controlled study, older patients (>65 years) in the exercise group demonstrated significant improvements in exercise capacity, subjective feelings of well-being, and quality of life measures compared with the control group. Exercise capacity improved an average of 17.3% in 3 months ($p < .001$) in the exercise group compared with 2.9% in the control group.[116]

In older women with CHD, Hung and colleagues[117] used two exercise training approaches—aerobic exercise only and a combination of aerobic and strength training. They reported significant improvements in both groups for $\dot{V}O_2$peak, 6-min walk distance, lower-extremity strength, and emotional and global quality of life. The combined training group also had improvements in upper-extremity strength and social and physical quality of life.

The physiologic characteristics of aging and the superimposed limitations caused by cardiovascular disease must be considered in formulating physical activity recommendations. Exercise recommendations must be individualized, avoiding excessive fatigue or exhaustion and limiting musculoskeletal injury by restriction of running, jumping, and other high-impact activities.[35] Brisk walking is an excellent physical activity recommendation that decreases the overall mortality rate in older persons.[118]

Both physical activity[119] and correct nutrition, including weight control, contribute to the maintenance of cardiovascular function at elderly age. Strength training can improve muscular strength, endurance, and neuromuscular function.[120] High-intensity resistance exercise can counteract muscle weakness and physical frailty even in very elderly persons.[121] Although exercise training effects on coronary morbidity and mortality rates have not been studied at elderly age, a British study of men (mean age 63 years) with CHD showed decreased all-cause mortality at 5 years associated with light to moderate physical activity.[122]

Despite the recommendation of cardiac rehabilitation as an essential component of the contemporary management of patients with CHD and with heart failure,[32,123] referral and participation of elderly patients, and particularly elderly women,[124] have been unacceptably low. Elderly patients need improved access to cardiac rehabilitation services, because exercise training can enhance functional capacity and limit disability and dependency, and comprehensive approaches to risk reduction can be implemented.

Summary

Secondary prevention of CHD in elderly persons was recently summarized in a scientific statement by the American Heart Association.[96] Elderly patients with CHD often have comorbidities and receive fewer beneficial therapies. The referral rate of elderly persons to cardiac rehabilitation programs is poor, even though exercise training and risk factor interventions improve survival and quality of life. To realize the benefits of secondary prevention, increased numbers of elderly patients have to be referred to and participate in cardiac rehabilitation and secondary prevention programs.

Diabetes Mellitus

Neil F. Gordon, MD, PhD, MPH

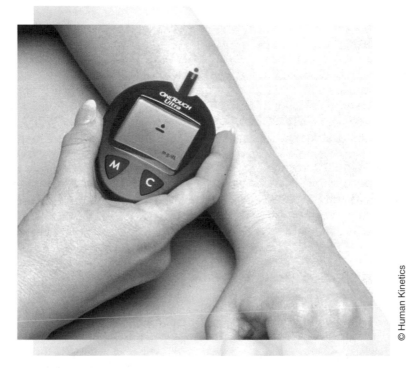

© Human Kinetics

Diabetes mellitus is a group of metabolic diseases characterized by hyperglycemia resulting from defects in insulin secretion, insulin action, or both. The chronic hyperglycemia of diabetes is associated with long-term damage, dysfunction, and failure of various organs, especially the eyes, kidneys, nerves, heart, and blood vessels.[1]

Diabetes is one of the most common chronic diseases in the United States and one of the major public health issues facing the world in the 21st century. At least 10.3 million Americans carry a diagnosis of diabetes mellitus, and another 5.4 million are estimated to have undiagnosed diabetes.[2] The human toll of diabetes can be gauged not only by medical statistics, which show it to be the leading cause of end-stage renal disease and new cases of visual loss in persons under age 65 years and a major cause of macrovascular disease, but also by the quantity of health care resources consumed. Moreover, although the prevalence of type 1 diabetes is increasing slowly, the prevalence of type 2 diabetes is increasing explosively.[3]

More than 20% of participants in cardiac rehabilitation programs are likely to suffer from diabetes. In this chapter, the major types of diabetes, complications of diabetes, and medical management of patients with diabetes are briefly reviewed together with exercise guidelines.

GUIDELINES, 4TH EDITION

- Chapter 9, pages 165-167

Classification, Diagnosis, and Screening

In 1997, the American Diabetes Association (ADA) revised its classification and diagnostic criteria.[1] The revised classification includes four major clinical classes of diabetes:

- Type 1 diabetes
- Type 2 diabetes
- Other specific types of diabetes mellitus
- Gestational diabetes mellitus

For the clinician and patient, it is less important to label the particular type of diabetes than it is to understand the pathogenesis of the hyperglycemia and to manage it effectively.[1]

The vast majority of cases of diabetes fall into two broad etiopathogenetic categories, namely, type 1 diabetes and type 2 diabetes. Type 1 diabetes, previously known as insulin-dependent diabetes or juvenile-onset diabetes, typically results from a cellular-mediated autoimmune destruction of the β-cells of the pancreas. In this form of diabetes, the rate of β-cell destruction is quite variable, being rapid in some individuals (mainly children) and slow in others (mainly adults). Autoimmune destruction of β-cells has multiple genetic predispositions and is also related to environmental factors that are poorly understood. In type 1 diabetes, hyperglycemia results from an absolute deficiency of insulin secretion.[1] People with type 1 diabetes usually present with acute symptoms of diabetes and marked hyperglycemia.

Type 2 diabetes, previously known as non-insulin-dependent diabetes or adult-onset diabetes, is a term used for individuals who have insulin resistance and usually have relative (rather than absolute) insulin deficiency. Type 2 diabetes is far more prevalent than type 1 diabetes. Type 2 diabetes is often associated with a strong genetic predisposition (more so than the autoimmune form of type 1 diabetes). The risk of developing type 2 diabetes increases with age, obesity, and lack of physical activity. This form of diabetes frequently goes undiagnosed for many years because the hyperglycemia develops gradually and, at earlier stages, is often not severe enough for the patient to notice any of the classic symptoms of diabetes. Unfortunately, this relatively

symptom-free undiagnosed period of diabetes is not benign—approximately 20% of newly diagnosed patients with type 2 diabetes already have evidence of chronic complications.[3]

Criteria for the diagnosis of diabetes in nonpregnant adults are shown in figure 11.1. Three ways to diagnose diabetes are available, and each must be confirmed on a subsequent day. Because of ease of use, acceptability to patients, and lower cost, fasting plasma glucose is the preferred test.[1] Hyperglycemia not sufficient to meet the diagnostic criteria for diabetes is categorized as impaired fasting glucose, impaired glucose tolerance, or prediabetes.

Many reasons preclude the recommendation to test individuals routinely for the presence of any of the immune markers for type 1 diabetes.[4] Criteria for screening for type 2 diabetes in asymptomatic adults are outlined in figure 11.2.

Symptoms of marked hyperglycemia include polyuria, polydipsia, weight loss (sometimes with polyphagia), and blurred vision. Susceptibility to certain infections may also accompany chronic hyperglycemia.

Complications

Acute, potentially life-threatening consequences of untreated or poorly managed diabetes are hyperglycemia with ketoacidosis or the nonketotic hyperosmolar syndrome. Ketoacidosis seldom occurs spontaneously in persons with type 2 diabetes, but when present it usually arises in association with the stress of another illness such as acute infection. Hypoglycemia is most likely to occur in patients with diabetes who receive treatment with insulin and, to

---

1. Symptoms of diabetes plus casual plasma glucose concentration ≥ 200 mg·dl⁻¹. Casual is defined as any time of day without regard to time since last meal. The classic symptoms of diabetes include polyuria, polydipsia, and unexplained weight loss.

or

2. Fasting plasma glucose ≥ 126 mg/dl. Fasting is defined as no caloric intake for at least 8 hours.

or

3. Two-hour plasma glucose ≥ 200 mg·dl⁻¹ during an oral glucose tolerance test. The test should be performed as described by the World Health Organization with a glucose load containing the equivalent of 75 g anhydrous glucose dissolved in water.

In the absence of unequivocal hyperglycemia with acute metabolic decompensation, these criteria should be confirmed by repeat testing on a different day.

Figure 11.1   Criteria for the diagnosis of diabetes mellitus.
Adapted from American Diabetes Association 2002.

1. Testing for diabetes should be considered in all individuals aged ≥45 years and, if normal, it should be repeated at 3-year intervals.

2. Testing should be considered at a younger age or be carried out more frequently in individuals-who

   ■ are overweight (body mass index ≥25 kg·m^{-2}),

   ■ have a first-degree relative with diabetes,

   ■ are members of a high-risk ethnic population (e.g., African American, Hispanic American, Native American, Asian American, Pacific Islander),

   ■ have delivered a baby weighing >9 lb or have been diagnosed with gestational diabetes mellitus,

   ■ are hypertenisve (≥140/90 mm Hg),

   ■ have a high-density lipoprotein cholesterol level ≤35 mg·dl^{-1} or a triglyceride level ≥250 mg·dl^{-1}, and

   ■ on previous testing, had impaired glucose tolerance or impaired fasting glucose.

The oral glucose tolerance test or fasting plasma glucose test may be used to diagnose diabetes; however, in clinical settings the fasting plasma glucose test is greatly preferred because of ease of administration, convenience, acceptability to patients, and lower cost.

Figure 11.2   Criteria for testing for diabetes in asymptomatic, undiagnosed individuals.

Adapted, by permission, from American Diabetes Association, 2002, "Screening for diabetes," 2002, *Diabetes Care* 25(suppl 1): S21-S49.

a lesser degree, insulin secretagogues (i.e., sulfonyl-ureas or meglitinides).

Some of the major long-term complications of chronic diabetes include retinopathy with potential loss of vision; nephropathy leading to renal failure; peripheral neuropathy with risk of foot ulcers, amputation, and Charcot joints; and autonomic neuropathy causing gastrointestinal, genitourinary, and cardiovascular symptoms and sexual dysfunction. Glycation of tissue proteins and other macromolecules and excess production of polyol compounds from glucose are among the mechanisms thought to produce tissue damage from chronic hyperglycemia.[1,5]

Most important, a large body of epidemiological and pathological data document that both type 1 and type 2 diabetes are independent risk factors for atherosclerotic cardiovascular disease in both men and women. Women with diabetes seem to lose most of their inherent protection against the development of atherosclerosis. In patients with diabetes, myocardial ischemia caused by coronary atherosclerosis commonly occurs without symptoms. Consequently, multivessel atherosclerosis often is present before ischemic symptoms occur and before treatment is instituted. A delayed recognition of coronary heart disease (CHD) undoubtedly worsens the prognosis for survival for many patients with diabetes. The American Heart Association (AHA) has formally designated diabetes a major risk factor for cardiovascular disease.[6]

In addition to the previously mentioned acute and chronic complications of diabetes, the emotional and social impact of diabetes and the demands of therapy may cause significant psychosocial dysfunction in patients and their families.

Medical Management

A cardinal feature in preventing the complications of diabetes is early diagnosis and management. People with diabetes should receive medical care from a physician-coordinated team including (but not limited to) physicians, nurses, dietitians, exercise physiologists, and mental health professionals with expertise and special interest in diabetes. The treatment plan should recognize diabetes self-management education as an integral component of care. Although glycemic control is fundamental to the management of diabetes, diabetes care is complex and requires that many issues (beyond glycemic control) be addressed. In this respect, a large body of evidence exists that supports a range of interventions to improve diabetes outcomes. The standards recommended by the ADA are briefly summarized in the sidebar on p. 130.[5]

Standards of Medical Care for Patients With Diabetes

Glycemic control

- Recommended glycemic goals for nonpregnant individuals are shown in table 11.1.
- Perform hemoglobin A1c (HbA1c) testing at least two times a year in patients who meet treatment goals (and who have stable glycemic control) and quarterly in patients whose therapy has changed or who are not meeting glycemic goals.
- Develop or adjust the management plan (i.e., lifestyle interventions and insulin therapy or oral antidiabetic medications) to achieve normal or near-normal glycemia with an HbA1c test goal of 7% or less.
- Instruct the patient in self-monitoring of blood glucose and routinely evaluate the patient's technique and ability to use data to adjust therapy.

Medical nutrition therapy (MNT)

- People with diabetes should receive individualized MNT as needed to achieve treatment goals, preferably provided by a registered dietitian familiar with the components of MNT.[7]

Physical activity

- A program of regular physical activity, adapted to the presence of complications, is recommended for all patients with diabetes who are capable of participating.[8]

Blood pressure (BP) control

- A target BP goal of less than 130/80 mm Hg is recommended if it can be safely achieved.
- BP should be measured at every routine diabetes visit (including orthostatic measurement to assess for the presence of autonomic neuropathy).
- Patients with a systolic BP of 130 to 139 mmHg or a diastolic BP of 80 to 89 mmHg should be given lifestyle and behavioral therapy alone for a maximum of 3 months and then, if targets are not achieved, in addition, should be treated pharmacologically.
- Patients with hypertension (systolic BP ≥140 mmHg or diastolic BP ≥90 mmHg) should receive drug therapy in addition to lifestyle and behavioral therapy.
- In hypertensive patients with microalbuminuria or clinical albuminuria or nephropathy, an angiotensin-converting enzyme (ACE) inhibitor or angiotensin receptor blocker (ARB) should be strongly considered.

Lipid management

- Lower low-density lipoprotein cholesterol to less than 100 mg·dl^{-1} as the primary goal of therapy for adults.
- Lower triglycerides to less than 150 mg·dl^{-1} and raise HDL cholesterol to greater than 40 mg·dl^{-1} in men and greater than 50 mg·dl^{-1} in women.

Aspirin therapy

- Use aspirin therapy (75-325 mg·day^{-1}) in all adult patients with macrovascular disease.
- Consider beginning aspirin therapy for primary prevention in patients 40 years of age or older with diabetes and one or more cardiovascular risk factors.

Smoking cessation

- Include smoking cessation counseling and other forms of treatment as a routine component of diabetes care.

CHD screening and treatment

- Use a risk factor-based strategy for the diagnosis of CHD that might include exercise stress testing, stress echocardiography, or perfusion imaging.
- Refer patients with signs or symptoms of cardiovascular disease or with positive noninvasive tests for CHD to a cardiologist.

(continued)

(continued)

Nephropathy screening and management

- Perform an annual test for the presence of microalbuminuria in type 1 diabetic patients who have had diabetes more than 5 years and all type 2 diabetic patients starting at diagnosis.

- In the treatment of albuminuria and nephropathy, both ACE inhibitors and ARBs can be used.

- With the onset of overt nephropathy, initiate protein restriction to 0.8 g·kg body weight^{-1}·day^{-1} or less (approximately 10% of daily calories); further restriction may be useful in selected patients.

Foot care

- Perform a comprehensive foot examination annually on patients with diabetes to identify risk factors predictive of ulcers and amputations. Perform a visual inspection of patients' feet at each routine visit.

- Educate all patients, especially those with risk factors or prior lower-extremity complications, about the risk and prevention of foot problems, and reinforce self-care behavior.

- Use a multidisciplinary approach for persons with foot ulcers and high-risk feet, especially those with a history of prior ulcer or amputation.

- Refer patents with claudication for further vascular assessment, and consider exercise training and surgical options.

Diabetic retinopathy screening and treatment

- Patients with type 1 diabetes should have an initial dilated and comprehensive eye examination by an ophthalmologist or optometrist within 3 to 5 years after the onset of diabetes.

- Patients with type 2 diabetes should have an initial dilated and comprehensive eye examination by an ophthalmologist or optometrist shortly after the diagnosis of diabetes is made.

- Subsequent examinations for type 1 and type 2 diabetic patients should be repeated annually.

Immunization

- Provide an annual influenza vaccine to all adult diabetic patients.

- Provide at least one lifetime pneumococcal vaccine for adults with diabetes. A one-time revaccination is recommended for individuals older than 64 years previously immunized when they were less than 65 years of age if the vaccine was administered more than 5 years ago.

Table 11.1 Glycemic Control for People With Diabetes

Biochemical index	Nondiabetic	Goal	Additional action suggested
Preprandial plasma glucose (mg·dl^{-1})	<100	90-130	<90 >150
Bedtime plasma glucose (mg·dl^{-1})	<120	110-150	<110 >180
HbA1c (%)	<6	<7	>8

Note. HbA1c = hemoglobin A1c. Values are by necessity generalized to the entire population of individuals with diabetes. Patients with comorbid diseases, the very young and older adults, and others with unusual conditions or circumstances may warrant different treatment goals. These values are for nonpregnant adults. "Additional action suggested" depends on individual patient circumstances. Such actions may include enhanced diabetes self-management education, comanagement with a diabetes team, referral to an endocrinologist, change in pharmacological therapy, initiation of or increase in self-monitored blood glucose (SMBG), or more frequent contact with the patient. HbA1c is referenced to a nondiabetic range of 4.0-6.0% (mean 5.0%, *SD* 0.5%).

From American Diabetes Association, 2002, *Therapy for diabetes mellitus and related disorders,* edited by H.E. Lebovitz (Alexandria, VA: American Diabetes Association).

Exercise Prescription

Recent advances in basic and clinical exercise physiology have facilitated a more precise approach to exercise prescription for healthy people and those with diabetes mellitus. However, the existing body of scientific information is not so extensive as to warrant its application in a highly rigid fashion. Although the principles for exercise prescription for people with diabetes that are outlined in this chapter are based on a solid foundation of scientific knowledge, they should not be construed as being theorems or laws. Rather, the recommended procedures should be viewed as guidelines that may be applied to a given person in a flexible manner.[9] See chapter 7 for more information on exercise prescription.

To optimize the likelihood of a safe and effective response, the exercise prescription for people with

---

Screening

- Search for vascular and neurological complications, including silent ischemia.
- Exercise electrocardiogram (ECG) is recommended for patients with one or more of the following: (a) known or suspected coronary artery disease, (b) type 1 diabetes of >15 years duration or type 2 diabetes of >10 years duration, (c) age >35 years, (d) any additional risk factor for coronary artery disease, (e) microvascular disease (proliferative retinopathy or nephropathy, including microalbuminuria), (f) peripheral vascular disease, or (g) autonomic neuropathy. In the absence of an exercise ECG, light to moderate rather than vigorous exercise should be prescribed for these patients.

Exercise program

- Type: Aerobic
- Frequency: 3-5 times per week
- Duration: 20-60 min of continuous or intermittent (minimum of 10-min bouts) exercise
- Intensity: 55-79% of maximum heart rate or 40-74% of $\dot{V}O_2$ reserve or heart rate reserve
- Energy expenditure: Modulate type, frequency, duration, and intensity to attain an energy expenditure of 700-2,000 kcal·week^{-1}
- Timing: Time participation so that it does not coincide with peak insulin absorption

Avoid complications

- Have the patient perform warm-up and cool-down
- Carefully select exercise type and intensity
- Educate the patient
- Choose proper footwear
- Avoid exercise in extreme heat or cold
- Inspect feet daily and after exercise
- Avoid exercise when metabolic control is poor
- Maintain adequate hydration
- Monitor blood glucose if the patient is taking insulin or insulin secretagogues, and follow guidelines to prevent hypoglycemia

Compliance

- Make exercise enjoyable
- Choose a convenient location
- Provide positive feedback from involved medical personnel and family

Figure 11.3 Summary of exercise recommendations for patients with diabetes.

diabetes should consider safety aspects as well as the mode, frequency, duration, intensity, rate of progression, and timing of physical activity. These fundamental components are interrelated and partly dependent on the purposes for which exercise is prescribed in a given person. The purposes will vary depending on the individual's interests, needs, background, and health status. For people with diabetes, the major potential benefits of a physically active lifestyle include increased physical fitness, improved glycemic control, reduced risk for cardiovascular disease, decreased adiposity, and enhanced psychological well-being.[8,10] The various components of the exercise prescription should be developed with these purposes in mind. However, the purposes need not carry equal or consistent weight in all people with diabetes. In some instances, for example, in an overweight person with type 2 diabetes, decreased adiposity and improved insulin sensitivity may be the central concerns. In other instances, for example, in a young person with type 1 diabetes, enhancement of physical fitness and psychological well-being may be the primary goals. Thus, the exercise prescription should focus on achieving the potential health-related benefits of exercise while at the same time reflecting the specific outcomes that are sought by a particular person with diabetes.

Exercise is a normal human function that can be undertaken with a high level of safety by most people, including those with diabetes. However, exercise is not without risks, and the recommendation that people with diabetes participate in an exercise program is based on the premise that the benefits outweigh these risks. Therefore, the foremost priority when developing the exercise prescription is to minimize the potential adverse effects of exercise via appropriate screening, program design, monitoring, and patient education (figure 11.3).

As is the case for the general population, the major potential health hazards of exercise for people with diabetes include musculoskeletal injury and sudden cardiac death. Other potential adverse effects that apply specifically to people with diabetes are listed in figure 11.4. Health professionals who counsel patients with diabetes on exercise should be familiar with these adverse effects and how to prevent them.

Depending on the severity of diabetes complications and other coexisting medical conditions, certain patients may need to participate in a medically supervised exercise program. However, before starting an

---

Cardiovascular

- Cardiac dysfunction and arrhythmias attributable to ischemic heart disease (often silent)
- Excessive increments in blood pressure during exercise
- Postexercise orthostatic hypotension

Microvascular

- Retinal hemorrhage
- Increased proteinuria
- Acceleration of microvascular lesions

Metabolic

- Worsening of hyperglycemia and ketosis
- Hypoglycemia in patients on insulin or insulin secretagogues

Musculoskeletal and traumatic

- Foot ulcers (especially in presence of neuropathy)
- Orthopedic injury related to neuropathy
- Accelerated degenerative joint disease
- Eye injuries and retinal hemorrhage

Figure 11.4 Potential adverse effects of exercise in patients with diabetes.

exercise program, all people with diabetes should undergo a complete medical history, usually the most important part of the pre-exercise evaluation, and physical examination. The physical examination should focus on the identification of macrovascular, microvascular, and neurological complications as well as other medical conditions that contraindicate exercise or require special consideration.[8] Untreated high-risk proliferative retinopathy, recent significant retinal hemorrhage, and acute or inadequately controlled renal failure are absolute contraindications to exercise. Relative contraindications to exercise include blood glucose greater than 300 mg·dl^{-1} or greater than 270 mg·dl^{-1} with urinary ketones and severe autonomic neuropathy with exertional hypotension.[11]

Because diabetes is potentially a progressive chronic disease, a continuing-care plan with follow-up medical evaluations is also necessary. Follow-up evaluations may be integrated into the patient's regular office visits, which should be scheduled at least quarterly until achievement of treatment goals and at least semiannually thereafter. The precise frequency and nature of follow-up physician visits, of course, will also depend on other factors, such as changes in the treatment regimen and the presence of complications or other medical conditions.[5]

From a pre-exercise evaluation perspective, the most serious complication of exercise participation is sudden cardiac death. Although habitual physical activity is associated with an overall reduction in the risk of sudden cardiac death in the general adult population, and the chances of sustaining a fatal cardiac event during exercise training are extremely small, it is well established that exercise can precipitate sudden cardiac death.[12-14] Moreover, several studies have now shown that in adults, the transiently increased risk of cardiac arrest that occurs during exercise results primarily from the presence of preexisting CHD.[15,16] In view of this, and because diabetes increases the risk for CHD by about threefold in men and possibly even more in women and is associated with a high prevalence of silent ischemia, certain individuals with diabetes should perform a graded exercise test with ECG monitoring as part of a medical evaluation before beginning an exercise program (see figure 11.3). Graded exercise testing in these individuals generally should be conducted in accordance with traditional guidelines that have been outlined in detail elsewhere.[9]

It may not be possible, for a variety of reasons, for many individuals with diabetes to perform an exercise test before beginning an exercise program. In patients for whom an exercise electrocardiogram (ECG) is recommended but not performed, light to moderate rather than vigorous exercise should be prescribed.

Specific safety precautions for people with diabetes who participate in exercise have been addressed in detail elsewhere.[17,18] Table 11.2 provides a brief overview of risks, recommendations, and special precautions that are associated with three of the more common and challenging chronic complications of diabetes: retinopathy, nephropathy, and neuropathy.[19]

Individuals with type 2 diabetes not treated with insulin or insulin secretagogues can generally exercise with no more concern for exercise-induced hypoglycemia than individuals without diabetes. In contrast, persons with type 1 or type 2 diabetes who take insulin should take a number of precautions to minimize their risk for exercise-induced hypoglycemia. Some general guidelines for the prevention of exercise-induced hypoglycemia in persons treated with insulin are provided in figure 11.5. However, as can be seen in figure 11.6, the precise hormonal and metabolic response to an acute bout of exercise is influenced by many factors. It is impossible, therefore, to give precise guidelines for insulin and diet therapy that will be suitable for all persons with diabetes who take insulin.[20] Although data on incidence rates are not available, exercise-induced hypoglycemia has been reported in sulfonylurea-treated patients. Reports suggest that during and after long-duration exercise in persons with type 2 diabetes who take insulin secretagogues, the prevention of hypoglycemia may require a dose reduction of the medication in question or additional carbohydrate intake.[21] Because of their particular modes of action, biguanides and other classes of oral antidiabetic agents, such as α-glucosidase inhibitors or thiazolidinediones, are not expected to precipitate exercise-induced hypoglycemia.[21]

As is evidenced in figure 11.7, whereas persons who are overinsulinized are at heightened risk for exercise-induced hypoglycemia, those who are underinsulinized are at heightened risk for becoming hyperglycemic during exercise.[20] Following is a discussion of important issues related to the exercise prescription for persons with diabetes. For comprehensive information related to exercise prescription methodologies, refer to chapter 7.

Mode

A key goal of the exercise prescription for patients with diabetes is caloric energy expenditure.[9,22] To accomplish this, activities that use large muscle groups, that can be maintained for a prolonged period, and are rhythmic and aerobic in nature are preferred. Typical examples include walking, jogging, swimming, cycling, cross-country skiing, rowing, dancing, skating, rope skipping, stair climbing, and various endurance game activities. For a given level of energy expenditure, the health-related benefits of exercise appear to

Table 11.2 Exercising With Diabetic Complications: Risks, Recommendations, and Precautions

| | Retinopathy | Nephropathy | NEUROPATHY | |
			Autonomic	Peripheral
Risks	• Elevations in blood pressure • Possible retina detachment from jarring of head	• Marked changes in hemodynamics • Marked elevations in blood pressure • Presence of retinopathy likely	• Hypoglycemia • Abnormal blood pressure response • Abnormal heart rate response • Impaired sympathetic or parasympathetic nerves • Abnormal thermoregulation (prone to dehydration)	• Superficial pain • Impaired balance or reflexes • Numbness or weakness in hands • Decreased proprioception • Weakness or atrophy of thigh muscles (when severe)
Recommendations	• Use heart rate and RPE based on blood pressure response (which should not exceed 170 mm Hg systolic; >200 increases damage to retina). • Use low-impact activities. • Use submaximal exercise testing. • If possible, monitor blood pressure during exercise. • Consider stationary cycling, walking, swimming, and low-intensity rowing.	• Include dynamic, weight-bearing, low-impact activity. • Use submaximal isometric or light weightlifting when blood pressure is controlled and left ventricular function is normal. • Develop specific programs for hemodialysis patients.	• Use submaximal exercise testing. • Use RPE to gauge exercise intensity. • Include water activities, stationary cycling, or both.	• Use RPE to monitor exercise intensity. • Include non-weight-bearing activities. • Use activities to improve balance.
Precautions	• Avoid Valsalva maneuvers. • Avoid heavy weightlifting, breath holding stretches, high-intensity exercise, and strenuous upper-arm exercise. • Avoid exercise if recent photocoagulation treatment or surgery has occurred.	• Avoid lifting heavy weights, intense aerobic activities, and Valsalva maneuvers. • Use cushioned shoes (gel or air). • Maintain hydration.	• Avoid high-intensity activity. • Avoid rapid changes in body position. • Avoid extremes of temperature.	• Examine feet frequently. • Use proper footwear. • Perform gentle, pain-free stretching.

Note. RPE = rating of perceived exertion.

Before exercise

1. Estimate intensity, duration, and the energy expenditure of exercise.
2. Eat a meal 1-3 hr before exercise.
3. Administer insulin correctly.
   a. Administer insulin >1 hr before exercise.
   b. Decrease the dose of insulin that has peak activity coinciding with the exercise period.
4. Assess metabolic control.
   a. If blood glucose is <5 mmol·L^{-1} (90 mg·dl^{-1}), extra calories before exercise will likely be required.
   b. If blood glucose is 5-15 mmol·L^{-1} (90-270 mg·dl^{-1}), extra calories may not be required.
   c. If blood glucose is >15 mmol·L^{-1} (270 mg·dl^{-1}), delay exercise and measure urine ketones. If urine ketones are negative, exercise can be performed, and extra calories are not required. If urine ketones are positive, take insulin and delay exercise until ketones are negative.
5. Do not use an exercising extremity as an injection site.

During exercise

1. Monitor blood glucose during long sessions.
2. Always adequately replace fluid losses.
3. If required, use supplemental carbohydrate feedings (30-40 g for adults, 15-25 g for children) every 30 min during extended periods of exercise.

After exercise

1. Monitor blood glucose, including overnight, if amount of exercise is not habitual.
2. Adjust insulin therapy to decrease immediate and delayed insulin action (intensive therapy regimes provide increased flexibility in adjusting insulin).
3. If required, increase calorie intake for 12-24 hr after activity, depending on the intensity and duration of exercise and risk of hypoglycemia.

Figure 11.5 Prevention of hypoglycemia or hyperglycemia during exercise in patients with diabetes on insulin.

Adapted from M. Berger, 2002, Adjustment of insulin and oral agent therapy. In *American Diabetes Association: Handbook of exercise in diabetes,* edited by N. Rudeman et al. (Alexandria, VA: American Diabetes Association), 365-376.

General population (including individuals with diabetes)

- Exercise intensity, duration, and type
- Fitness level
- Nutritional state
- Temporal relationship to meal
- Calories and content of meal
- Environmental factors

Factors specific to individuals with diabetes

- Temporal relationship to insulin or oral hypoglycemic agents
- If insulin is used, temporal relationship to last treatment, type of insulin, site of administration, or mode of delivery
- Metabolic control
- Presence of complications

Figure 11.6 Factors that influence the hormonal and metabolic response to acute exercise.

Reprinted, by permission, from D.H. Wasserman et al., 2002, Fuel metabolism during exercise in health and disease. In *American Diabetes Association: Handbook of exercise in diabetes,* eidted by N. Rudeman et al. (Alexandria, VA: American Diabetes Association), 66-99.

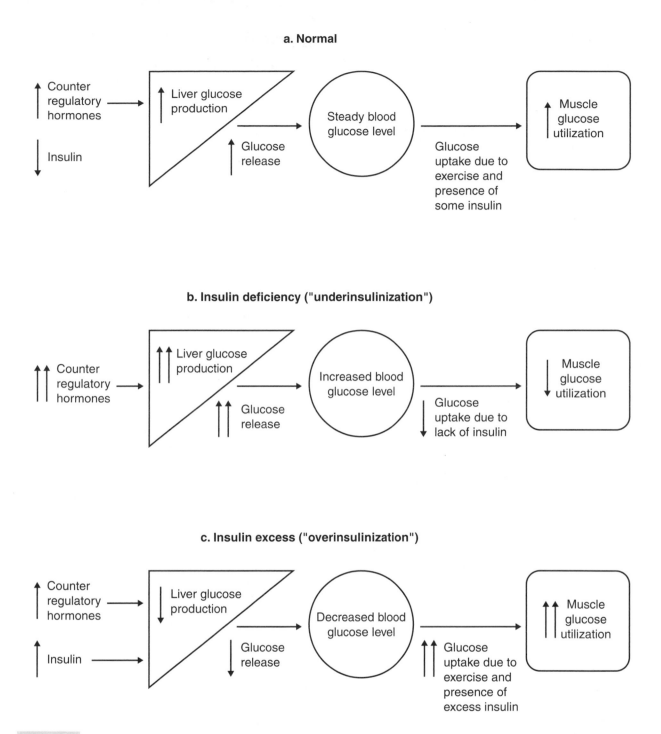

a. Normal

b. Insulin deficiency ("underinsulinization")

c. Insulin excess ("overinsulinization")

Figure 11.7   *(a)* Normal insulin level. How *(b)* insulin deficiency ("underinsulinization") and *(c)* insulin excess ("overinsulinization") affect blood glucose levels during an acute bout of exercise.

be independent of the mode of aerobic activity. Therefore, provided no contraindications exist, the types of aerobic exercise a patient performs are a matter of personal preference.

Aerobic activities that require running and jumping are considered high-impact types of exercise. Such activities are more likely to traumatize the feet in patients with peripheral neuropathy and precipitate vitreous hemorrhage or traction retinal detachment in patients with active diabetic retinopathy.[8,10] Thus, these factors must be considered when the exercise modality is prescribed for people with diabetes.

When precise control of exercise intensity is needed, as in the early stages of an exercise program for patients with diabetes complications, preferred activities are those that can be readily maintained at a constant intensity and for which interindividual variability in energy expenditure is relatively low.[9] Such activities include walking and stationary cycling.

Recent studies suggest that appropriately designed resistance training programs may be safe and effective for patients with diabetes, provided they do not have contraindications to such exercise.[23-25] Although additional research is needed, existing data suggest that strenuous resistance exercise is often associated with hyperglycemia during and shortly after acute training sessions.[25] These observations are consistent with findings of hyperglycemic responses to intense aerobic exercise in persons with diabetes. Acute increases in blood glucose with resistance exercise are frequently followed by hypoglycemia in patients on insulin, which may occur several hours postexercise. Patients on insulin or insulin secretagogues who participate in resistance training should be advised to monitor their blood glucose before, during, and after resistance exercise and should be instructed to take appropriate action in response to undesirable glycemic effects.[25]

Frequency

Available evidence suggests that the duration of glycemic improvement after the last bout of exercise in patients with diabetes is greater than 12 but less than 72 hr.[26] In view of this, it is recommended that aerobic exercise be performed on at least 3 nonconsecutive days each week and ideally on 5 days·week^{-1}. Patients on insulin who experience difficulty in balancing their daily insulin and caloric needs may find it preferable to exercise daily. Similarly, obese patients who also have diabetes may need to exercise more frequently (i.e., 6-7 days·week^{-1}) to optimize caloric expenditure and weight loss.

Multiple shorter bouts of exercise spread throughout the day may produce improvements in exercise capacity similar to a single longer session.[27] Although more comprehensive scientific inquiry is needed, multiple short bouts of exercise closely resemble the physical activity that typically has been measured in epidemiological studies.[28] In these studies, the accumulation of energy expenditure has been found to be inversely related to the risk for CHD and the development of type 2 diabetes. Therefore, although additional confirmatory data are needed, it is thought that if the total daily energy expenditure is the same, comparable health benefits should accrue with multiple versus single bouts of exercise. For multiple bouts of exercise, a minimum of 10 min per bout is recommended by the ACSM.[29]

Intensity

Prescribing the appropriate exercise intensity is the most difficult aspect of designing exercise programs. Programs emphasizing low- to moderate-intensity exercise may be preferable for most people with diabetes. If the complications of diabetes permit, exercise generally should be prescribed at an intensity corresponding to 55% to 79% of maximum heart rate (HRmax), 40% to 74% of oxygen consumption reserve ($\dot{V}O_2R$) or heart rate reserve (HRR), or a rating of perceived exertion (RPE) of 12 to 15 (intensities between 55% and 65% of HRmax, between 40% and 50% of VO_2R or HRR, or eliciting an RPE of 12 are most appropriate for individuals who are quite unfit). For patients for whom an exercise ECG is recommended but not performed, it may be prudent not to exceed an exercise intensity corresponding to 69% of HRmax, 59% of VO_2R or HRR, or an RPE of 13.[11] Generally for people with diabetes complications, both heart rate and RPE should be monitored. Although the use of heart rate as an estimate of intensity of exercise is the recommended approach, for those without diabetes complications or coexisting medical conditions that may be worsened by exercise, RPE may be used on its own.

If exercise training intensity is going to be prescribed using heart rate, ideally target heart rates should be prescribed using the individual's HRmax determined during graded exercise testing. This is particularly important for patients with cardiovascular complications or autonomic neuropathy or those receiving medications, such as β-blockers, that may alter the heart rate response to exercise.

Duration

Beyond the general guidelines for exercise duration, there are no special considerations for persons with diabetes. The appropriate duration of each exercise session is inversely related to the intensity at which the exercise is performed. Longer exercise sessions may result in a higher incidence of musculoskeletal injury and difficulty with compliance.

Timing

Ideally, exercise training should be performed at the time of day that is most convenient for the participant. However, because exercise can potentiate the effects of insulin, hypoglycemia during or after exercise is a definite risk for individuals receiving treatment with insulin and, to a lesser degree, insulin secretagogues.

Therefore, patients using insulin should time participation so that it does not coincide with periods of peak insulin absorption and should decrease the dose of insulin that has peak activity coinciding with the exercise period. Initially, to enhance blood glucose control, it may be preferable for patients on insulin to exercise at a similar time each day. However, this is not absolutely necessary, especially once the patient gains adequate experience with hypoglycemia prevention.

12

Chronic Heart Failure

Terence Kavanagh, MD

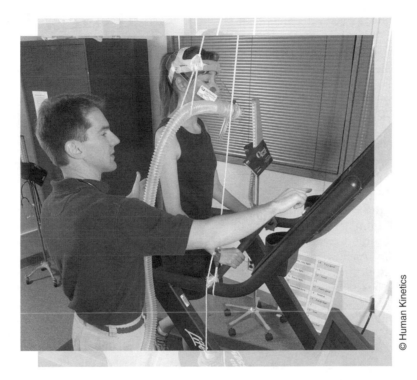

© Human Kinetics

The prevalence and incidence of chronic heart failure (CHF) have increased dramatically over the past 4 decades, the product of an aging population and an improved survival rate for patients with severe ischemic heart disease. In North America, it is estimated that some 5 million patients suffer from CHF, with 550,000 new cases diagnosed every year. Annually, CHF is the primary cause of death in 52,828 individuals.[1] It is estimated that 15 million individuals worldwide suffer from this condition.[2]

Chronic heart failure is a complex clinical syndrome, initiated by the inability of the heart to pump blood at a rate commensurate with the requirements of the metabolizing tissues. In an attempt to reverse the effect of declining cardiac output, circulating levels of renin, arginine, vasopressin, catecholamines, and atrial natriuretics are elevated, systems that are designed to increase sodium and water retention and vasoconstrictor drive. In the short term, these compensating mechanisms are effective, but they ultimately become counterproductive. Vasoconstriction increases total peripheral resistance and thus afterload, adding further to the burden on the failing heart. In short, failure begets failure.

Heart failure is most commonly caused by systolic dysfunction arising from impaired myocardial contractility, for example, secondary to extensive myocardial ischemia. Left ventricular ejection fraction is reduced, generally to less than 40%. The diagnosis carries both a bleak prognosis and the prospect of a rapidly deteriorating quality of life, with easy fatigue, excessive breathlessness, muscle wasting, weakness, and poor exercise tolerance.

Whereas systolic failure is attributable to the inability of the heart to adequately eject blood, diastolic failure results from problems arising from the heart's inability to fill properly. Abnormalities such as slow left ventricular relaxation or filling, reduced left ventricular diastolic distensibility, and increased left ventricular chamber stiffness result in elevated diastolic filling pressures, which are transmitted to the pulmonary and systemic venous circulations. Systolic and diastolic dysfunctions frequently coexist, and a clinical diagnosis of pure diastolic failure requires that the clinical features of CHF be present, but with a normal or only mildly abnormal ejection fraction and a normal left ventricular end-diastolic volume. During exercise, the resultant increase in left ventricular pressure fails to increase end-diastolic volume, stroke volume cannot increase by way of the Frank–Starling mechanism, and exercise capacity is severely limited. Diastolic failure is often associated with left ventricular hypertrophy and is preceded by elevation of systolic blood pressure. Myocardial ischemia is another frequent accompaniment. Less common causes are hypertrophic cardiomyopathy, constrictive pericardial disease, and valvular heart disease. Many elderly patients (≥70 years) with CHF, as many as 50% in some series, have diastolic dysfunction.[3,4] In this population, limitation of exercise capacity by exertional dyspnea rather than muscle fatigue may be an early feature of diastolic failure.

GUIDELINES, 4TH EDITION

- Chapter 9, pages 151-157

The mainstays of CHF treatment have been enforced rest, a salt-free diet, and digoxin; subsequent additions to the drug armamentarium are vasodilators, inotropes, angiotensin-converting enzyme inhibitors, and β-blockers. However, in recent years there has been increasing evidence that encouraging rest and restricting physical activity can be counterproductive and that a medically prescribed exercise training regimen helps to alleviate symptoms, improve exercise tolerance, and enhance quality of life.[5]

The previous reluctance of physicians to prescribe exercise for heart failure patients is understandable, because an acute bout of exercise not only can increase wall stress but also can trigger an abrupt increase in the secretion of neurohormones and thus have a negative effect on myocardial remodeling. This concern was fuelled by an early publication from Jugdutt and coworkers,[6] who concluded that prescribing exercise to patients who had reduced ventricular function following a large anterior infarct could lead to wall thinning, infarct expansion, further asynergy, and a reduction in ejection fraction. Subsequently, however, two well-designed randomized clinical trials by Giannuzzi and coworkers[7] failed to substantiate these findings. The first, the Exercise in Anterior Myocardial Infarction (EAMI) study[7] demonstrated that beneficial training effects could be obtained without adversely affecting remodelling, whereas the second, the Exercise in Left Ventricular Dysfunction (ELVD) study,[8] showed that a structured exercise rehabilitation program could actually attenuate the remodeling process. Analysis of the data from these and other studies confirmed that the finding applied to patients with ischemic and nonischemic cardiomyopathy and with both moderate and severe left ventricular dysfunction.[9,10] Furthermore, in those cases where training has been shown to improve peak cardiac output, this has been

achieved without deleterious effects on central hemodynamic pressures at rest or during exercise.[11] Thus, the weight of evidence strongly favors the view that exercise training is safe and effective in patients with stable chronic heart failure. This being said, we need to consider the benefits of training, the mechanisms by which they are achieved, training protocols, and the selection of suitable patients.

Exercise Benefits

A number of studies have established that a medically prescribed and supervised exercise program can improve exercise capacity and relieve the symptoms of dyspnea and fatigue in patients with stable CHF. Many, if not all, of these benefits appear to be attributed to peripheral training responses.

In the late 1980s, Sullivan and coworkers[12,13] from Duke University published the first reports of their experience with training patients who had a documented diagnosis of chronic heart failure. These authors were able to show a significant improvement in exercise tolerance, as evidenced by an increase in exercise duration and peak oxygen intake ($\dot{V}O_2$peak). Shortness of breath was relieved and was demonstrated by a reduction in minute ventilation at submaximal work rates, an increase in the anaerobic threshold, and a reduction in submaximal lactate levels. There was also an increase in leg blood flow. The first randomized crossover trial of exercise training in CHF was carried out by Coats and the Oxford group.[14] Patients performed 8 weeks of home-based cycle ergometry exercise, followed by 8 weeks of no exercise. Following the 8 weeks of exercise training, there was a significant improvement in exercise duration and $\dot{V}O_2$peak as well as alleviation of the symptoms of breathlessness and fatigue.[14]

Because the primary cause for the syndrome of chronic heart failure is an impairment of the heart's pumping capacity, it seems reasonable to assume that (a) the symptoms of fatigue and breathlessness are central in origin, and (b) any therapy, including exercise, that relieves symptoms, acts by improving ventricular function. However, this does not appear to be the case. Increasing cardiac output by the use of inotropes fails to be matched by an increase in exercise capacity.[15] Similarly, heart transplantation recipients, despite normal systolic function, continue to show a reduced peak power output and oxygen intake on cycle ergometry for as long as 12 months after surgery.[16] Also, although left ventricular ejection fraction is frequently used as an index of myocardial systolic function, it has been shown to have a poor correlation with exercise capacity.[17] Finally, training-induced significant improvement in $\dot{V}O_2$peak has been shown not to be accompanied by changes in resting or exercise stroke volume, cardiac output, or left ventricular ejection fraction.[14] Thus, although two separate studies have shown some improvement in myocardial perfusion[18] and diastolic filling rate[19] in response to 8 weeks of moderate training, it appears that most of the reasons for training-induced symptom relief must be sought elsewhere.

Subsequently, a series of trials confirmed these results. They also described beneficial changes in autonomic control, skeletal muscle metabolism, and endothelial function and, more recently, improvement in myocardial perfusion, improvement in diastolic function, reduced morbidity and mortality rates, less hospital readmissions, and an enhanced quality of life.

Amelioration of Decreased Skeletal Muscle Mass

Loss of muscle mass and endurance is a feature of chronic heart failure, and muscle biopsies show a decrease in slow-twitch type I fibers, an increase in fast-twitch type IIb fibers, and a decrease in the oxidative enzymes succinate dehydrogenase and citrate synthetase.[12] Studies using phosphorous-31 magnetic resonance spectroscopy (^{31}P-MRS) have demonstrated that CHF patients, unlike healthy normal people, show a progressive decrease in pH at all submaximal workloads and a more rapid depletion and slower resynthesis of phosphocreatine,[20] further indications of impaired oxidative metabolism.

There seems little doubt that these changes are at least partially caused by deconditioning, with other factors superimposed. For example, in cardiac cachexia, the most extreme form of muscle wasting that occurs in CHF, there are increased levels of norepinephrine, human growth hormone, insulin, and tumor necrosis factor (TNF)-α,[21-24] all of which may play a role in muscle wasting of lesser degree.

A number of exercise training studies have shown that these abnormalities can at least be partially reversed. Belardinelli and colleagues[25] reported on the effects of a low-intensity (below anaerobic threshold) exercise training program on a group of CHF patients and observed that although $\dot{V}O_2$peak increased and submaximal work lactate levels decreased, there was no change in resting or exercise hemodynamics, indicating that the origin of the changes are in the periphery. Muscle histology, however, revealed an increase in fiber size and mitochondrial volume density, with a high correlation between changes in the latter and changes in $\dot{V}O_2$peak and anaerobic threshold.[25]

Stratton and coworkers,[26] using ^{31}P-MRS and one-limb forearm training, were able to show an increase in exercise duration accompanied by higher muscle pH at submaximal workloads and a reduced depletion as well as a more rapid resynthesis of phosphocreatine (i.e., an enhanced muscle enzyme activity). Similar results were obtained by Hambrecht and colleagues[27] using cycle ergometer aerobic training. Thus, there is a convincing body of evidence to support the hypothesis that some of the symptomatology encountered in CHF originates in skeletal muscle and that this can be partially corrected by exercise training.

Improved Pulmonary Function

Early investigators attempted to attribute the severe dyspnea seen during exercise in CHF patients to changes in the lung. Arguably, this is the case in *acute* heart failure, where poor systolic function is associated with elevated left atrial pressure, pulmonary venous pressure, and ultimately pulmonary edema. In this situation, dyspnea can be explained on the basis of the pulmonary changes and correlates with increases in pulmonary wedge pressure. In the case of nonedematous chronic heart failure, however, the evidence fails to support this interpretation. Pulmonary wedge pressure correlates poorly with exercise tolerance,[28] and arterial blood gases are normal during a bout of exercise.[29] Furthermore, the same patient may be forced to stop by dyspnea while undergoing a rapid incremental exercise test but by fatigue when the test is more prolonged.[30] This indicates that both symptoms are interrelated and that the stimulus for the dyspnea lies elsewhere than in the lungs. Weakness and easy fatigability of respiratory muscle have been observed in CHF patients,[31] and specific respiratory muscle training has been reported to improve exercise tolerance and breathlessness as measured by the Borg and Guyatt dyspnea scales and the Transitional Dyspnea Index.[32] Furthermore, a study by Beniaminovitz and colleagues[33] demonstrated a marked improvement in exercise performance and alleviation of dyspnea following 3 months of low-level cycle ergometry and treadmill exercise.

The precise mechanism by which muscle activity triggers dyspnea remains unclear. One possibility is increased lactate production at low level of exercise. Reducing lactate production in CHF patients by infusing dichloroacetate, however, fails to increase exercise capacity.[34] A more likely possibility can be found in the work of Piepoli and colleagues.[35] They described small work-sensitive receptors (ergoreceptors) within skeletal muscle. Activation of these receptors by exercise metabolites stimulates unmyelinated and small myelinated affront nerves, which travel up the lateral spinothalamic tract to the brain stem. Piepoli and colleagues[36] were able to demonstrate that the ergoreflex controls ventilation, is hyperactive in CHF patients, and can be down-regulated by a 5-week period of forearm training.

Improved Hormonal System Regulation

The failing heart triggers a series of compensatory mechanisms that are designed to maintain an adequate circulation but are ultimately self-defeating. Prominent among these is a marked activation of various neurohumoral mechanisms, including diminished sensitivity of arterial and cardiac baroreceptors[37] as well as activation of the renin–angiotensin system with increased norepinephrine secretion and adrenergic receptor responsiveness.[38] These changes reduce arterial compliance, increase vascular resistance, and decrease peripheral blood flow. Elevated norepinephrine levels have also been shown to be an adverse prognostic indicator for survival.[39] Studies carried out in the 1970s demonstrated that training could reduce both resting and exercise norepinephrine levels in both healthy adults and individuals recovering from a myocardial infarction.[40,41] Later, a group from Oxford described a training-induced reduction in norepinephrine in CHF patients.[42] Using power spectral analysis, they also reported an increase in heart rate variability, indicating a reduction in sympathetic and an increase in vagal (parasympathetic) tone. A study by Shemesh and coworkers[43] supported these findings, reporting decreases in norepinephrine and atrial natriuretic peptide levels both at rest and during exercise in CHF patients exposed to exercise rehabilitation. Braith and colleagues,[44] in a randomized controlled trial, demonstrated significant reductions in angiotensin II, aldosterone, arginine vasopressin, and atrial natriuretic peptide following 16 weeks of exercise training.

More recently, Larsen and colleagues[45] entered a group of 28 CHF patients into a 12-week aerobic training program consisting of 30 min of calisthenics, walking, and jogging at an approximate intensity of 80% of maximal capacity at least three times weekly. Initial and final assessments included a cardiopulmonary exercise test on the cycle ergometer, a 6-min walk test, and blood sampling for plasma levels of the cytokines TNF-α, interleukin-8, and interleukin-6. There was a 45% increase in peak power output on the cycle ergometer, an 8% improvement in the 6-min walk, and a significant decrease in TNF-α levels—from 28.7 ± 19.0 to 25.1 ± 14.4 pg·ml^{-1} (p = .013). At 4-year follow-up, it was found that those patients who had the greatest reduction in TNF-α had the greatest survival rate. Furthermore, among survivors, there was a significant correlation between increase in $\dot{V}O_2$peak and reduction in TNF-α (r = –.643, p = .013).

Improved Endothelial Function

Chronic heart failure is associated with poor delivery of blood to the periphery during exercise, the result of reduced flow and impaired arteriolar vasodilation. There is a decline in the production of nitric oxide, attributable in part to a degradation of nitric oxide by superoxide anion and in part to a decrease in endothelial shear stress associated with prolonged inactivity.

There is increasing evidence that exercise training can correct endothelial function. Hornig and coworkers[46] exposed a group of patients to 4 weeks of hand-grip exercises and found that this restored flow-dependent vasodilatory capacity in the radial artery. Hambrecht and colleagues,[47] using cycle ergometry at an intensity of 70% $\dot{V}O_2$peak, demonstrated improved nitric oxide formation in the femoral artery. Subsequently, Linke and colleagues[48] corrected endothelial dysfunction in the upper limbs using cycle ergometry training, clear evidence of a systemic effect of local chronic exercise. Finally, Hambrecht and colleagues[49] reported a cycle ergometer training–induced improvement in endothelium-dependent vasodilation in both epicardial coronary vessels and resistance vessels in patients with coronary artery disease.

Reduced Cardiovascular Mortality

To date 17 randomized controlled trials have assessed the effects of exercise training in CHF. In all, they involved only 775 subjects and none were designed to demonstrate whether the benefits of exercise included a reduction in mortality rate. Nevertheless, Belardinelli and colleagues[50] provided some encouraging evidence in that direction. Subjects were exercised on the cycle ergometer at 60% $\dot{V}O_2$peak for up to 1 year.[50] Both $\dot{V}O_2$peak and thallium activity score improved at 8 weeks (18% and 24%, respectively). Follow-up continued for approximately 3 years, during which time there were nine deaths (all cardiac) and five hospital readmissions for heart failure in the trained group compared with 20 and 14, respectively, in the controls (relative risk = 0.37, p = .01, and relative risk = 0.29, p = .02, respectively). The only independent predictor of events was ventilatory threshold at baseline and post-training thallium activity score. A recent collaborative meta-analysis studied the effect of exercise training on all-cause mortality in patients with CHF compared to patients not receiving exercise training. A total of 801 patients were include in this meta-analysis and results demonstrated a significant reduction in mortality in the exercise training group (p = .015).[138]

Exercise Testing

Cardiopulmonary exercise testing plays a major role in evaluating functional capacity in CHF patients. The addition of gas exchange analysis to the test allows for direct measurement of $\dot{V}O_2$peak and the ventilatory equivalent of the anaerobic threshold. Both values are reduced in asymptomatic and symptomatic CHF and are a measurement of the disease severity. Weber and Janicki[51] classified functional impairment in CHF into four categories, based on $\dot{V}O_2$peak and ventilatory equivalent of the anaerobic threshold, and these are shown to correlate with cardiac index (table 12.1). Measured $\dot{V}O_2$peak also plays a role in the prognosis and is an independent predictor of mortality over 5 years of follow-up.[52] More recently, the slope of minute ventilation versus the rate of carbon dioxide production ($\dot{V}_E/VCO_2$) has also been shown to be a powerful independent prognostic indicator.[53-55] Mancini and colleagues[56] also used the $\dot{V}O_2$peak value to determine the need for and timing of cardiac transplantation.

Before starting an exercise program, all CHF patients should undergo a full physical assessment including exercise testing. Patients should be stable and free from exercise-induced complex ventricular arrhythmias, severe ischemia, or exertional hypertension. The addition of respiratory gas exchange measurements allows for precise, reproducible measurements of $\dot{V}O_2$peak and thus an accurate determination of a safe and effective training intensity. Whether the test is carried out on a treadmill or cycle ergometer will depend on the preference of the individual laboratory. The cycle ergometer uses less muscle mass than the treadmill, and therefore the $\dot{V}O_2$peak attained is approximately 10% to 15% below the treadmill value. Older, frail patients generally feel more secure on the cycle, and gas collection, blood pressure measurements, and invasive hemodynamic data are easier to obtain. On the other hand, walking is a natural skill and part of normal activities of daily living, so the treadmill may appeal to many patients. Again the choice will be made on the basis of the exercise testing personnel's preference and experience. The exercise test protocol is generally incremental in type and should be tailored to the patient's physical capabilities. The initial work rate should be low and the increments small, but the aim should be to reach peak effort in 8 to 10 min.

Exercise Training

The use of exercise training in patients with stable heart failure has been recommended for about 10 years.[57] However, the recommended components of the exercise prescription have not been well defined. Various studies have used a variety of aerobic or resistance training protocols with no standard intensity, duration, or frequency. The length of training has ranged from several weeks to 1 year. In the absence of a standardized training protocol, the exercise prescription should be individualized and based on data from a recent exercise test, preferably including gas exchange data.

Mode

Most CHF training programs have used aerobic-type exercise, most commonly stationary cycling and walking (table 12.2). The former affords accurate reproducibility of prescribed power outputs, whereas walking is a natural everyday activity, adaptable to all ranges of disability.

Table 12.1   Functional Classification Based on Peak Exercise Oxygen Uptake and Anaerobic Threshold

Functional class	$\dot{V}O_2$peak (ml·kg^{-1}·min^{-1})	$\dot{V}O_2$ at anaerobic threshold (ml·kg^{-1}·min^{-1})
A	>20	>14
B	16-20	11-14
C	10-15	8-11
D	<10	<8

Table 12.2   Training Protocols in Reported Clinical Trials of Exercise in Chronic Heart Failure

Mode (in order of use)	Cycle ergometer, walking, stair machine, rowing machine, calisthenics, resistance exercises
Intensity	40-70% $\dot{V}O_2$peak 40-70% heart rate reserve 11-13 rating of perceived exertion (Borg scale 6-20)
Frequency	3-7 times per week (average 3-5)
Duration	8-52 weeks (average 12)

Interval training permits a greater training workload to be placed on the peripheral musculature without an accompanying increase in cardiovascular stress. A typical protocol calls for 30 s of work at 50% of exercise capacity, followed by a 60-s rest, repeated 10 times for a total of 15 min.[58] So-called short-term peak exercise capacity is determined using a steep ramp test on the cycle ergometer; after 3 min of warm-up, the power output is increased by 25 W every 10 s until voluntary fatigue or clinical indications to stop. Using 50% of this value, Meyer and colleagues[59] reported an approximate 20% increase in ventilatory threshold and peak oxygen intake after 3 weeks of training, a similar improvement seen in patients completing up to 24 weeks of steady-state training.

Intensity

Intensity is a critical component of the CHF exercise prescription and is generally expressed as a percentage of the $\dot{V}O_2$peak (or the heart rate at which this value occurs), which in most reported studies has been measured directly by a cardiopulmonary exercise test. Values in the range of 40% to 70% $\dot{V}O_2$peak have been reported to be safe and effective, with the lower end being a prudent choice for the initial stages of the exercise program or for the severely deconditioned patient. Intensities above 70% $\dot{V}O_2$peak have an adverse effect on left ventricular systolic function. Similarly, caution should be used when exercising CHF patients above the ventilatory derived anaerobic threshold; this can be associated with depressed systolic function and an abrupt increase in plasma norepinephrine.

In the absence of facilities to carry out cardiopulmonary exercise testing, peak heart rate may be a viable alternative, with 40% to 70% of heart rate reserve approximating the same training range of $\dot{V}O_2$peak. This also correlates with a perceived exertion of 11 to 13 on the Borg scale (6-20). Regardless of the method chosen to measure training intensity, the clinician must carefully monitor symptoms, blood pressure, heart rate, and rhythm in the initial stages of the exercise program, generally for 12 weeks, and the program may have to be modified or temporarily suspended in the face of adverse signs and symptoms (see the sidebar). After this it may be deemed safe to permit unsupervised exercise sessions. McKelvie and colleagues,[60] reporting on the Exercise Rehabilitation Trial (EXERT), in which patients received 3 months of supervised exercise training followed by 9 months of home-based exercise, found that the unsupervised exercise resulted in an additional 40% increment in $\dot{V}O_2$peak, although adherence to the training regimen decreased.

Duration and Frequency

As with intensity, duration and frequency are determined by the patient's clinical condition. Where the functional capacity is low, short workouts of 10 min repeated three or four times daily are appropriate. Sessions are gradually increased to 30 min as fitness improves, repeated three to five times weekly.

To date, only two studies have attempted to determine the program length at which optimal improvement occurs.[50,61] In the Toronto study, cardiorespiratory and quality of life measurements were made initially and then at 4, 8, 12, 16, 26, and 52 weeks of a 1-year walking program. Maximal improvement in peak power output, $\dot{V}O_2$peak, and $\dot{V}_E/VCO_2$ slope occurred at 16 weeks, resting heart rate at 26 weeks, and ventilatory equivalent of the anaerobic threshold at 52 weeks. Peak improvements in quality of life measures (Chronic Heart Failure Questionnaire) showed improvement over the first 4 weeks of training but continued to progress over at least 26 weeks of observation.[61] Belardinelli and colleagues,[50] in their randomized controlled trial examining the effects of a 12-month training program on functional capacity and quality of life, reported similar findings.

Indications to Stop or Modify Exercise Program in CHF Patients

- Excessive exercise-induced fatigue (>14 rating of perceived exertion on the Borg scale) or dyspnea (>40 breaths·min^{-1})
- Weight increase of 1 kg or more body weight within 24 hr
- Development of pulmonary rales or gallop rhythm
- Failure of systolic blood pressure to increase more than 10 mmHg with exercise
- Development of exercise-induced complex ectopy
- Pulse pressure less than 10 mm Hg
- Resting heart rate 100 beats·min^{-1} or more

Apart from one study that demonstrated an improvement in left ventricular diastolic filling after exercise rehabilitation in patients with dilated cardiomyopathy,[19] there is little evidence that training is of benefit in isolated diastolic failure. However, given that exercise exerts a favorable influence on myocardial ischemia and hypertension, the two most common accompaniments of diastolic failure, it seems a reasonable therapeutic option. Furthermore, there are grounds to believe that aerobic training can improve diastolic function in healthy older (≥60 years) subjects.[5] The program mode, intensity, frequency, and duration need not differ from those used in systolic failure patients.

Resistance Training

Increasing recognition of the importance of skeletal muscle abnormalities in the production of CHF symptoms has led to an interest in resistance training, and there is evidence that this can be both safe and effective when properly prescribed. McKelvie and colleagues,[62] using a rhythmic one-leg press exercise, with 10 repetitions at 70% of 1 repetition maximum, reported that the systolic blood pressure, ejection fraction, and diastolic and systolic volume responses were no greater than those found during stationary cycling exercise at an intensity of 70% of $\dot{V}O_2$peak. Others have demonstrated an enhanced contractile function of the left ventricle as shown by an increased cardiac index and left ventricular stroke index during rhythmic two-leg press exercise at loads of 60% and 80% of one maximum voluntary contraction.[63] An interval type protocol was used, with 60-s work phases of 12 repetitions each and 120-s rest phases. However, although rhythmic strength exercise seems very promising, more experience is needed and therefore advice regarding its use in CHF patients must be guarded.

Contraindications

Exercise training is advisable only in stable chronic heart failure and is contraindicated in aortic stenosis, obstructive cardiomyopathy, myocarditis, significant ischemia at low work rates (<2 metabolic equivalents), recent-onset atrial fibrillation, and probably in the case of a measured peak oxygen intake less than 8 ml·kg^{-1}·min^{-1}. Wilson and coworkers[64] delineated a subset of patients who failed to obtain benefit from training because their major limiting feature was a poor cardiac output response to exercise rather than poor peripheral function.

New York Heart Association class IV patients have rarely been included in training studies, although they comprise 20% of a group that Belardinelli and colleagues[50] reported as having lower mortality and morbidity rates following a 1-year moderate (60% $\dot{V}O_2$peak) aerobic training program.

Risks

Although there are no reports of adverse events directly associated with exercise training in CHF patients, published studies have been relatively few and the subjects highly selected. Therefore, it is advisable to initiate the training program in a supervised setting, where individual responses to physical activity can be observed and modified accordingly.

Once a safe and effective level of training has been established, most patients can be advanced to a combined supervised and nonsupervised program. Nevertheless, continued clinical vigilance is necessary to detect signs and symptoms that indicate the need to adjust or at least temporarily discontinue the program.

Summary

Substantial training benefits can be achieved in patients with stable chronic heart failure. However, the number of patients involved in randomized clinical exercise trials is still relatively small, and there is need for a large multiple-center trial, preferably international in scope, to determine appropriate training regimens, precise selection of patients, mortality benefits, and cost benefits.

13

Cardiac Transplantation

Terence Kavanagh, MD

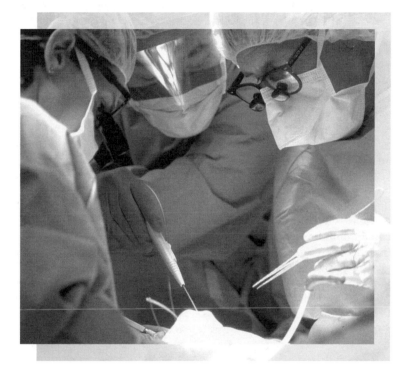

With 5- and 12-year survival rates of 60% and 35%, respectively, there is no doubt that cardiac transplantation has emerged as the treatment of choice in selected patients in the terminal stages of congestive heart failure.[65] The procedure improves not only the length but also the quality of life. At the same time, it also commits the patient to a lifelong rigorous medical follow-up protocol—one that can seriously strain vocational, family, interpersonal, and social relationships. In addition, severe deconditioning frequently follows months of debilitating ill health. Thus, one can readily appreciate the need for formal postsurgical rehabilitation. This should include not only physical training but also a prudent diet, weight control, guidance in smoking cessation, advice on the effects and side effects of medication, and psychological and possibly vocational counseling. This chapter deals with the exercise training component as well as relevant aspects of the pathophysiology of the transplanted heart.

GUIDELINES, 4TH EDITION

- Chapter 9, pages 159-165

Physiology of the Denervated Heart

Orthotopic heart transplantation involves removing the native heart at the level of the atrioventricular junction, leaving an atrial cuff, and transecting the aorta and pulmonary artery just above the semilunar valves. The native atria remains innervated, but effectively there is no conduction across the suture line and the donor heart is denervated.

In the immediate postsurgical stage, cardiac right- and left-side chamber filling pressures are elevated as a result of myocardial anoxia associated with graft transfer. However, within weeks the myocardium recovers, pulmonary hypertension regresses, and the intravascular pressures normalize. These abnormalities return only after the onset of an episode of transplant rejection. The following description therefore pertains to the status of the patient who has recovered from surgery and is free from manifestations of rejection.

In general, resting systolic performance is within normal limits as measured by left ventricular ejection fraction, myocardial contractility, and contractile reserve.[66-68] However, some impairment of diastolic function may persist in the long-term cardiac transplant patient.[69] In such cases, there is increased myocardial stiffness resulting in uncoordinated contraction and relaxation, possibly attributable to lack of sympathetic control, repeated episodes of mild rejection, prolonged graft ischemic time, accelerated coronary atherosclerotic disease, or the side effects of immunosuppressant therapy.[67,70,71]

The most prominent clinical finding observed in the heart transplant patient is the rapid resting heart rate, usually 15 to 25 beats·min^{-1} above age- and sex-matched controls.[72-76] This is attributable to the intrinsic rate of the transplanted heart's sinoatrial node, now free from customary vagal inhibition.[77,78] The heart rate does not alter in response to the Valsalva maneuver, carotid sinus massage, or a change in body position from lying to standing.[76] Any minor fluctuations in heart rate that occur over a 24-hr period are the result of variations in the levels of circulating catecholamines.[79,80] The resting tachycardia is associated with

a reduced stroke volume resulting in a normal,[16,81] or only mildly impaired, cardiac output at rest.[69]

Resting hypertension is a common finding.[16] It is characteristically associated with an elevated peripheral vascular resistance, which may be a persistent response to the preoperative state of congestive heart failure and its resultant chronic elevation of plasma norepinephrine[68] or an increased myocardial sensitivity to circulating catecholamines.[82,83] Cyclosporine therapy may also be a factor,[84,85] and some have suggested that the hypertensive effect is increased by the concomitant use of steroids.[86,87]

Exercise Responses

The transplanted heart's limitations become more obvious during a bout of exercise, largely as a result of its denervated state (figure 13.1). Beating at the high intrinsic rate of the sinoatrial node and lacking any neural influence, the transplanted heart cannot respond to physical exertion by immediate acceleration and relies entirely on the Frank–Starling mechanism to augment cardiac output. Increased venous return associated with the action of the skeletal–muscle pump and an increase in blood volume result in an elevated left ventricular end-diastolic volume, which in turn results in an increase in stroke volume.[81,88] With continuing effort, the heart rate, contractility, and ejection fraction increase in response to endogenously released catecholamines and their direct effect on the

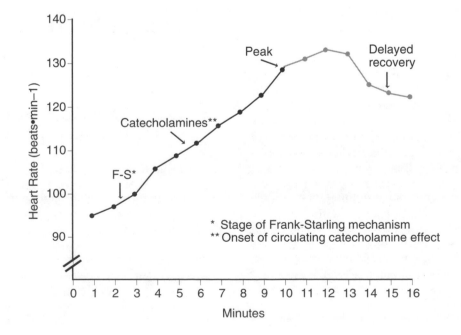

Figure 13.1   The limitations of transplanted hearts.

sinus node and myocardium.[89] The tendency of the heart rate to continue to increase after the cessation of exercise, and its delayed return to resting levels in the recovery period, mirror the gradual decrease in catecholamine concentrations.[90] Thus, the heart transplant patient may be considered to be sequentially "preload dependent" during the initial stages of effort and then "catecholamine dependent" during prolonged exercise, unlike the normal response in which both events occur simultaneously.

Peak heart rate and peak systolic blood pressure are both reduced to approximately 80% of normal because of the loss of sympathetic stimulation of the sinus node and impairment of myocardial contractility. As a result, cardiac output is reduced by approximately 25%. The heart rate reserve (maximum heart rate minus resting heart rate), normally 90 to 110 beats·min^{-1}, is reduced to 30 to 50 beats·min^{-1}.

Most investigators report that peak work rate and peak oxygen intake are lower in heart transplant patients than in age-matched controls. This is probably attributable to a combination of central and peripheral limitations. Kao and colleagues,[69] studying exercise responses in a group of cardiac transplant patients at regular intervals for up to 72 months after their surgery, confirmed that patients continued to show a significantly reduced peak work rate and peak oxygen intake.[67] Pulmonary capillary wedge, right atrial, and mean pulmonary arterial pressures were elevated and the arteriovenous oxygen difference was 24% lower at peak effort. The authors attributed the limited exercise tolerance to a combination of chronotropic incompetence and diastolic dysfunction limiting the appropriate compensatory use of the Frank-Starling mechanism. The limiting effect of reduced heart rate on exercise capacity was elegantly demonstrated by Braith and coworkers.[91] A heart transplant patient who had received a pacemaker for chronotropic incompetence underwent two maximal treadmill exercise tests, one in which the pacemaker was programmed to be rate responsive and the other in which it was not. Peak heart rate and peak oxygen intake were significantly improved by 15% and 20%, respectively, as a result of rate responsive pacing.[91]

Abnormal pulmonary diffusion has been reported in some heart transplant patients;[91] this may be caused by cyclosporine therapy[93] or the residual effects of congestive heart failure. Abnormal pulmonary diffusion could account for at least some part of the reduction in peak oxygen intake. [94,95]

If the reduction in exercise capacity were attributable to cardiac abnormalities, then the heart transplant recipient could be expected to regain full function shortly after surgery. In fact this is not the case, suggesting that the problem may reside in the periphery. As a result, increasing attention has been focused on the role of skeletal muscle. In my experience, the heart transplant patient has a 10% to 15% reduction in lean body mass, likely the result of a prolonged period of preoperative physical inactivity, aggravated by the side effects of immunosuppressant steroid or cyclosporine therapy.[16] The ensuing weakness would discourage physical activity, leading to further muscle loss, greater weakness, and increasing disinclination to exercise. In fact, Braith and coworkers[96] demonstrated reduced leg strength in a group of heart transplant recipients and showed that this correlated highly (r = .9) with the reduction in peak oxygen intake.[96]

The preexisting heart failure state is associated with abnormalities in skeletal muscle metabolism, and this may persist for some time after heart transplantation. Stratton and colleagues, using magnetic resonance spectroscopy, studied forearm exercise in groups of patients awaiting transplantation and at approximately 4 and 15 months after surgery.[26] Skeletal muscle abnormalities persisted up to 4 months posttransplantation. At 15 months, there was a significant improvement in phosphocreatine resynthesis rate and a trend to improvement in phosphocreatine concentration, but these did not reach normal levels. Bussières and coworkers[97] took muscle biopsies from the vastus lateralis muscle in 12 patients at 3 and 12 months postsurgery and found that the ratio of type I to type II fibers did not change. However, cross-sectional area increased by 35% in all fiber types at 12 months, although dimensions still remained below normal. There was no change in the number of capillaries per fiber. Oxidative and glycolytic enzymes increased significantly at 12 months, as did peak oxygen intake, but the latter still remained less than normal.[97]

The early onset of anaerobiosis gives rise to higher than normal lactate levels during submaximal effort, with increased frequency of breathing. The absolute ventilatory threshold is lower than normal, but because of the reduced peak oxygen intake, the relative ventilatory threshold is similar to age-matched controls.

Evidence for Reinnervation

Early experiments established that over time, reinnervation could occur in the denervated transplanted dog heart. Naturally, such an outcome in the human heart would be highly desirable, and a number of workers have addressed this issue over the years, only to arrive at the conclusion that, for all practical purposes, the human transplanted heart remains denervated. Nevertheless, there is some evidence that autonomic reinnervation may occur. Stark and colleagues[98] were the first to report chest pain typical of angina in two cardiac transplantation patients who were subsequently discovered to have developed severe coronary atherosclerosis. Both also had significant release of myocardial norepinephrine in response to a tyramine challenge, indicating some level of afferent sympathetic activity. As a result, various techniques have been used to detect autonomic reinnervation, including analysis of heart rate variability,[99-101] positron emission tomography,[102] measurement of myocardial norepinephrine release,[103-105] and immunohistochemical examination of myocardial tissue for evidence of neuron growth.[106] From these data, one can conclude that, over a 2- to 8-year period following surgery, (a) there is evidence of limited sympathetic reinnervation in the transplanted heart but that it is inconsistent, and (b) there is no evidence of vagal reinnervation. One study, however, suggested that when sympathetic reinnervation does take place, it may confer practical benefit in terms of improved exercise capacity. Lord and colleagues[107] reported on eight orthotopic heart transplant patients in whom intracoronary injection of tyramine resulted in an increase in heart rate, an associated higher work rate and peak heart rate, and a more rapid recovery rate than patients in whom response to tyramine was less marked. The authors concluded that sympathetic efferent sinus node reinnervation can occur and can increase exercise time and total work rate, although not to normal levels.

Exercise Training

By the time patients undergo cardiac transplantation surgery, they are typically very deconditioned, and exercise training is recommended following surgery.[57] Studies have documented an increase in $\dot{V}O_2$peak of 18% to 20%.[16,108] As with heart failure patients, there has been limited experience with exercise training of cardiac transplantation patients, and there is no standardized approach to training.

Inpatient

Most units follow a regimen similar to that used at the Mayo Clinic and so well described by McGregor.[109] After 24 to 48 hr of intensive care monitoring, patients commence the customary breathing, postural, and mobilization exercises. By the fifth day patients are walking in the ward, and they may then begin to use a cycle ergometer, pedaling at zero resistance for 3 to 5 min at a perceived exertion of 12 to 14 on the Borg scale (6-20). As performance improves, the duration of exercise and the power outputs on the ergometer are increased progressively. Corridor walking is also introduced, and by the time of discharge from hospital, usually about 3 weeks after surgery, a low-level incremental exercise test may be carried out on the cycle ergometer or the treadmill. This test allows for the prescription of a walking or stationary cycling program, which can be carried out during the early (4-8 weeks) outpatient phase.

Extra vigilance is necessary in the early postoperative weeks to monitor development of transplant rejection, infection, arrhythmias in the donor heart, neurological deficits, and renal dysfunction.

Outpatient

The preliminary exercise test can be carried out on either a treadmill or a cycle ergometer, the protocol in general calling for progressive increments in work rate of 1 to 2 metabolic equivalents (METs) until peak or maximal effort is achieved, ideally within 10 to 14 min. Suitable protocols include the modified Naughton[110] or the modified Bruce[111] or that proposed by Savin and colleagues.[112] A common incremental cycle ergometer protocol uses power outputs of 100 kp·m·min^{-1} (16.4 W) every minute or, in the case of the more severely deconditioned individual, 50 kp·m·min^{-1} (8.2 W).[16] Predicting peak oxygen intake from heart rate following transplantation is invariably inaccurate, because of the atypical heart rate response to exercise. Therefore, direct measurement of oxygen intake at peak power output is essential for precise functional evaluation.

Whatever the protocol, it is customary to monitor the exercise electrocardiogram, the rating of perceived exertion on the Borg scale (6-20), and the blood pressure. Expired air is collected and analyzed to measure ventilation, oxygen intake, carbon dioxide production, and the ventilatory equivalent of the anaerobic threshold. The ventilatory threshold is usually attainable even by patients who are unable or unwilling to exert maximal effort.[113] It is the preferred training intensity for cardiac patients and poorly conditioned subjects and generally occurs at an oxygen intake of between 50% and 65% of maximal oxygen intake. This relationship was investigated by Brubaker and colleagues,[114] who compared the invasive (blood lactates) and noninvasive (ventilatory) determination of anaerobic threshold in cardiac transplant patients and normal control participants. There was no significant difference between the oxygen intake at which the ventilatory and lactate thresholds occurred in heart transplant patients. The same was true for control participants, although the absolute values were higher than in the transplant patients. Neither was there any difference between the relative oxygen intake (percentage peak) at which lactate threshold and ventilatory threshold occurred in transplant and normal participants.

Allograft coronary atherosclerosis is a major complication following heart transplantation,[115] but unfortunately one cannot rely on angina or exercise-induced ST-segment depression as an indicator of myocardial ischemia.[116] Particular attention has to be paid, therefore, to the symptoms of dyspnea, lightheadedness, and faintness as well as to the development of ischemia-related arrhythmias.

The modalities generally used for aerobic training include walking, stationary cycling, rowing machine, arm ergometry, stair stepping, and calisthenics. Heart rate generally cannot be used for prescribing intensity of exercise because of its atypical response to effort. Instead, the intensity is based on the work rate or peak power output occurring at 60% of peak oxygen intake, supported by the ventilatory threshold, and a perceived exertion of 12 to 14 on the Borg scale. In the Toronto–Harefield program,[16] the initial exercise prescription called for the patient to walk 1.6 km, five times weekly, at a walking pace of between 11 and 14 min·km^{-1}. The distance was then increased by 1.6 km every 2 weeks, maintaining the same pace until, by 6 weeks, the patient was walking 4.8 km, five times weekly. The pace was then quickened by 1 min per 1.6 km until the 4.8 km was accomplished in 45 min (typically within 4 months of starting the program). Thereafter, 50-m bouts of slow jogging were introduced until ultimately the entire 4.8 km was completed in 36 min. After the first 6 weeks, if the patient was "stuck" at a given pace, the exercise prescription was adjusted to obtain a training session lasting 30 to 60 min.

Accurate pacing is emphasized, as well as thorough familiarity with the concept of perceived exertion and correct interpretation of such symptoms of myocardial ischemia as excessive dyspnea, unusual fatigue, light-headedness, and extrasystoles. Rejection episodes or intercurrent infections may interrupt the training program from time to time, and patients should be advised of this possibility at the outset of their program.

Initially, some patients may need regular supervision or even electrocardiographic monitoring during the exercise sessions, but these are a minority. Most will be able to train at home without risk, attending a supervised class only once a week, or even once monthly. During the first 6 to 12 months there are frequent return visits to the transplant unit or the local hospital for routine follow-up testing, and this gives ample oppor-tunity for the appropriate rehabilitation team to carry out exercise testing and to assess the patient's progress and adherence to the training regimen.

Resistance training is now accepted as an integral part of a cardiac rehabilitation program, and heart transplantation regimens are no exception to this. I believe that much of the training effect is attributable to an increase in lean body mass or an improved skeletal muscle metabolism. Braith and colleagues[96] reported a correlation between leg strength and peak oxygen intake in heart transplant recipients and also demonstrated the beneficial effect of biweekly sessions of resistance training for 6 months on steroid-induced bone loss.[117,118] These authors, however, warn against the possibility of transient hypotension during resistance exercise, a problem they find is exaggerated when the exercise requires lifting above the level of the heart. To prevent this occurrence they advise (a) alternating upper-body exercises with lower-body exercises, (c) having symptomatic participants walk 2 min between exercises, and (c) concluding each resistance training session with a 5-min cool-down walk at low intensity.[119]

Risks

As pointed out previously, the development of hypertension is always a potential problem in the management of heart transplant patients. Although likely to be a side effect of immunosuppressant cyclosporine therapy, it may also be a persistent response to the preoperative state of congestive heart failure and its resultant chronic elevation of plasma norepinephrine. If this is so, then exercise training should help, because it has been shown to reduce catecholamine levels[120] and to have an antihypertensive effect, particularly in hyperadrenergic individuals.[121] In any event, a resting systolic blood pressure greater than 210 mmHg or a diastolic pressure greater than 120 mmHg is a contraindication to exercise testing or training. Furthermore,

Recommended Exercise Prescription Parameters for Cardiac Transplantation Patients

Exercise intensity

- 50% to 75% V̇O$_2$peak or equivalent METs
- Rating of perceived exertion 11 to 15 (6-20 scale)
- Ventilatory threshold
- Dyspnea scale

Exercise duration

- 15 to 60 min

Exercise frequency

- Four to six times per week

Adapted from: Franklin BA (ed). ACSM's Guidelines for Exercise Testing and Training (6th edition). Baltimore: Lippincott Williams and Wilkins, 2000. p.193

an exaggerated inotropic exercise response in which the systolic pressure exceeds 260 mmHg or the diastolic pressure exceeds 115 mmHg[122] is enough to preclude entry into a training program, at least until the hypertension is controlled.

Rejection of the graft occurs most frequently in the first 6 months following surgery, affecting some 85% of all heart transplant recipients. Thereafter, the incidence decreases. Nevertheless, acute episodes of graft rejection are an ever-present threat and are detected most accurately by endomyocardial biopsy. Rejection may be accompanied by episodes of ventricular arrhythmias. Maintaining the training level at or below the ventilatory threshold should ensure that the arrhythmia threshold is not reached. Major rejection episodes are a contraindication to training. Intercurrent infections attributable to immunosuppression, particularly cytomegalovirus infection, are another hazard. Despite the formidable list of potential problems, total abstinence from physical activity is seldom required, and even then only for relatively brief periods.

By the fifth post-operative year, some 50% of patients show angiographic evidence of coronary atherosclerosis. Because anginal pain is absent, one has to be particularly vigilant for such signs of ischemia as undue exertional breathlessness, lightheadedness, and arrhythmias.

Benefits

The earliest exercise training report was from Squires and coworkers,[123] who demonstrated that the training regimen could be both effective and safe. Since that time, a series of reports have confirmed these findings and described further training-induced benefits.[124-133] There is general agreement that an aerobic-type of training program results in significant improvement in cardiopulmonary fitness. Heart transplant patients compete regularly in the World Transplant Games, and some have taken part in long-distance road runs, from 20 km to the 42-km marathon.[108,134,135] $\dot{V}O_2$peak is increased, and the onset of anaerobiosis is delayed; the latter is reflected in an increase in the absolute ventilatory threshold and a reduction in blood lactates at equivalent submaximal work rates. Decreases in resting and submaximal heart rates have also been reported, together with an increase in maximal rate–pressure product, the extent of these changes depending to some degree on the intensity and duration of the training program. The shorter programs have all resulted in appreciable gains in cardiorespiratory fitness, but the reduction in resting heart rate has been noted only after a longer training period.[16] There have been no reports of training-induced changes in cardiac dimensions or function. All programs use a training intensity corresponding to 12 to 14 on the Borg rating scale of perceived exertion, the ventilatory threshold, 50% to 70% $\dot{V}O_2$peak, or some combination. See sidebar on p. 153.

Long-Term Effects

There is minimal information on the long-term effects of an exercise training program following heart transplantation. However, a recent report collected data on a group of 36 patients who had completed 16 months of aerobic training 12 years after the program.[136] There were 23 survivors at 12 years. Findings were compared with a group of age-matched controls who were followed over the same period of time, and factors influencing survival were also examined.

The survivors' $\dot{V}O_2$peak increased 26% after training and then declined from the posttraining value of 28 $ml\cdot kg^{-1}\cdot min^{-1}$ at the rate of 0.39 $ml\cdot kg^{-1}\cdot min^{-1}$ per year. There was no difference in the rate of decline between those participants who continued to exercise regularly and those who failed to do so. Neither was there any significant difference in the rate of decline experienced by the control participants (0.37 $ml\cdot kg^{-1}\cdot min^{-1}$ per year from a $\dot{V}O_2$peak of 34 $ml\cdot kg^{-1}\cdot min^{-1}$). Thus, although most of the gains in exercise capacity resulting from the training program were lost over 12 years, this was commensurate with normal aging. Furthermore, the final $\dot{V}O_2$peak of 24 $ml\cdot kg^{-1}\cdot min^{-1}$ remained slightly higher than the initial pretraining value (22 $ml\cdot kg^{-1}\cdot min^{-1}$), a level of aerobic function well above the threshold of 18 $ml\cdot kg^{-1}\cdot min^{-1}$ that frail, elderly persons need to perform many of the activities of daily living, and one which the participants would conceivably have reached within 10 years had they not had the benefit of an exercise program.

As for prognostic indicators, those who died had reduced training responses in $\dot{V}O_2$peak and lean body mass compared with those who survived. However, the small sample size weakens the inferences drawn regarding markers for survival. On the other hand, Braith and colleagues[96] reported a significant correlation between leg strength and $\dot{V}O_2$peak, and Kavanagh and colleagues[137] identified $\dot{V}O_2$peak as an important independent marker of prognosis, findings which, taken in concert, tend to support the predictive value of these two measures in heart transplant patients.

Summary

The routine use of a comprehensive exercise rehabilitation program following heart transplantation maximizes the benefits of surgery and can induce a good training effect, although complete restoration of physiological functioning may not be possible. The prescription of exercise must take into account the denervated heart's peculiar response to effort and must rely heavily on perceived exertion and metabolic measurements rather than on target heart rates for defining the intensity of training.

Appendix A

Risk Factors for CHD

John C. Ashworth, MA; Suzanne Hughes, RN, MSN; Maureen E. Mays, MD; and Patrick E. McBride, MD, MPH

A risk factor is defined as "a clearly defined characteristic that has been associated with the increased rate of a subsequently occurring disease."[1(p. 1581)] Cardiovascular research has focused on risk factors for many years, and the lists of modifiable risk factors and those that cannot be changed is well established. According to the American Heart Association, clinical and statistical studies have identified several factors that increase coronary heart disease (CHD) risk. Current estimates on the burden of CHD predicted by known risk factors is approximately 90%.[2]

Individuals with known CHD are at high risk of a future cardiovascular event. In fact, more than 90% of those patients will die of a cardiovascular event. Therefore, the goal for those people is to reduce premature death and disability to the greatest extent possible, by treating both the underlying disease and CHD risk factors. Treatment of risk factors is as important as revascularization in reducing risk of future CHD. This is especially true for tobacco cessation, cholesterol treatment, antiplatelet treatments, and blood pressure therapy.[3]

The well-known Framingham database is a valuable tool in preventive cardiology and primary care, but it is not used in cardiac rehabilitation or secondary prevention. Framingham risk assessment scores are for primary prevention; that is, they are used to establish the level of risk in persons with no prior CHD diagnosis or event. Because some cardiac rehabilitation programs also treat patients for primary prevention of CHD, these risk assessment tools can be applied to those primary prevention patients but should not be extrapolated to secondary prevention.[4]

Reduction of CHD risk factors is vital to both primary and secondary prevention of CHD events. Substantial reductions in premature death and disability are possible through the treatment of established risk factors. Patients and health professionals must form a partnership to identify all risk factors, use effective treatments, and reach risk factor goals. A knowledgeable and supportive cardiac rehabilitation staff is an invaluable part of the efforts.

Established Risk Factors

Age

Male gender

Family history of premature atherosclerosis[a]

Smoking

Diabetes mellitus

Hypertension

Dyslipidemia

Elevated LDL

Elevated VLDL (triglycerides)

Low HDL

Elevated non-HDL

Obesity or overweight

Sedentary lifestyle

Psychosocial stressors

Emerging Risk Factors

Homocysteine

Lipoprotein(a)

High-sensitivity C-reactive protein

Fibrinogen

Interleukin-6

Note. LDL = low-density lipoprotein; VLDL = very low-density lipoprotein; HDL = high-density lipoprotein.
[a]Parent, sibling, grandparent, or child with CHD diagnosis at age <60 years.

CHD

Over the past 50 years, a large body of epidemiologic evidence has been amassed linking both biological and lifestyle risk factors to the development of cardiovascular disease (CHD). Subsequent clinical research into the effects of modifying these factors on cardiovascular events and cardiovascular mortality rate has followed. This body of knowledge has provided the basis for guidelines for prevention of CHD and for the development of pharmacological interventions that, when used optimally, have the potential for increasing both length and quality of life. In particular, the causal link between high blood cholesterol level and CHD is well known. Potent and safe pharmacological agents have been developed to reduce cholesterol levels, and these agents have been demonstrated in multiple large, randomized trials to reduce cardiovascular events, cardiovascular mortality rate, and all-cause mortality rate.[5-10]

From the Framingham Heart Study, however we know that 50% of myocardial infarctions in the United States occur in persons with below-average cholesterol levels.[11] Research into the "novel," "emerging," or "nontraditional" cardiovascular risk factors strives to discover other factors that may have a causal relationship with the development of atherosclerosis. These factors under investigation, like the traditional cardiac risk factors, may be associated with physical characteristics (short stature,[12] abdominal adiposity[13]), or may be biological. The following review summarizes what is known about two of the biological factors currently under study. Certain biological factors may be associated with cardiovascular disease without a cause–effect relationship.

In 1981, Hopkins and Williams[14] listed 246 postulated causes of cardiovascular disease. Now, more than 20 years later, the list would certainly have grown. By the time this book is seen in print, new findings will have superseded this commentary. Print media, television, and the Internet provide the lay public with current medical research findings almost concurrently with the appearance of such findings in the medical literature. This poses a challenge for clinicians when advising patients. To process this rapidly growing body of literature and to advise patients in a credible and timely fashion, clinicians can use a framework with which to critically review the literature. The criteria posed by Sir Austin Bradford Hill in 1965 provide a suitable framework from an epidemiologic perspective.

From a clinical prespective, the following queries are added for consideration.

- Is a valid and accurate measurement tool used?
- Is the intervention proven to modify the factor?
- Does selective modification alter outcomes?

Inflammation and Infection as Risk Factors for CHD

Two possible risk factors for CVD that have been emphasized in the recent past are inflammation and infection. Following is a discussion of both of these factors.

Inflammatory Factors

Since 1990, there has been a growing appreciation for the integral role played by inflammation in the development and progression of atherosclerosis. Atherosclerosis is clearly an inflammatory disease, not simply a "bland lipid storage disease."[15] Inflammatory processes play a role not only in chronic atherosclerosis but in acute coronary syndromes as well. Large epidemiologic studies have provided solid evidence that elevated baseline levels of several inflammatory factors, including systemic cytokines such as interleukin-6[16] and tumor necrosis factor-α[17], and adhesion molecules such as intercellular adhesion molecule-1,[18] predict the development of atherosclerotic disease. Likewise, what we know as the "downstream" inflammatory markers, such as C-reactive protein (CRP) and fibrinogen (see hemostatic factors for discussion of fibrinogen), predict risk of future cardiovascular events. These downstream factors are produced by the liver in response to systemic

Bradford Hills Criteria for Causation

- Strength of association—the stronger the association the more likely the relation is casual.
- Dose-response relation—as the dose of exposure to a factor increases, the risk of disease also increases. Exceptions may exist (i.e., a threshold effect).
- Consistency—similar findings from different studies and in different populations.
- Specificity—a specific exposure is associated with only one disease (possibly the weakest of all the criteria).
- Temporal relation—if a factor is believed to be a cause of disease, exposure to the factor must precede the development of the disease.

cytokines. Obesity, particularly central obesity, is associated with increased levels of CRP. Adipocytes, in fact, produce proinflammatory cytokines.

CRP has emerged as the most clinically useful inflammatory marker. CRP (actually "highly sensitive [hs]" or ultrasensitive [us]" CRP) is easily measured. CRP has a long half-life, and levels do not undergo circadian changes.[15] Current assays measure small gradations of CRP that previously were considered within the normal range. Multiple large population-based studies have demonstrated that elevated baseline CRP levels predict risk of future cardiovascular disease in both men and women. Similar associations are noted between baseline CRP and the development of peripheral vascular disease.[19]

Measurement of CRP appears to add to the coronary risk profile, when considered in combination with the lipid profile.[20,21] Certain members of the HMG coenzyme A reductase inhibitor group of lipid-lowering agents (statins) have been shown to decrease CRP.[22] It is likely that the anti-inflammatory action of the statins (perhaps the entire class) contributes to their benefit in cardiovascular risk reduction. It has been speculated that CRP could ultimately become a target of therapy. At the least, it appears to identify those who would most benefit from aggressive treatment of their lipid disorders. It has been found that hormone replacement therapy (estrogen alone or estrogen with progesterone) increases CRP.[23,24] The clinical significance of this is not yet known. It was recently found that higher levels of physical activity (by self-report) in a healthy elderly population were associated with lower levels of several inflammatory markers, CRP and fibrinogen among them.[25]

In January 2003, the Centers for Disease Control and the American Heart Association published a scientific statement regarding inflammatory markers and their application to clinical and public health practice.[26] In summary, these organizations identified a role for hs-CRP in assessing patients at moderate risk (10-20% 10-year risk). For this subgroup, measurement of hs-CRP was identified as an optional adjunct to help guide further evaluation and risk factor management. With regard to secondary prevention, risk reduction strategies in patients with established CHD should not be contingent on hs-CRP levels.

Infection

Various infectious processes have been implicated as causal factors for atherosclerosis. The possible culprits include cytomegalovirus (CMV), *Chlamydia pneumoniae*, *Helicobacter pylori*, and certain herpes viruses. More recently, periodontitis[27] has been implicated. Infection and cardiovascular disease have many overlapping risk factors, namely, age, low socioeconomic status, and smoking.

CMV, herpesvirus hominis, and *C. pneumoniae* have each been identified in human atheromae. There are several mechanisms by which these infectious processes may cause or amplify the atherothrombotic process. These can be divided into the direct effects of infection on the endothelium and the indirect systemic effects secondary to chronic inflammation, via an autoimmune-mediated process, or potential interactions with other CHD risk factors including lipids, homocysteine, or hemostatic factors.[28]

Results from a trial by Gupta and colleagues[29] examining the benefit of antichlamydial antibiotics as secondary prevention of CHD in a *C. pneumoniae*-exposed group indicated a decrease in cardiovascular end points in the macrolide antibiotic–treated group. The ROXIS (Roxithromycin Ischemic Syndromes) trial compared outcomes post-non-Q-wave coronary syndromes in a group treated with roxithromycin versus placebo for 30 days. Clinical benefit was noted in the treatment group at 30 days and at 90 days. Benefit was no longer seen at 180 days.[30] In a Finnish study of 148 patients randomized to clarithromycin or placebo for 3 months, clarithromycin appeared to reduce the risk of CHD events, and the benefit was sustained over 18 months.[31]

In 1996, a consensus panel was convened to issue a scientific statement regarding a causal relationship between infection and atherosclerosis.[32] Specifically, the evidence implicating *C. pneumoniae* and CMV was evaluated. The framework used by this panel was an evaluation of the current knowledge in light of Koch's three postulates required to prove causality. The panel concluded that thus far, only one of the three criteria had been satisfied: The agent had been identified in the lesion. Thus far, the organism had not been isolated from the host, nor, in humans, had the agent produced the disease when transferred to a susceptible host. At this time, it remains unclear whether infectious agents participate in or amplify atherothrombotic process or are innocent bystanders. Prophylactic treatment with antibiotics as CVD prevention (primary or secondary) may require long-term administration of antimicrobial agents with the attendant public health concern of the emergence of drug-resistant organisms.[33]

Two recent studies focused on the use of antibiotics for the secondary prevention of CHD. Grayston and colleagues34 investigated the use of azithromycin for 1 year in persons with documented CHD and found a non-significant reduction of 1% in CHD mortality and morbidity compared to patients in the control group. Another study used gatifloxacin for an average of 2 years in persons with documented CHD and the authors reported no significant difference in all-cause mortality and CHD morbidity between the treated group and the group using a placebo.35 Finally, the reader is directed to a comprehensive review concerning the role of inflammation in the development of CHD.36

Appendix B

Patient Education Example for Cardiac Rehabilitation

Timothy R. McConnell, PhD, and Troy A. Klinger, MS

The educational component of comprehensive cardiac rehabilitation programs must provide patients with relevant and understandable information. Education is typically implemented using an individualized and group approach. Individualized instruction is usually completed during one-on-one sessions or during individual discussions during exercise. The group didactic approach consists of programs on different topics that all participants have an opportunity to attend during their program tenure. The group sessions are open to family members and friends and have handouts or other support materials.

Following is a suggested structure for patient education on atherosclerosis, including the purpose, objectives, and content outline.

Purpose

To provide patients, families, and significant others with information regarding the cardiac anatomy (specifically the coronary circulation), the development of coronary heart disease, which can lead to angina or a heart attack, and the proper use of nitroglycerin.

Learner Objectives

I. The patient will learn the basics of coronary anatomy and physiology.

A. Anatomy

1. Using diagram or heart model, the patient will locate right, left main, left anterior descending, and circumflex coronary arteries.

B. Angina (the pain or discomfort associated with coronary heart disease) versus myocardial infarction or heart attack

1. Angina occurs when the heart muscle is not receiving an adequate blood supply to meet its metabolic needs; it usually occurs during physical exertion or increased stress or emotional upset.

   a. The decreased blood flow is caused by a buildup of fat, cholesterol, calcium, and blood platelets and a blockage or near blockage of one or more of the coronary arteries.

   b. Angina differs from person to person. It can be pain or discomfort in the chest, arm, jaw, neck, or shoulders.

   c. Some may not experience the "traditional" heart attack pain or discomfort but may have an "anginal equivalent" such as shortness of breath, tightness, indigestion, or others.

   d. Angina will usually be relieved with rest or nitroglycerin.

C. Myocardial infarction or heart attack pain, caused by a total blockage of a coronary artery (no blood flow through the artery)

1. Heart attack pain will present itself much like angina (described previously); however, the pain is usually more severe and associated with one or more of the following: nausea, vomiting, diaphoresis, cold and clammy skin, and shortness of breath.

2. Heart attack pain is usually not relieved by rest or using nitroglycerin.

II. The patient will be introduced to the currently available treatment and management modalities.

   A. Management by medication

   B. Percutaneous interventions

      1. Percutaneous transluminal angioplasty

      2. Stent

      3. Atherectomy

   C. Coronary artery revascularization bypass surgery

III. The patient will learn how to use nitroglycerin.

   A. When the chest discomfort or pain begins (suspected angina), the patient should immediately sit down and place one nitroglycerin underneath his or her tongue. If the pain or discomfort is not relieved after 5 min, the patient should use another nitroglycerin up to a total of no more than three nitroglycerin pills or until the pain is relieved. If the pain or discomfort is not relieved after the third nitroglycerin, the patient should call 911.

   B. Special considerations

      1. Nitroglycerin is to be carried by the patient at all times.

      2. Nitroglycerin is to be kept in the brown glass bottle (or a stainless steel nitroglycerin pendant, which is light- and water-resistant and airtight).

      3. A new prescription of nitroglycerin should be obtained at least every 6 months.

      4. Cotton should be removed from new bottles so that the medication is "ready to go."

   C. The patient will be instructed in prophylactic use of nitroglycerin. Should the patient find that a particular activity routinely causes him or her to have angina, he or she should be instructed to take nitroglycerin before that activity.

   D. Report to physician

      1. Change in anginal pattern—increased frequency, intensity, duration—and decreased activity tolerance

      2. Change from exertional angina to rest angina

      3. Awakened with angina

Outcome Goals: Guidelines and Recommendations for Risk Factor Management

Jeffrey L. Roitman, EdD, and Thomas P. LaFontaine, PhD

GUIDELINE

RECOMMENDATION	JNC VII 2003[54]	AHA Diet Guidelines 2000[34]	NCEP III 2001[23]	AHA/ACC Guidelines for Secondary Prevention:2001 update[33]	2nd Joint TF of European Society on Coronary Prevention 1998[4]	Guide to Preventive Cardiology in Women 1999[85]	Secondary Prevention in Elderly (>75 yrs) 2002[165]	ADA Clinical Practice Recommendation 2003[62]	ACSM Position Stand on Weight Loss[81]
Smoking	Complete cessation	Complete cessation	NR	Complete cessation	Complete cessation	Complete cessation	Complete cessation	Complete cessation	NR
SBP (mm Hg)	<120	NR	NR	<140 or <130 (if CHF or CRF) or <130 (if DM)	<140	<140 or optimal ≤120	<140 or <130 (if CHF or CRF) or <130 (if DM)	<130	NR
DBP (mm Hg)	<80	NR	NR	<90 or <85 (if CHF or CRF) or <80 (if DM)	<90	<90 or optimal. ≤80	<90 or <85 (if CHF or CRF) or <80 (if DM)	<80	NR
Cholesterol (mg/dL)	NR	NR	<200	<200	<190	<200	<200	NR	NR
LDL (mg·dL⁻¹)	NR	Achieve desirable level	<70	Primary goal <100	<115	<100 (NCEP III)	<100	<100	NR
HDL (mg·dL⁻¹)	NR	Achieve desirable level	>40 men; >45 women	Secondary goal >40	NR	>35	>40	>45	NR
Triglycerides (mg·dL⁻¹)	NR	Achieve desirable level	<150	Secondary goal <150	NR	<200; if DM <150	<200	<200	NR
Dietary fat	NR	<30% (but no specific recommendation for CHD)	25-35% of total calories	NR	<30% of total calories	<30% of total calories	NR	NR	<30% total calories
Dietary SAFA	Reduce	<7% total calories	<7% of total calories	NR	Reduce through replacing with MUFA	<7% of total calories	NR	<10% total calories; if LDL >100, then <7%	NR

(continued)

161

(continued)

	GUIDELINE								
RECOMMENDATION	JNC VII 2003[54]	AHA Diet Guidelines 2000[34]	NCEP III 2001[23]	AHA/ACC Guidelines for Secondary Prevention: 2001 update[33]	2nd Joint TF of European Society on Coronary Prevention 1998[4]	Guide to Preventive Cardiology in Women 1999[85]	Secondary Prevention in Elderly (>75 yrs) 2002[165]	ADA Clinical Practice Recommendation 2003[62]	ACSM Position Stand on Weight Loss[81]
Dietary cholesterol (mg·day⁻¹)	Reduce	<200	<200	NR	<300	<200	NR	<300; if LDL >100, then <200	NR
Exercise/activity	30 min·day⁻¹ most days	30-60 min·day⁻¹ on most days; expend 100-200 kcal per session	Increase physical activity	Minimum goal: 30-40 min, 3-4 days per week; optimal: daily	Increase physical activity	>30 min on all or most days	Increase activity and exercise	NR	>2000 kcal·week⁻¹ (200-300 min·week⁻¹)
Blood glucose (mg/dL) or HbA1c	NR	NR	NR	HbA1c <7%	FBG: type 1: 91-120; pp pk: 136-160; HbA1c = 6.2-7.5%; type 2: lower goals	FBG = 80-120; HbA1c <7.0%;	HbA1c <7.0%;	NR	NR
Body weight and obesity	BMI = 18.5-24.9 kg·m⁻²	Maintain a healthy body weight	Reduce body weight	BMI = 18.5-24.9 kg·m⁻²	BMI <25.0 kg·m⁻² or waist circumference <94cm in men; <80 cm in women	BMI <18.5-24.9 kg·m⁻²	Reduce body weight	NR	BMI <25.0 kg·m⁻²
Sodium (mg·day⁻¹)	2,400	2,400	NR	NR	NR	<2,400	NR	NR	NR

162

RECOMMENDATION									
Alcohol	<2 drinks per day or 1 drink per day for women or low weight	2 drinks per day for men; 1 drink per day for women	NR	NR	NR	NR	NR	NR	NR
Other (see reference for specifics)	DASH eating plan	1. High unsaturated fat diets 2. Folic acid, vitamin B_6 3. Soy protein and isoflavones 4. Omega-3 fatty acids 5. Increased fiber 6. Stanol–sterol ester-containing foods	Medications	1. Antiplatelet-anticoagulants 2. ACE inhibitors 3. β-blockers	1. ASA 2. β-blockers 3. ACE inhibitors 4. Anticoagulation	1. HRT: individual (no longer recommended) 2. Antiplatelet-anticoagulation 3. β-blockers 4. ACE inhibitors 5. Oral contraception	1. Psychosocial intervention 2. Cardiac rehab participation 3. Angina, MI, intervention, CABG, arrhythmias	NR	1. Lose 5-10% body weight if obese 2. Change eating and exercise behavior 3. Reduce energy intake by 500-1,000 kcal·day^{-1} 4. Supplement endurance exercise with resistance training

Note. This table includes published statements and guidelines about risk factor modification as well as recommendations for levels of specific risk factors related to the specific topic covered in the statement. All of the recommendations are specific to "secondary prevention" (individuals with clinical evidence of disease) if the statement makes specific recommendations. Otherwise, "optimal" levels are selected for goals. References indicated correspond to chapter three. JNC VII = Joint National Committee on Prevention, Detection, Evaluation and Treatment of High Blood Pressure; AHA = American Heart Association; NCEP = National Cholesterol Education Program; ACC = American College of Cardiology; TF = Task Force; ADA = American Diabetes Association; ACSM = American College of Sports Medicine; NR = no recommendation; SBP = systolic blood pressure; CHF = congestive heart failure; CRF = chronic renal failure; DM = diabetes mellitus; DBP = diastolic blood pressure; HDL = high-density lipoprotein; CHD = coronary heart disease; SAFA = saturated fat; MUFA = monounsaturated fat; LDL=low-density lipoprotein; HbA1c = Hemoglobin A1c; FBG = fasting blood glucose; pp pk = postprandial peak; BMI = body mass index; DASH= Dietary Approaches to Stop Hypertension; ACE = angiotensin-converting enzyme; ASA = acetylsalicylic acid; HRT= hormone replacement therapy; MI = myocardial infarction; CABG = coronary artery bypass graft.

Appendix D

Exercise Prescription Case Studies

Adam T. de Jong, MA, and Barry A. Franklin, PhD

Case Study 1

Mr. K is a 56-year-old investment banker who presented to the hospital emergency center complaining of moderate (5/10) midsternal chest pain with radiation to his left jaw. The symptoms were similar to those he had been experiencing while jogging over the past 2 weeks, only slightly more severe. The patient's medical history, as summarized in table D.1, included mild elevations in total and low-density lipoprotein (LDL) cholesterol and triglycerides, borderline systolic hypertension, and a 20-pack year history of smoking, including a current consumption of 1 pack per day. In addition, he had a strongly positive family history of premature heart disease, with both his father and a brother having had a myocardial infarction before age 45.

Serial electrocardiograms (ECGs) performed during the initial examination in the emergency center revealed non-specific ST-segment depression in the anterolateral leads. These ECG changes resolved spontaneously following administration of sublingual nitroglycerine. In addition, patient was given 325 mg of aspirin. An urgent cardiac catheterization was ordered to assess his coronary morphology.

Coronary angiography revealed an ejection fraction of 65%. A 95% stenosis in the midportion of the left anterior descending (LAD) artery was noted, with an additional 60% to 70% stenosis in the distal circumflex artery. The remainder of the coronary vasculature was unremarkable. The LAD stenosis was treated with percutaneous transluminal coronary angioplasty (PTCA) and stenting, resulting in a residual blockage of 10%. Medical management of the circumflex stenosis was deemed the most viable option. Mr. K's hospital stay was uneventful and he was discharged 2 days post-PTCA on the following medications: Atenolol (25 mg·day^{-1}), aspirin (81 mg·day^{-1}), and Lipitor (20 mg·day^{-1}).

Two weeks following hospital discharge, Mr. K underwent a follow-up examination with his cardiologist, at which time he completed a peak or symptom-limited graded exercise test with concomitant myocardial perfusion imaging. The results of his treadmill stress test are summarized in the sidebar.

Table D.1	Selected Demographic Data and Coronary Risk Factors for Mr. K*	
	Demographics	**Current data**
	Weight	180 lb (81.8 kg)
	Height	73 in. (185 cm)
	Total cholesterol	210 mg·dl^{-1}
	LDL cholesterol	134 mg·dl^{-1}
	HDL cholesterol	40 mg·dl^{-1}
	Triglycerides	180 mg·dl^{-1}
	Resting blood pressure	142/80 mm Hg

Note. Values were determined during his most recent physical examination. LDL = low-density lipoprotein; HDL = high-density lipoprotein.

Treadmill Stress Test Results

Protocol: Bruce

Resting values

- Heart rate (HR): 65 beats·min^{-1}
- Blood pressure (BP): 110/80 mmHg

End point

- Stage 3 (3.4 mph/14% grade) for 3 min
- Metabolic equivalent (MET) level achieved: 10.0 (estimated)
- Peak *HR: 1442 beats·min^{-1}
- Peak BP: 188/76 mm Hg
- Test was terminated secondary to volitional fatigue.
- 1.0 mm horizontal ST-segment depression (V$_5$ and V$_6$) was noted at a heart rate of 124 beats·min^{-1}.
- Myocardial perfusion imaging demonstrated a lateral-wall reversible perfusion abnormality.

Because of his class B risk stratification, according to the criteria of the American Heart Association, Mr. K was referred for ECG telemetry monitored exercise therapy. His exercise intensity range was calculated as seen in the sidebar.

Target Heart Rate (THR)

THR = 144 beats·min^{-1} − 65 beats·min^{-1} × (40-60%) + 65 beats·min^{-1}

THR = 79 beats·min^{-1} × (40-60%) + 65 beats·min^{-1}

THR = 32 + 65 = 97 beats·min^{-1} (for 40% heart rate reserve [HRR])

47 + 65 = 112 beats·min^{-1} (for 60% HRR)

Based on the exercise-induced ST-segment depression and reversible perfusion abnormality noted during the entry stress test, the prescribed exercise intensity should be at least 10 beats·min^{-1} below the ischemic ECG threshold (124 beats·min^{-1}).

Initial exercise intensity should be based on the estimated oxygen uptake reserve determined from the graded exercise test completed before cardiac rehab entry.

Training Range

An estimated reserve of 9 METs would suggest a training range of

4.6 METs ([9 × 40%] + 1 = 4.6 METs or 16.1 ml·kg^{-1}·min^{-1})

to

6.4 METs ([9 × 60%] + 1 = 6.4 METs or 22.4 ml·kg^{-1}·min^{-1}).

Mr. K enjoys treadmill walking and would like to maintain this activity. In addition, he would like to begin using a cycle ergometer. Given that he can comfortably walk 4 mph, a grade must be established on the treadmill to allow for adequate training and progression. In addition, workloads for the cycle ergometer must also be established (see the sidebar for these calculations). Accordingly, he would initiate his training program (40% V̇O$_2$ reserve) at 4 mph and 1.0% grade and progress to 60% V̇O$_2$ reserve, or 22.4 ml·kg^{-1}·min^{-1} (corresponding to 4.0 mph and 4.0% grade).

Workload Calculations

Treadmill

- 26.8 m·min^{-1} = 1 mph
- Meters × mph = 26.8 m·min^{-1} × 4 mph = 107.2 m·min^{-1}

thus,

- 16.1 ml·kg^{-1}·min^{-1} = (0.1 × speed) + (1.8 × speed × grade) + 3.5
- 16.1 ml·kg^{-1}·min^{-1} = (0.1 × 107.2) + (1.8 × 107.2 × grade) + 3.5
- 16.1 ml·kg^{-1}·min^{-1} = (0.1 × 107.2) + (193.0 × grade) + 3.5
- 16.1 ml·kg^{-1}·min^{-1} = 10.72 + (193.0 × grade) + 3.5
- 12.6 ml·kg^{-1}·min^{-1} = 10.72 + (193.0 × grade)
- 1.88 ml·kg^{-1}·min^{-1} = 193.0 (grade)
- 0.009 or (1%) = grade

Progressing to:

- 22.4 ml·kg^{-1}·min^{-1} = (0.1 × speed) + (1.8 × speed × grade) + 3.5
- 22.4 ml·kg^{-1}·min^{-1} = (0.1 × 107.2) + (1.8 × speed × grade) + 3.5

(continued)

(continued)

Progressing to *(continued)*:

- $18.9 \text{ ml·kg}^{-1}\text{·min}^{-1} = 10.72 + (193.0 \times \text{grade})$
- $8.18 \text{ ml·kg}^{-1}\text{·min}^{-1} = 193.0 \text{ (grade)}$
- $8.18 \div 193.0 = 0.04 \text{ or } (4\%) = \text{grade}$

Cycle Ergometer

- $\dot{V}O_2 = 7.0 + 1.8 \text{ (work rate)/(body mass)}$
- $16.1 \text{ ml·kg}^{-1}\text{·min}^{-1} = 7.0 + 1.8 \text{ (work rate)/(body mass)}$
- $16.1 \text{ ml·kg}^{-1}\text{·min}^{-1} = 7.0 + 1.8 \text{ (work rate)/81.8 kg}$
- $9.1 \text{ ml·kg}^{-1}\text{·min}^{-1} = 1.8 \text{ (work rate)/81.8}$
- $744.4 = 1.8 \text{ (work rate)}$
- $744.4 \div 1.8 = 413.6 = 414 \text{ kg·m·min}^{-1} = \text{work rate}$
- $\dot{V}O_2 = 7.0 + 1.8 \text{ (work rate)/(body mass)}$
- $22.4 \text{ ml·kg}^{-1}\text{·min}^{-1} = 7.0 + 1.8 \text{ (work rate)/(body mass)}$
- $22.4 \text{ ml·kg}^{-1}\text{·min}^{-1} = 7.0 + 1.8 \text{ (work rate)/81.8 kg}$
- $15.4 \text{ ml·kg}^{-1}\text{·min}^{-1} = 1.8 \text{ (work rate)/81.8}$
- $1259.7 = 1.8 \text{ (work rate)}$
- $700 \text{ kg·m·min}^{-1} = \text{work rate}$

The prescribed exercise intensity should fall within a rating of perceived exertion (RPE) level of "fairly light" to "somewhat hard" (11-13 on the 6-20 scale), especially during the initial weeks of an outpatient exercise training program.

A recommended starting duration is approximately 15 to 30 min, which should be complemented by 5- and 10-min warm-up and cool-down periods, respectively. Additional emphasis could also be placed on flexibility exercises during the cool-down period on 2 or 3 days of the week.

This exercise program should be followed for a minimum of 3 days per week, emphasizing progression to 5 days per week within 3 to 6 months. This patient should also be counseled to increase physical activity in daily living. As with the progression in frequency and duration, an increase in exercise intensity should occur over time, depending on the patient's response to training. This prescription should be reevaluated after 6 months.

Case Study 2

Mrs. L is a 67-year-old retired waitress who was admitted to the hospital emergency center with severe dyspnea and mild (3/10) left-sided chest pressure. Her medical history includes a previous inferior and lateral-wall myocardial infarction (7 years ago) and coronary artery bypass surgery (also 7 years ago) involving a left internal mammary artery graft to the LAD artery and saphenous vein grafts to the circumflex and obtuse marginal branches, respectively. She completed 18 sessions of an exercise-based outpatient cardiac rehabilitation program at that time and was discharged with no complications.

The patient has a history of elevated cholesterol, obesity (BMI = 31.3 kg·m^{-2}), and chronic heart failure (New York Heart Association class III). She is currently sedentary and had a 30-pack-year history of smoking before quitting 10 years ago.

Echocardiographic studies in the emergency center revealed a left ventricular ejection fraction of 30% with akinesis in the apical and lateral ventricular walls. Mild mitral and tricuspid valve regurgitation were also noted.

A peak or symptom-limited graded exercise test with concomitant measures of peak oxygen consumption was performed (at her physician's request) while she was in the hospital. The results of the test are outlined in the sidebar.

Symptom-Limited Graded Exercise Test Results

Protocol: Modified Bruce

Current Medications

furosemide, metroprolol, enalapril, potassium, digoxin

Resting Values

- HR: 50 beats·min^{-1}
- Supine BP: 110/64 mm Hg
- Standing BP: 106/68 mm Hg
- Resting ECG: normal sinus rhythm, left axis deviation, left anterior fascicular block, significant lateral Q waves, poor R-wave progression in the anterior leads with nonspecific lateral ST-segment depression

(continued)

End Point

- Peak workload: 2.5 mph/12% grade
- Total walking time: 10 min
- Peak HR = 120 beats·min^{-1} (78% predicted maximum)
- Peak BP = 135/60 mm Hg
- Peak oxygen consumption (measured): 15.8 ml·kg^{-1}·min^{-1} (4.5 METs)
- Test was terminated secondary to moderately severe dyspnea and fatigue.
- No chest pressure was reported.

No additional ST-segment depression was noted during exercise or in recovery. Isolated premature ventricular contractions (PVCs) at peak exercise and occasional premature atrial contractions were noted, primarily during submaximal exercise.

Mrs. L would like to begin exercise therapy using the treadmill that she has purchased for her home. She prefers adding an incline to a comfortable 2.0 mph walking pace and typically walks at a grade of 3.5%. She wants to know if this grade is still appropriate for her.

On her recent stress test, Mrs. L demonstrated a functional capacity of 4.5 METs. It is recommended that she exercise at an intensity corresponding to 40% to 60% of her maximal oxygen uptake reserve, or 2.4 to 3.1 METs. Walking at her desired pace would approximate the aerobic requirements as seen in the sidebar.

Aerobic Requirements

- $\dot{V}O_2 = (0.1 \times \text{speed}) + (1.8 \times \text{speed} \times \text{grade}) + 3.5$
- $= (0.1 \times 53.6) + (1.8 \times 53.6 \times 0.035) + 3.5$
- $= 5.36 + 3.38 + 3.5$
- $\dot{V}O_2 = 12.2$ ml·kg^{-1}·min^{-1} or 3.5 METs

Thus, this workload (i.e., 2 mph, 3.5% grade) would be slightly higher than the desired intensity, corresponding to approximately 70% of her maximal oxygen uptake reserve. Reducing the grade from 3.5% to 2.0% would achieve the desired upper limit (60% of maximal oxygen uptake reserve). In addition, Mrs. L should focus on adequate warm-up and cool-down periods, approximating 10 min each, and avoid pure isometric exercises.

Training should occur a minimum of 3 days per week, with an ultimate goal of daily exercise. In addition, multiple short-duration exercise bouts, lasting approximately 20 to 25 min, should be used to accommodate for initial deconditioning and dyspnea. Progression of exercise should focus on the lengthening of exercise sessions to approximately 30 to 40 min per session, while increasing the number of exercise days per week to 4 or 5.

Emphasis should be placed on using perceived exertion and dyspnea scales to modulate the exercise intensity, rather than relying solely on the chronotropic response to exercise. Target work levels should range between "fairly light" and "somewhat hard," corresponding to 11 to 13 on the Borg scale (6-20), using moderate dyspnea (+2/4) as the upper intensity limit for training.

Abbreviations

ACC—American College of Cardiology

ACE—angiotensin-converting enzyme

ACS—acute coronary syndrome

ACSM—American College of Sports Medicine

ADA—American Diabetes Association

AHA—American Heart Association

AHCPR—Agency for Health Care Policy and Research

ARB—angiotensin receptor blocker

ARIC—Atherosclerosis in Communities

AT—anaerobic threshold

ATP—adenosine triphosphate

ATP III— Adult Treatment Panel III

ATP-PCr—adenosine triphosphate-phosphocreatine

AV—atrioventricular

AVNRT—AV nodal reentry tachycardia

$(a-\bar{v})O_2$—difference between arterial and venous oxygen

AVRT—AV reciprocating tachycardia

BARI—Bypass Angioplasty Revascularization Investigation

BBB—bundle branch block

BMI—body mass index

BP—blood pressure

CABG—coronary artery bypass graft

CAD—coronary artery disease

CARE—Cholesterol and Recurrent Events

CASS—Coronary Artery Surgery Study

CHD—coronary heart disease

CHF—congestive heart failure

CMV—cytomegalovirus

CO_2—carbon dioxide

COPD—chronic obstructive pulmonary disease

CPB—cardiopulmonary bypass

CR—cardiac rehabilitation

CRP—C-reactive protein

CVD—cardiovascular disease

CVR—cardiovascular rehabilitation

DART—Diet and Reinfarction Trial

DASH—Dietary Approaches to Stop Hypertension

DCA—directional coronary atherectomy

DM—diabetes mellitus

EAMI—Exercise in Anterior Myocardial Infarction

ECAT—European Concerted Action on Thrombosis and Disabilities Study

ECG—electrocardiogram

ELVD—Exercise in Left Ventricular Dysfunction

ERA—Estrogen Replacement and Atherosclerosis

EXERT—Exercise Rehabilitation Trial

F_EO_2—fractional amount of oxygen in expired air

FEV_1—forced expiratory volume in 1 s

F_IO_2—fractional amount of oxgen in inspired air

4S—Scandinavian Simvastatin Survival Trial

FRISC II—Fragmin and Fast Revascularization During Instability in Coronary Artery Disease II

GISSI—Gruppo Italiano per lo Studio della Sopravvivenza nell'Infarto Miocardico

Hb—hemoglobin

Hcy—homocysteine

HDL—high-density lipoprotein

HERS—Heart and Estrogen/Progestin Replacement Study

HR—heart rate

HRmax—maximum heart rate

HRR—heart rate reserve

HRrest—resting heart rate

HRT—hormone replacement therapy

hs-CRP—high sensitive C-reactive protein

ICS—intercostal space

IDL—intermediate-density lipoprotein

JNC VII—Seventh Report of the Joint National Committee on Prevention, Detection, Evaluation and Treatment of High Blood Pressure

LA—left arm

LAD—left anterior descending

LAFB—left anterior fascicular block

LBBB—left bundle branch block

LCA—left circumflex artery

LDL—low-density lipoprotein

LIMA—left internal mammary artery

LIPID—Long-Term Intervention With Pravastatin in Ischemic Disease

LL—left leg

Lp(a)—lipoprotein(a)
LPFB—left posterior fascicular block
LV—left ventricular
MASS—Medicine, Angioplasty, or Surgery Study
METs—metabolic equivalents
MI—myocardial infarction
MIDCAB—minimally invasive direct coronary artery bypass
MILIS—Multicenter Investigation of the Limitation of Infarct Size
MNT—medical nutrition therapy
MUFA—monounsaturated fats
NACI—Newer Approaches to Coronary Interventions
NCEP—National Cholesterol Education Program
NQMI—non-Q-wave myocardial infarction
NSTE-ACS—non-ST-segment-elevation acute coronary syndrome
NSTEMI—non-ST-elevation myocardial infarction
OM—obtuse marginal
PAC—premature atrial contraction
PAD—peripheral artery disease
PAI-1—plasminogen activator inhibitor
P_aO_2—partial pressure of alveolar oxygen
PCI—percutaneous coronary intervention
PCO_2—partial pressure of carbon dioxide
PDA— posterior descending artery
PET—positron emission tomography
^{31}P-MRS—phosphorous-31 magnetic resonance spectroscopy
PSVT—paroxysmal supraventricular tachycardia
PTCA—percutaneous transluminal coronary angioplasty
PUFA—polyunsaturated fats
PVC—premature ventricular contraction
RA—right arm
RBBB—right bundle branch block
RCA—right coronary artery

RCT—randomized controlled trial
RF—risk factor
RPE—rating of perceived exertion
RV—right ventricular
RVMI—right ventricular myocardial infarction
SA—sinoatrial
SAFA—saturated fats
SBP—systolic blood pressure
SCRIP—Stanford Coronary Risk Intervention Project
SES—socioeconomic status
SF—saturated fats
SHEP—Systolic Hypertension in the Elderly Program
STARS—St. Thomas Atherosclerosis Trial
STEMI—ST-elevation myocardial infarction
SVG—saphenous vein graft
SVT—supraventricular tachycardia
SYST-EUR—Systolic Hypertension Europe
TdP—torsade de pointes
THR—target heart rate
TIMI IIIB—Thrombosis in Myocardial Ischemia IIIB
TNF—tumor necrosis factor
TONE—Trial of Nonpharmacologic Intervention in the Elderly
tPA—tissue plasminogen activator
TPR—total peripheral resistance
$T\dot{V}O_2$—target $\dot{V}O_2$
VANQWISH—Veterans Affairs Non-Q-Wave Infarction Strategies in Hospital
VCO_2—carbon dioxide production
$\dot{V}_E$—minute ventilation
VLDL—very low density lipoprotein
$\dot{V}O_2$—oxygen uptake
$\dot{V}O_2$max—maximal oxygen uptake
$\dot{V}O_2$peak—peak oxygen uptake
$\dot{V}O_2$R—oxygen consumption reserve
VT—ventricular tachycardia
WISE—Women's Ischemia Syndrome Evaluation

References

Chapter 1

1. Enos WF, Holmes RH, Beyer J. Coronary disease among United States soldiers killed in action in Korea: Preliminary report. *JAMA* 1953;152:1090-1093.

2. Kadar A, Mozes G, Illyes G, et al. WHO-ISFC pathological determinants of atherosclerosis in youth study. *Nutr Metab Cardiovasc Dis* 1999;9:220-227.

3. McGill HC. Origin of atherosclerosis in childhood and adolescence. *Am J Clin Nutr* 200;72:1307S-1315S.

4. Stary HC, Blankenhorn DH, Chandler AB, et al. A definition of advanced lesions and classification of arteriosclerosis. *Circulation* 1995;92:1355-1374.

5. Stary HC, Chandler AB, Glagov S, et al. A definition of initial, fatty streak and intermediate lesions of atherosclerosis. *Circulation* 1994;89:2462-2478.

6. American Heart Association. *ACLS Provider Manual.* Dallas: American Heart Association, 2001, p. 125.

7. Kadar A, Glasz T. Development of atherosclerosis and plaque biology. *Cardiovasc Surg* 2001;9:109-121.

8. Ross R. The pathogenesis of arteriosclerosis: A perspective for the 1990s. *Nature* 1993;362:801-809.

9. Glagov S, Bassiouny HS, Giddens DP, et al. Pathobiology of plaque modeling and complication. *Surg Clin North Am* 1995;75:545-556.

10. Ridker PM. Inflammation, atherosclerosis, and cardiovascular risk: An epidemiologic view. *Blood Coagul Fibrinolysis* 1999;10:S9-S12.

11. Albert NM. Inflammation and infection in acute coronary syndromes. *J Cardiovasc Nurs* 2000;15:13-26.

12. Libby P. Atherosclerosis: The new view. *Scientific American* May 2002:46-55

13. Frothingham C. The relationship between acute infectious diseases and arterial lesions. *Arch Intern Med* 1911;8:153-162.

14. Epstein SE, Zhou YF, Zhu J. Infection and atherosclerosis. Emerging mechanistic paradigms. *Circulation* 1999;100:1-9.

15. Braunwald E. Shattuck Lecture—Cardiovascular medicine at the turn of the millennium: Triumphs, concerns, and opportunities. *N Engl J Med* 1997;337:1360-1369.

16. Zhou YF, Laon MB, Waclawiw MA, et al. Association between prior cytomegalovirus infection and the risk of restenosis after coronary atherectomy. *N Engl J Med* 1996;335:624-630.

17. Valentine HA, Gao SZ, Menon SG, et al. Impact of prophylactic immediate post-transplant ganclivor on development of transplant atherosclerosis: A post hoc analysis of a randomized, placebo controlled study. *Circulation* 1999;100:61-66.

18. Ventura HO, Mehra MR, Smart FW, Stapleton DD. Cardiac allograft vasculopathy: Current concepts. *Am Heart J* 1995;129:791-798.

19. Mawhorter SD, Lauer MA. Is atherosclerosis an infectious disease? *Cleve Clin J Med* 2001;68:449-458.

20. Ross R. Atherosclerosis—An inflammatory disease. *N Engl J Med* 1999;340:115-126.

21. Libby P, Egan D, Skarlatos S. Roles of infectious agents in atherosclerosis and restenosis: An assessment of the evidence and need for future research. *Circulation* 1997;96:4094-4103.

22. Torgano G, Costentini R, Mandelli C, et al. Treatment for *Helicobacter pylori* and *Chlamydia pneumoniae* infections decreases fibrinogen plasma level in patients with ischemic heart disease. *Circulation* 1999;99:1555-1559.

23. Schmitz G, Aslanidis C, Lackner KJ. Recent advances in molecular genetics of cardiovascular disorders. Implications for atherosclerosis and diseases of cellular lipid metabolism. *Pathol Oncol Res* 1998;4:152-160.

24. Wenzel K, Blackburn A, Ernst M, et al. Relations of polymorphism in the renin-angiotensin system and E-selectin of patients with early severe coronary heart disease. *J Mol Med* 1997;75:57-61.

25. Wang XL, Sim AS, Badenhop RF, et al. A smoking dependent risk of coronary artery disease associated with a polymorphism of the endothelial nitric oxide synthase gene. *Nat Med* 1996;2:41-45.

26. Wenzel K, Felix S, Kleber FX, et al. E-selectin polymorphism and arteriosclerosis: An association study. *Hum Mole Genet* 1994;11:1935-1937.

Chapter 2

1. Westaby S. *Landmarks in Cardiac Surgery.* Oxford, UK: Isis Medical Media, 1997.

2. Gruntzig AR, Senning A, Siegenthaler WE. Nonoperative dilation of coronary artery stenosis: Percutaneous transluminal coronary angioplasty. *N Engl J Med* 1979;301:61-68.

3. American Heart Association. *Heart Disease and Stroke Statistics–2005 Update.* Dallas: American Heart Association, 2005.

4. Rogers WJ, Coggin CJ, Gersh BJ, et al. Ten-year follow-up of quality of life in patients randomized to receive medical therapy or coronary artery bypass graft surgery: The coronary artery surgery study (CASS). *Circulation* 1990;82:1647-1658.

5. Bypass Angioplasty Revascularization Investigation (BARI) Investigators. Comparison of coronary bypass surgery with angioplasty in patients with multivessel disease. *N Engl J Med* 1996;335:217-225.

6. CABRI Trial Participants. First-year results of CABRI (coronary angioplasty versus bypass revascularization investigation). *Lancet* 1995;346:1179-1184.

7. Eagle KA, Guyton RA, Davidoff R, et al. ACC/AHA guidelines for coronary artery bypass graft surgery. *J Am Coll Cardiol* 1999;34:1262-1346.

8. Hamm CW, Reimers J, Ischinger T, et al. A randomized study of coronary angioplasty compared with bypass surgery in patients with symptomatic multivessel coronary disease: German angioplasty bypass surgery investigation. *N Engl J Med* 1994;331:1037-1043.

9. Hueb WA, Bellotti G, de Oliveira SA, et al. The medicine, angioplasty, or surgery study (MASS): A prospective, randomized trial of medical therapy, balloon angioplasty or bypass surgery for single proximal left anterior descending artery stenoses. *J Am Coll Cardiol* 1995;26:1600-1605.

10. King, SBI, Lembo NJ, Weintraub WS, et al. A randomized trial comparing coronary angioplasty with coronary bypass surgery: Emory angioplasty versus bypass trial (EAST). *N Engl J Med* 1994;331:1044-1050.

11. RITA Trial Participants. Coronary angioplasty versus coronary artery bypass surgery: The Randomized Intervention Treatment of Angina (RITA) trial. *Lancet* 1993;341:573-580.

12. Rodriguez A, Boullon F, Periez-Balino N, et al. Argentine randomized trial of percutaneous transluminal coronary angioplasty versus coronary artery bypass surgery in multivessel disease (ERACI): In-hospital and 1-year follow-up. *J Am Coll Cardiol* 1993;22:1060-1070.

13. Chaitman BR, Fisher LD, Bourassa MG, et al. Effect of coronary bypass surgery on survival patterns in subsets of patients with left main coronary artery disease: Report of the Collaborative Study in Coronary Artery Surgery (CASS). *Am J Cardiol* 1981;48:765-777.

14. Detre KM, Guo P, Holubkov R, et al. Influence of diabetes on 5-year mortality and morbidity in a randomized trial comparing CABG and PTCA in patients with multivessel disease: The Bypass Angioplasty Revascularization Investigation (BARI). *Circulation* 1997;96:1761-1769.

15. Roach GW, Kanchuger M, Mangano CM, et al. Adverse cerebral outcomes after coronary bypass surgery: Multicenter study of perioperative ischemia research group and the ischemia research and education foundation investigators. *N Engl J Med* 1996;335:1857-1863.

16. Newman MF, Kirchner JL, Phillips-Bute B, et al. Longitudinal assessment of neurocognitive function after coronary bypass surgery. *N Engl J Med* 2001;344:395-402.

17. Van Dijk D, Jansen EW, Hijman R, et al. Cognitive outcome after off-pump and on-pump coronary artery bypass graft surgery: A randomized trial. *JAMA* 2002;287:1448-1450.

18. Milano CA, Kesler K, Archibald N, et al. Mediastinitis after coronary artery bypass graft surgery: Risk factors and long-term survival. *Circulation* 1995;92:2245-2251.

19. Nagachinta T, Stephens M, Reitz B, et al. Risk factors for surgical-wound infection following cardiac surgery. *J Infect Dis* 1987;156:967-973.

20. Fitzgibbon GM, Kafka HP, Leach AJ, et al. Coronary bypass fate and patient outcome: Angiographic follow-up of 5,065 grafts related to survival and reoperation in 1,388 patients during 25 years. *J Am Coll Cardiol* 1996;28:616-626.

21. Angelini GD, Taylor FC, Reeves BC, et al. Early and midterm outcome after off-pump and on-pump surgery in Beating Heart Against Cardioplegic Arrest Studies (BHACAS 1 and 2): A pooled analysis of two randomised controlled trials. *Lancet* 2002;359:1194-1199.

22. Borst C, Santamore W, Smedira NG, et al. Minimally invasive coronary artery bypass grafting: On the beating heart and via limited access. *Ann Thorac Surg* 1997;63(suppl):S1-S5.

23. Diegeler A, Hirsh R, Schneider F, et al. Neuromonitoring and neurocognitive outcome in off-pump versus conventional coronary bypass operation. *Ann Thorac Surg* 2000;69:1162-1166.

24. Lloyd CT, Ascione R, Underwood MJ, et al. Serum S-100 protein release and neuropsychological outcome during coronary revascularization on the beating heart: A prospective randomized study. *J Thorac Cardiovasc Surg* 2000;119:148-154.

25. American Association of Cardiovascular and Pulmonary Rehabilitation. *Guidelines for Cardiac Rehabilitation and Secondary Prevention Programs.* Fourth Edition. Champaign, IL: Human Kinetics, 2004.

26. Pollock ML, Franklin BA, Balady GJ, et al. AHA Science Advisory. Resistance exercise in individuals with and without cardiovascular disease. *Circulation* 2000;101:828-833.

27. Mintz GS, Pichard AD, Kent KM, et al. Axial plaque redistribution as a mechanism of percutaneous transluminal coronary angioplasty. *Am J Cardiol* 1996;77:427-430.

28. Potkin BN, Keren G, Mintz GS, et al. Arterial responses to balloon coronary angioplasty: An intravascular ultrasound study. *J Am Coll Cardiol* 1992;20:942-951.

29. Elliot JM, Berdan LG, Holmes DR, et al. One year follow-up in the coronary angioplasty versus excisional atherectomy trial (CAVEAT). *Circulation* 1995;91:2158-2166.

30. Holmes DR, Topol EJ, Califf RM, et al. A multicenter, randomized trial of coronary angioplasty versus directional atherectomy for patients with saphenous vein bypass graft lesions: Caveat II. *Circulation* 1995;91:1966-1974.

31. Lefkovits J, Holmes DR, Califf RM, et al. Predictors and sequelae of distal embolization during saphenous vein graft intervention from the CAVEAT-II trial. *Circulation* 1995;92:734-740.

32. Giri S, Ito S, Lansky AJ, et al. Clinical and angiographic outcome in the Laser Angioplasty for Restenotic Stents (LARS) multicenter registry. *Catheter Cardiovasc Interv* 2001;52:24-34.

33. Koster R, Kahler J, Terres W, et al. Six-month clinical and angiographic outcome after successful excimer laser angioplasty for in-stent restenosis. *J Am Coll Cardiol* 2000;36:69-74.

34. Mehran R, Mintz GS, Satler LF, et al. Treatment of in-stent restenosis with excimer laser coronary angioplasty: Mechanisms and results compared with PTCA alone. *Circulation* 1997;96:2183-2189.

35. Topaz O. Holmium laser angioplasty. *Semin Interv Cardiol* 1996;1:149-161.

36. Levine GN, Ali MN. The role of percutaneous revascularization in the treatment of ischemic heart disease. *Chest* 1997;112:805-821.

37. Danchin N, Brengard A, Etheveno G, et al. Ten year follow up of patients with single vessel coronary artery disease that was suitable for percutaneous transluminal coronary angioplasty. *Br Heart J* 1988;59:269-275.

38. Mark DB, Nelson CL, Califf RM, et al. Continuing evolution of therapy for coronary artery disease: Initial results from the era of coronary angioplasty. *Circulation* 1994;89:2015-2035.

39. Parisi AF, Folland ED, Hartigan P. A comparison of angioplasty with medical therapy in the treatment of single-vessel coronary artery disease. *N Engl J Med* 1992;326:10-16.

40. Straus WE, Fortin T, Hartigan P, et al. A comparison of quality of life scores in patients with angina pectoris after angioplasty compared with after medical therapy: Outcomes of a randomized clinical trial. *Circulation* 1995;92:1710-1719.

41. Folland ED, Hartigan PM, Parisi AF. Percutaneous transluminal coronary angioplasty versus medical therapy for stable angina pectoris: Outcomes for patients with double-vessel versus single-vessel coronary artery disease in a Veterans Affairs Cooperative randomized trial. *J Am Coll Cardiol* 1997;29:1512-1514.

42. Folland ED, Parisi AF, Hartigan P, et al. PTCA vs medicine for double vessel disease: Initial results of the randomized VA ACME trial. *Circulation* 1991;84(suppl):II-252.

43. The TIMI IIIB Investigators. Effects of tissue plasminogen activator and a comparison of early invasive and conservative strategies in unstable angina and non-Q-wave myocardial infarction: Results of the TIMI IIIB trial: Thrombolysis in Myocardial Ischemia. *Circulation* 1994;89:1545-1556.

44. FRagmin and Fast Revascularization during InStability in Coronary artery disease (FRISC) Investigators. Invasive compared with non-invasive treatment in unstable coronary-artery disease: FRISC II prospective randomized multicentre study. *Lancet* 1999;354:708-715.

45. Cannon CP, Weintraub WS, Demopoulos LA, et al. Comparison of early invasive and conservative strategies in patients with unstable coronary syndromes treated with the glycoprotein IIb/IIIa inhibitor tirofiban. *N Engl J Med* 2001;344:1879-1887.

46. Wallentin L, Lagerqvist B, Husted S, et al. Outcome at 1 year after an invasive compared with a non-invasive strategy in unstable coronary-artery disease: The FRISC II invasive randomised trial. *Lancet* 2000;356:9-16.

47. Braunwald E, Antman EM, Beasley JW, et al. ACC/AHA guideline update for the management of patients with unstable angina and non-ST-segment elevation myocardial infarction. Available at: http://acc.org/clinical/guideline/unstable/unstable.pdf. Accessed November, 2000.

48. Michels KB, Yusuf, S. Does PTCA in acute myocardial infarction affect mortality and reinfarction rates? A quantitative overview (meta-analysis) of the randomized clinical trials. *Circulation* 1995;91:476-485.

49. Nasser TK, Mohler ER, Wilenksy RL, et al. Peripheral vascular complications following coronary interventional procedures. *Clin Cardiol* 1995;18:609-614.

50. Moscucci M, Mansour KA, Kent C, et al. Peripheral vascular complications of directional atherectomy and stenting: Predictors, management, and outcome. *Am J Cardiol* 1994;74:448-453.

51. Cutlip DE, Baim DS, Kalon KL, et al. Stent thrombosis in the modern era: A pooled analysis of multicenter coronary stent clinical trials. *Circulation* 2001;103:1967-1971.

52. Karrillon GJ, Morice MC, Benveniste E, et al. Intracoronary stent implantation without ultrasound guidance and with replacement of conventional anticoagulation by antiplatelet therapy: 30-day clinical outcome of the French Multicenter Registry. *Circulation* 1996;94:1519-1527.

53. Moussa I, Mario CD, Reimers B, et al. Subacute stent thrombosis in the era of intravascular ultrasound-guided coronary stenting without anticoagulation: Frequency, predictors and clinical outcome. *J Am Coll Cardiol* 1997;29:6-12.

54. Fischman DL, Leon M, Baim DS, et al. A randomized comparison of coronary stent placement and balloon angioplasty in the treatment of coronary artery disease. *N Engl J Med* 1994;331:496-501.

55. Haude M, Erbe R, Issa H, et al. Subacute thrombotic complications after intracoronary implantation of Palmaz-Schatz stents. *Am Heart J* 1993;126:15-22.

56. Nath FC, Muller DWM, Ellis SG, et al. Thrombosis of a flexible coil coronary stent: Frequency, predictors and clinical outcome. *J Am Coll Cardiol* 1993;21:622-627.

57. Schatz RA, Baim DS, Leon M, et al. Clinical experience with the Palmaz-Schatz coronary stent: Initial results of a multicenter study. *Circulation* 1991;83:148-161.

58. Serruys PW, de Jaegere P, Kiemeneij F, et al. A comparison of balloon-expandable stent implantation with balloon angioplasty in patients with coronary artery disease. *N Engl J Med* 1994;331:489-495.

59. Serruys PW, Strauss BH, Beatt KJ, et al. Angiographic follow-up after placement of a self-expanding coronary-artery stent. *N Engl J Med* 1991;324:13-17.

60. Colombo A, Hall P, Nakamura S, et al. Intracoronary stenting without anticoagulation accomplished with intravascular ultrasound guidance. *Circulation* 1995;91:1676-1688.

61. Goldberg SL, Colombo A, Nakamura S, et al. The benefit of intracoronary ultrasound in the deployment of Palmaz-Schatz stents. *J Am Coll Cardiol* 1994;24:996-1003.

62. Nakamura S, Hall P, Gaglione A, et al. High pressure assisted coronary stent implantation accomplished without intravascular ultrasound guidance and subsequent anticoagulation. *J Am Coll Cardiol* 1997;29:21-27.

63. Albiero R, Hall P, Itoh, A, et al. Results of a consecutive series of patients receiving only antiplatelet therapy after optimized stent implantation. *Circulation* 1997;95:1145-1156.

64. Berger PB, Bell MR, Hasdai D, et al. Safety and efficacy of ticlopidine for only 2 weeks after successful intracoronary stent placement. *Circulation* 1999;99:248-253.

65. Berger PB, Bell MR, Rihal CS, et al. Clopidogrel versus ticlopidine after intracoronary stent placement. *J Am Coll Cardiol* 1999;34:1891-1894.

66. Bertrand ME, Rupprecht HJ, Urban P, et al. Double-blind study of the safety of clopidogrel with and without a loading dose in combination with aspirin compared with ticlodipine in combination with aspirin after coronary stenting: The Clopidogrel Aspirin Stent International Cooperative Study (CLASSICS). *Circulation* 2000;102:624-629.

67. Leon MD, Baim DS, Popma JJ, et al. A clinical trial comparing three antithrombotic-drug regimens after coronary-artery stenting. *N Engl J Med* 1998;339:1665-1671.

68. Schomig A, Neumann FJ, Kastrati A, et al. A randomized comparison of antiplatelet and anticoagulant therapy after the placement of coronary-artery stents. *N Engl J Med* 1996;334:1084-1089.

69. Schuhlen H, Kastrati A, Pache J, et al. Incidence of thrombotic occlusion and major adverse cardiac events between two and four weeks after coronary stent placement: Analysis of 5,678 patients with a four-week ticlopidine regimen. *J Am Coll Cardiol* 2001;37:2066-2073.

70. Bertrand ME, Legrand V, Boland J, et al. Randomized multicenter comparison of conventional anticoagulation versus antiplatelet therapy in unplanned and elective coronary stenting: The full anticoagulation versus aspirin and ticlopidine (FANTASTIC) study. *Circulation* 2001;98:1597-1603.

71. Urban P, Macaya C, Rupprecht HJ, et al. Randomized evaluation of anticoagulation versus antiplatelet therapy after coronary stent implantation in high-risk patients: The Multicenter Aspirin and Ticlopidine Trial after Intracoronary Stenting (MATTIS). *Circulation* 1998;98:2126-2132.

72. Bhatt DL, Bertrand ME, Berger PB, et al. Meta-analysis of randomized and registry comparisons of ticlopi-dine with clopidogrel after stenting. *J Am Coll Cardiol* 2002;39:9-14.

73. Dangas G, Mehran R, Abizaid AS, et al. Combination therapy with aspirin plus clopidogrel versus aspirin plus ticlopidine for prevention of subacute thrombosis after successful native coronary stenting. *Am J Cardiol* 2001;87:470-472.

74. Mishkel GJ, Aguirre FV, Ligon RW, et al. Clopidogrel as adjunctive antiplatelet therapy during coronary stenting. *J Am Coll Cardiol* 1999;34:1884-1890.

75. Moussa I, Oetgen M, Roubin G, et al. Effectiveness of clopidogrel and aspirin versus ticlopidine and aspirin in preventing stent thrombosis after coronary stent implantation. *Circulation* 1999;99:2364-2366.

76. Muller C, Buttner HJ, Peterson J, et al. A randomized comparison of clopidogrel and aspirin versus ticlopidine and aspirin after the placement of coronary artery stents. *Circulation* 2000;101:590-593.

77. Smith SC, Dove JT, Jacobs AK, et al. ACC/AHA guidelines for percutaneous coronary intervention: A report of the American College of Cardiology/American Heart Association Task Force on Practice Guidelines (Committee to Revise the 1993 Guidelines for Percutaneous Transluminal Coronary Angioplasty). *J Am Coll Cardiol* 2001;37:2215-2238.

78. Kuntz RE, Gibson CM, Nobuyoshi M, et al. Generalized model of restenosis after conventional balloon angioplasty, stenting and directional atherectomy. *J Am Coll Cardiol* 1993;21:15-25.

79. Mintz GS, Popma JJ, Pichard AD, et al. Arterial remodeling after coronary angioplasty: A serial intravascular ultrasound study. *Circulation* 1996;94:35-43.

80. Sangiorgi G, Taylor AJ, Farb A, et al. Histopathology of postpercutaneous transluminal coronary angioplasty remodeling in human coronary arteries. *Am Heart J* 1999;138:681-687.

81. Levine GN, Chodos AP, Loscalzo J. Restenosis following coronary angioplasty: Clinical presentations and therapeutic options. *Clin Cardiol* 1995;18:693-703.

82. Rose B, Pepine CJ. Restenosis following coronary angioplasty: Patterns, recognition, and results of repeat angioplasty. *Cardiovasc Clin* 1988;9:233-251.

83. Serruys PW, Luijten HE, Beatt KJ, et al. Incidence of restenosis after successful coronary angioplasty: A time-related phenomenon. *Circulation* 1988;77:361-371.

84. Currier JW, Leitschuh ML. The management of patients following successful coronary angioplasty. In: *Practical Angioplasty*. Faxon DP (ed). New York: Raven Press, 1994, pp. 173-178.

85. Glazier JJ, Varricchione TR, Ryan TJ, et al. Outcome in patients with recurrent restenosis after percutaneous transluminal balloon angioplasty. *Br Heart J* 1989;61:485-488.

86. Holmes DR, Vliestra RE, Smith H, et al. Restenosis after percutaneous coronary transluminal angioplasty (PTCA): A report from the PTCA registry of the National Heart, Lung, and Blood Institute. *Am J Cardiol* 1984;53(suppl):77C-81C.

87. Joelson JM, Becker DJ, Most AS, et al. Initial presentation predicts clinical manifestations of restenosis after successful coronary angioplasty. *Circulation* 1988;78(suppl II):II-633.

88. Miller JM, Ohman EM, Moliterno DJ, et al. Restenosis: The clinical issues. In: *Textbook of Interventional Cardiology*. Third Edition. Topol EJ (ed). Philadelphia: Saunders, 1999, pp. 379-415.

89. Piessens JH, Stammen F, Desmet W, et al. Immediate and 6-month follow-up results of coronary angioplasty for restenosis: Analysis of factors predicting recurrent clinical restenosis. *Am Heart J* 1993;126:565-570.

90. Quigley PJ, Hlatky MA, Hinohara T, et al. Repeat percutaneous transluminal coronary angioplasty and predictors of recurrent restenosis. *Am J Cardiol* 1989;63:409-413.

91. Weintraub WS, Ghazzal ZMB, Douglas JS, et al. Initial management and long-term clinical outcome of restenosis after initially successful percutaneous transluminal coronary angioplasty. *Am J Cardiol* 1992;70:47-55.

92. Joelson JM, Most AS, Williams DO. Angiographic findings when chest pain recurs after successful percutaneous transluminal coronary angioplasty. *Am J Cardiol* 1987;60:792-795.

93. Al Suwaidi J, Berger PB, Holmes DR. Coronary artery stents. *JAMA* 2000;284:1828-1836.

94. Antoniucci D, Santoro GM, Bolognese L, et al. A clinical trial comparing stenting of the infarct-related artery with optimal primary angioplasty for acute myocardial infarction. *J Am Coll Cardiol* 1998;31:1234-1239.

95. Betriu A, Masotti M, Serra A, et al. Randomized comparison of coronary stent implantation and balloon angioplasty in the treatment of de novo coronary artery lesions (START). *J Am Coll Cardiol* 1999;34:1498-1506.

96. Buller CE, Dzavik V, Carere RG, et al. Primary stenting versus balloon angioplasty in occluded coronary arteries: The Total Occlusion Study of Canada (TOSCA). *Circulation* 1999;100:236-242.

97. Grines CL, Cox DA, Stone GW, et al. Coronary angioplasty with or without stent implantation for acute myocardial infarction. *N Engl J Med* 1999;341:1949-1956.

98. Hanekamp CCE, Koolen JJ, Den Heyer P, et al. A randomized comparison between balloon angioplasty and elective stent implantation in venous bypass grafts: The Venestent study. *J Am Coll Cardiol* 2000;35(suppl A):9A.

99. Hoher M, Wohrle J, Grebe OC, et al. A randomized trial of elective stenting after balloon recanalization of chronic total occlusions. *J Am Coll Cardiol* 1999;34:722-729.

100. Saito S, Hosokawa G, Tanaka S, et al. Primary stent implantation is superior to balloon angioplasty in acute myocardial infarction. *Catheter Cardiovasc Interv* 1999;48:262-268.

101. Savage MP, Douglas JS, Fischman DL, et al. Stent placement compared with balloon angioplasty for obstructed coronary bypass grafts. *N Engl J Med* 1997;337:740-747.

102. Serruys PW, van Hout B, Bonnier H, et al. Randomised comparison of implantation of heparin-coated stents with balloon angioplasty in selected patients with coronary artery disease. *Lancet* 1998;352:673-681.

103. Sirnes PA, Golf S, Myreng Y, et al. Stenting in chronic coronary occlusion (SICCO): A randomized, controlled trial of adding stent implantation after successful angioplasty. *J Am Coll Cardiol* 1996;28:1444-1451.

104. The EPISTENT Investigators. Randomised placebo-controlled and balloon-angioplasty-controlled trial to assess safety of coronary stenting with use of platelet glycoprotein-IIb/IIIa blockade. *Lancet* 1998;352:87-92.

105. Versaci F, Gaspardone A, Tomai F, et al. A comparison of coronary-artery stenting with angioplasty for isolated stenosis of the proximal left anterior descending coronary artery. *N Engl J Med* 1997;336:817-822.

106. Weaver WD, Reisman MA, Griffin JJ, et al. Optimum percutaneous transluminal coronary angioplasty compared with routine stent strategy trial (OPUS-1): A randomised trial. *Lancet* 2000;355:2199-2203.

107. Goldberg SL, Berger P, Cohen DJ, et al. Rotational atherectomy of balloon angioplasty in the treatment of intra-stent restenosis: BARASTER multicenter registry. *Catheter Cardiovasc Interv* 2000;51:407-413.

108. Topol EJ, Leya F, Pinkerton CA, et al. A comparison of directional atherectomy with coronary angioplasty in patients with coronary artery disease. *N Engl J Med* 1993;329:221-227.

109. Baim DS, Cutlip DE, O'Shaughnessy CD, et al. Final results of a randomized trial comparing the NIR stent to the Palmaz-Schatz stent for narrowings in native coronary arteries. *Am J Cardiol* 200;187:152-156.

110. Calcer AL, Blows LJ, Harmer S, et al. Clopidogrel for prevention of major cardiac events after coronary stent implantation: 30-day and 6-month results in patients with smaller stents. *Am Heart J* 2000;140:483-491.

111. Cremonesi A, Benit E, Carlier M, et al. Multicenter registry to evaluate the efficacy of the NIROYAL stent in de novo or restenotic coronary stenosis. *J Invasive Cardiol* 2000;12:233-235.

112. de Jaegere P, Mudra H, Figulla H, et al. Intravascular ultrasound-guided optimized stent deployment. Immediate and 6 month clinical and angiographic results from the Multicenter Ultrasound Stenting in Coronaries Study (MUSIC Study). *Eur Heart J* 1998;19:1214-1223.

113. Di Mario C, Moses JW, Anderson TJ, et al. Randomized comparison of elective stent implantation and coronary balloon angioplasty guided by online quantitative angiography and intracoronary Doppler. *Circulation* 2000;102:2938-2944.

114. Holmes DR, Lansky A, Kuntz R, et al. The PARAGON stent study: A randomized trial of a new martensitic nitinol stent versus the Palmaz-Schatz stent for treatment of complex native coronary arterial lesions. *Am J Cardiol* 2000;86:1073-1079.

115. Kastrati A, Schuhlen SH, Hausleiter J, et al. Restenosis after coronary stent placement and randomization to a 4-week combined antiplatelet or anticoagulant therapy:

Six-month angiographic follow-up of the Intracoronary Stenting and Antithrombotic Regimen (ISAR) Trial. *Circulation* 1997;96:462-467.

116. Kereiakes DJ, Midei M, Hermiller J, et al. Procedural and late outcomes following multi-link duet coronary stent deployment. *Am J Cardiol* 1999;84:1385-1390.

117. Kobayashi Y, De Gregorio J, Kobayashi N, et al. Comparison of immediate and follow-up results of the short and long NIR stent with the Palmaz-Schatz stent. *Am J Cardiol* 1999;84:499-504.

118. Manolis AS. Reduced incidence of clinical restenosis with newer generation stents, stent oversizing, and high-pressure deployment: single-operator experience. *Clin Cardiol* 2001;24:119-126.

119. O'Shea JC, Hafley GE, Greenberg S, et al. Platelet glycoprotein IIb/IIIa integrin blockade with eptifibatide in coronary stent intervention: The ESPRIT trial: A randomized controlled trial. *JAMA* 2001;285:2468-2473.

120. Park SJ, Park SW, Lee CW, et al. Immediate results and late clinical outcomes after new crossflex coronary stent implantation. *Am J Cardiol* 1999;83:502-506.

121. Rodriguez A, Ayala F, Bernardi V, et al. Optimal coronary balloon angioplasty with provisional stenting versus primary stent (OCBAS): Immediate and long-term follow-up results. *J Am Coll Cardiol* 1998;32:1351-1357.

122. Topol EJ, Moliterno DJ, Herrmann HC, et al. Comparison of two platelet glycoprotein IIb/IIIa inhibitors, tirofiban and abciximab, for the prevention of ischemic events with percutaneous coronary revascularizations. *N Engl J Med* 2001;344:1888-1894.

123. Sousa JE, Serruys PW, Costa MA. New frontiers in cardiology. Drug-eluting stents: Part I. *Circulation* 2003;107:2274-2279.

124. Sousa JE, Serruts PW, Costa MA. New frontiers in cardiology. Drug-eluting stents: Part II. *Circulation* 2003;107:2383-2389.

125. Chenu PC, Schroeder E, Kremer R, et al. Long-term outcome of patients with asymptomatic restenosis after percutaneous transluminal coronary angioplasty. *Am J Cardiol* 1993;72:1209-1211.

126. Hernandez RA, Macaya C, Iniguez C, et al. Midterm outcome of patients with asymptomatic restenosis after coronary balloon angioplasty. *J Am Coll Cardiol* 1992;19:1402-1409.

127. Kovac JD, Brack MJ, Harley A, et al. Longer term clinical outcome in patients presenting with asymptomatic restenosis at 4 month trial angiography. *Circulation* 1995;92(suppl):I-347.

128. Laarman G, Luijten HE, van Zeyl LG, et al. Assessment of "silent" restenosis and long-term follow-up after successful angioplasty in single vessel coronary artery disease: The value of quantitative exercise electrocardiography and quantitative coronary angiography. *J Am Coll Cardiol* 1990;16:578-585.

129. Ritchie JL, Batemen TM, Bonow RO, et al. Guidelines for clinical use of cardiac radionuclide imaging: Report of the American College of Cardiology/American Heart Association Task Force on Assessment of Diagnostic and Therapeutic Cardiovascular Procedures (Committee on Radionuclide Imaging). *J Am Coll Cardiol* 1995;25:521-547.

130. Gibbons RJ, Balady GJ, Beasley JW, et al. ACC/AHA guidelines for exercise testing: A report of the American College of Cardiology/American Heart Association Task Force on Practice Guidelines (Committee on Exercise Testing). *J Am Coll Cardiol* 1997;30:260-315.

131. Baladay GJ, Leitschuh ML, Jacobs AK, et al. Safety and clinical use of exercise testing one to three days after percutaneous transluminal coronary angioplasty. *Am J Cardiol* 1992;69:1259-1264.

132. Sheppard R, Schechter D, Azoulay A, et al. Results of a routine exercise treadmill testing strategy early after percutaneous transluminal coronary angioplasty. *Can J Cardiol* 2001;17:407-414.

133. Bresiblatt WM, Wieland FL, Spaccavento LJ. Stress thallium-201 imaging after coronary angioplasty predicts restenosis and recurrent symptoms. *J Am Coll Cardiol* 1988;15(suppl A):52A.

134. Hecht HS, Shaw, RE, Chin HL, et al. Silent ischemia after coronary angioplasty: Evaluation of restenosis and extent of ischemia in asymptomatic patients by tomographic thallium-201 exercise imaging and comparison with symptomatic patients. *J Am Coll Cardiol* 1991;17:670-677.

135. Bengtson JR, Sheikh KH, Aboul-Enein H, et al. Exercise echocardiography is a valuable adjunct to treadmill testing for detection of restenosis after coronary angioplasty. *J Am Coll Cardiol* 1990;15(suppl A):52A.

136. Heinle SK, Lieberman EB, Ancukiewicz M, et al. Usefulness of dobutamine echocardiography for detecting restenosis after percutaneous transluminal coronary angioplasty. *Am J Cardiol* 1993;72:1220-1225.

137. Boden WE, O'Rourke RA, Crawford MH, et al. Outcomes in patients with acute non-Q-wave myocardial infarction randomly assigned to an invasive as compared with a conservative management strategy: Veterans Affairs Non-Q-Wave Infarction Strategies in Hospital (VANQWISH) trial. *N Engl J Med* 338;1998:1785-1792.

138. Serruys PW, Unger F, Sousa JE, et al. Comparison of coronary-artery bypass surgery and stenting for the treatment of multivessel disease. *N Engl J Med* 2001;344:1117-1124.

Chapter 3

1. Oldridge NB, Guyatt GH, Fisher ME, Rimm AA. Cardiac rehabilitation after myocardial infarction: Combined experience of randomized clinical trials. *JAMA* 1988;260:945-950.

2. O'Connor GT, Buring JE, Usuf S, et al. An overview of randomized trials of rehabilitation with exercise after myocardial infarction. *Circulation* 1989;80:234-244.

3. Smith SC, Blair SN, Criqui MH, et al. AHA consensus panel statement: Preventing heart attack and sudden death in patients with coronary artery disease. *Circulation* 1995;92:3-4.

4. Prevention of coronary heart disease in clinical practice: Recommendations of the Second Joint Task Force of European and Other Societies on Coronary Prevention. *Eur Heart J* 1998;19:1434-1503.

5. Simes RJ, Marschner IC, Hunt D, et al. Relationship between lipid levels and clinical outcomes in the Long-Term Intervention With Pravastatin in Ischemic Disease (LIPID) Trial. *Circulation* 2002;105:1162-1169.

6. Kannel WB, Willerson JT, Cohn JN (eds). Coronary risk factors: An overview. In: *Cardiovascular Medicine.* New York: Churchill Livingstone, 1995, p. 1816.

7. Grundy SM, Pasternak R, Greenland P, et al. Assessment of cardiovascular risk by use of multiple-risk-factor assessment equations: A statement for healthcare professionals from the American Heart Association and the American College of Cardiology. *Circulation* 1999;100:1481-1492.

8. Yusuf S, Hawken S, Ounpuu S, et al. Effect of potentially modifiable risk factors associated with myocardial infarction in 52 countries (the INTERHEART study): Case-control study. *Lancet* 2004;364(9438):937-952.

9. Forrester JS, Merz NB, Bush TL, et al. Task Force 4. Efficacy of risk factor management. *J Am Coll Cardiol* 1996;27:991-1005.

10. Fletcher GF, Balady GJ, Vogel RA. 33rd Bethesda Conference: Preventive cardiology: How can we do better? *J Am Coll Cardiol* 2002;579-6001.

11. Haskell WL, Alderman EL, Fair JM, et al. Effects of intensive multiple risk factor reduction on coronary atherosclerosis and clinical cardiac events in men and women with coronary artery disease: The Stanford Coronary Risk Intervention Project (SCRIP). *Circulation* 1994;89:975-990.

12. Ornish D, Scherwitz LW, Billings JH, et al. Intensive lifestyle changes for reversal of coronary heart disease. *JAMA* 1998;280:2001-2007.

13. Executive Summary of the Third Report of the National Cholesterol Education Program (NCEP) Expert Panel on Detection, Evaluation, and Treatment of High Blood Cholesterol in Adults (Adult Treatment Panel III). *JAMA* 2001;285:2486-2497.

14. Nordmann A, Heilmbauer I, Walker T, Martina B, Battegay E. A case-management program of medium intensity does not improve cardiovascular risk factor control in coronary artery disease patients: The Heartcare I Trial. *Am J Med* 2001;110:543-550.

15. Pitt B, Waters D, Brown WV, et al. Aggressive lipid-lowering therapy compared with angioplasty in stable coronary artery disease. *Circulation* 1999;99:178-182.

16. Pearson TA. New tools for coronary risk assessment: What are their advantages and limitations? *Circulation* 2002;105:886-892.

17. Hammalainen H, Luurila OJ, Kallio V, Knuts LR. Reduction in sudden death and coronary mortality in myocardial infarction patients after rehabilitation: 15-year follow-up study. *Eur Heart J* 1996;16:1839-1844.

18. Wannamethee SG, Shaper AG, Walker M. Changes in physical activity, mortality, and incidence of coronary heart disease in older men. *Lancet* 1998;351(9116):1603-1608.

19. Steffen-Batey L, Nichaman, MZ, Goff DC, et al. Change in level of physical activity and risk of all-cause mortality or reinfarction. *Circulation* 2000;102:2204-2209.

20. Van Hees L, Fagard R, Thijs L, et al. Prognostic significance of peak exercise capacity in patients with coronary artery disease. *J Am Coll Cardiol* 1994;23:358-363.

21. Kavanagh T, Mertens DJ, Hamm LF, et al. Prediction of long-term prognosis in 12,169 men referred for cardiac rehabilitation. *Circulation* 2002;106:666-671.

22. La Rovere MT, Bersano C, Gnemmi M, et al. Exercise-induced increase in baroreflex sensitivity predicts improved prognosis after myocardial infarction. *Circulation* 2002;106:945-949.

23. Niebauer J, Hambrecht R, Velich T, et al. Attenuated progression of coronary artery disease after 6 years of multifactorial risk intervention. *Circulation* 1997;96:2534-2541.

24. *Smoking and Health. Report of the Advisory Committee to the Surgeon General of the Public Health Service.* Washington DC: U.S. Government Printing Office, 1964.

25. *Reducing the Health Consequences of Smoking: 25 Years of Progress.* Washington DC: U.S. Government Printing Office, 1989.

26. Pyorala K, DeBacker G, Graham I, Poole-Wilson P, Wood P. Prevention of coronary heart disease in clinical practice: Recommendations of the Task Force of the European Society of Cardiology, European Atherosclerosis Society and European Society of Hypertension. *Atherosclerosis* 1994;110:121-161.

27. *The Health Benefits of Smoking Cessation. A Report of the Surgeon General.* Washington DC: U.S. Department of Health and Human Services, 1990.

28. Office of the Surgeon General. *Tobacco Cessation Guideline.* Available at: www.surgeongeneral.gov/tobacco/. Accessed March 2001

29. Tashkin DP, Kanner R, Bailey W, et al. Smoking cessation in patients with chronic obstructive pulmonary disease: A double-blind, placebo-controlled, randomized trial. *Lancet* 2001;357:1571-1575.

30. The LIPID Study Group: Long term effectiveness and safety of pravastatin in 9014 patients with coronary heart disease and average cholesterol concentrations: The LIPID trial follow-up. *Lancet* 2002;359:1379-1387.

31. Pedersen TR, Olsson AG, Faergeman O, et al. Lipoprotein changes and reduction in incidence of major coronary heart disease events in the Scandinavian Simvastatin Survival Study (4S). *Circulation* 1998;97:1453-1460.

32. Sachs FM, Moye LA, Davis BR, et al. Relationship between plasma LDL concentrations during treatment with pravastatin and recurrent coronary events in the

Cholesterol and Recurrent Events Trial. *Circulation*. 1998;97:1446-1452.

33. Smith SC Jr, Blair SN, Bonow RO, Brass LM, et al. AHA/ACC Scientific Statement: AHA/ACC guidelines for preventing heart attack and death in patients with atherosclerotic cardiovascular disease: 2001 update: A statement for healthcare professionals from the American Heart Association and the American College of Cardiology. *Circulation* 2001;104:1577-1599.

34. Krauss RM, Eckel RH, Howard B, Appel LJ, et al. AHA Dietary Guidelines: Revision 2000: A statement for healthcare professionals from the Nutrition Committee of the American Heart Association. *Circulation* 2000;102:2284-2299.

35. Kris-Etherton PM. Monounsaturated fatty acids and the risk of cardiovascular disease. *Circulation* 1999;100:1253-1258.

36. Kris-Etherton P, Daniels SR, Eckel RH, et al. Summary of the scientific conference on dietary fatty acids and cardiovascular health: Conference summary from the Nutrition Committee of the American Heart Association. *Circulation* 2001;103:1034-1039.

37. Lichtenstein AH, Deckelbaum RJ, for the AHA Nutrition Committee. Stanol-sterol ester-containing foods and blood cholesterol levels: A statement for healthcare professionals from the Nutrition Committee of the American Heart Association. *Circulation* 2001;103:1177-1179.

38. Kris-Etherton P, Harris WS, Appel LJ, for the Nutrition Committee. Fish consumption, fish oil, omega-3 fatty acids and cardiovascular disease. *Circulation* 2002;106:2747-2757.

39. Sdringola S, Nakagawa K, Yusuf SW, et al. Combined intense lifestyle and pharmacologic lipid treatment further reduce coronary events and myocardial perfusion abnormalities compared with usual-care cholesterol-lowering drugs in coronary artery disease. *J Am Coll Cardiol* 2003;41:263-272.

40. Welty FK, Stuart E, O'Meara M, Huddleston J. Exercise boosts cholesterol-lowering diet effects. *Am J Cardiol* 2002;89:1201-1204.

41. Stefanick ML, Mackey S, Sheehan M, et al. Effects of diet and exercise in men and post menopausal women with low levels of HDL cholesterol and high levels of LDL cholesterol. *N Engl J Med* 1998;339:12-20.

42. Schaefer EJ. Lipoproteins, nutrition and heart disease. *Am J Clin Nutr* 2002;75:191-212.

43. Hu FB, Willett WC. Optimal diets for prevention of coronary heart disease. *JAMA* 2002;288:2569-2578.

44. Krumhout D, Menotti A, Kesteloot H, Sans S. Prevention of coronary heart disease by diet and lifestyle: Evidence from prospective cross-cultural cohort and intervention studies. *Circulation* 2002;105:893-898.

45. Kris-Etherton P, Eckel RH, Howard BV, et al. Lyon Diet Heart Study: Benefit of a Mediterranean-style, National Cholesterol Education Program/American Heart Association Step 1 dietary pattern on cardiovascular disease. *Circulation* 2001;103:1823-1825.

46. Burr ML, Gulbert JF, Holliday RM, et al. Effects of changes in fat, fish and fiber intakes on death and myocardial reinfarction: Diet and Reinfarction Trial (DART). *Lancet* 1989;2:757-761.

47. de Lorgeril M, Salen P, Martin JL, et al. Mediterranean diet, traditional risk factors, and the rate of cardiovascular complications after myocardial infarction: Final report of the Lyon Diet Heart Study. *Circulation* 1999;99:779-785.

48. Miller BD, Alderman EL, Haskell WL, et al. Predominance of dense low-density lipoprotein particles predicts angiographic benefit of therapy in the Stanford Coronary Risk Intervention Project. *Circulation*. 1996;94:2146-2153.

49. Grundy SM, Cleeman JI, Merz CNB, et al. Implications of recent clinical trials for the National Cholesterol Education Program Adult Treatment Panel III Guidelines. *Circulation* 2004;110:227-239.

50. Van Horn L. Fiber, lipids, and coronary heart disease: A statement for healthcare professionals from the Nutrition Committee, American Heart Association. *Circulation* 1997;95:2701-2704.

51. Bloomfield Rubins HR, Robins SJ. Conclusions from the VA-HIT study. *Am J Cardiol* 2000:86:543.

52. Cui Y, Blumenthal RS, Flaws JA, et al. Non-high-density lipoprotein cholesterol levels as a predictor of cardiovascular disease mortality. *Arch Intern Med* 2001;161:1413-1419.

53. Grundy SM, Howard B, Smith S Jr, Eckel R, et al. Prevention Conference IV: Diabetes and cardiovascular disease: Executive summary: Conference proceeding for healthcare professionals from a special writing group of the American Heart Association. *Circulation* 2002;105:2231-2239.

54. Clinical Practice Recommendations. *Diabetes Care* 2003;26(suppl):S1-S156.

55. Wilson PWF, D'Agostino RB, Sullivan L, et al. Overweight and obesity as determinants of cardiovascular risk. *Arch Intern Med* 2002;162:1867-1872.

56. Al Suwaidi S, Higano ST, Holmes DR, et al. Obesity is independently associated with coronary endothelial dysfunction in patients with normal or mildly diseased coronary arteries. *J Am Coll Cardiol* 2001;37:1523-1528.

57. Alexander JK. Obesity and coronary heart disease. *Am J Med Sci* 2001;321:215-224.

58. Stern MP, Haffner SM. Body fat distribution and hyperinsulinemia as risk factors for diabetes and cardiovascular disease. *Atherosclerosis* 1986;6:123-130.

59. Frayn KN. Visceral fat and insulin resistance—Causative or correlative? *Br J Nutr* 2000;83(suppl 1):S71-S77.

60. Chobanian AV, Bakris GL, Black HR, et al. The Seventh Report of the Joint National Committee on Prevention, Detection, Evaluation and Treatment of High Blood Pressure: The JNC 7 report. *JAMA* 2003;19:2560-2572.

61. Grundy SM, Brewer HB Jr, Cleeman JI, et al. Definition of metabolic syndrome. Report of the National Heart, Lung, and Blood Institute/American Heart Association

Conference on Scientific Issues Related to Definition. *Circulation* 2004;109:433-438.

62. Grundy SM, Hansen B, Smith SC, et al. Clinical management of metabolic syndrome. Report of the American Heart Association/National Heart, Blood, and Lung Institute/American Diabetes Association Conference on Scientific Issues Related to Management. *Circulation* 2004;109:551-556.

63. Jakicic JM, Clark K, Coleman E, et al. Appropriate intervention strategies for weight loss and prevention of weight gain for adults, ACSM position stand. *Med Sci Sports Exerc* 2001;33:2145-2156.

64. Despres JP, Moorjani S, Ferland M, et al. Adipose tissue distribution and plasma lipoprotein levels in obese women: Importance of intra-abdominal fat. *Arteriosclerosis* 1989;9:203-210.

65. Wing RR, Hill JO. Successful weight loss maintenance. *Ann Rev Nutr* 2001;21:323-341.

66. Knowler WC, Barrett-Connor E, Fowler SE, et al. Reduction in the incidence of type 2 diabetes with lifestyle intervention or metformin. *N Engl J Med* 2002;346:393-403.

67. Sacks FM, Svetkey LP, Vollmer WM, et al. Effects on blood pressure of reduced dietary sodium and the Dietary Approaches to Stop Hypertension (DASH) diet. DASH-Sodium Collaborative Research Group. *New Engl J Med* 2001;344:3-10.

68. Obarzanek E, Sacks FM, Vollmer WM, et al. Effects on blood lipids of a blood pressure-lowering diet: The Dietary Approaches to Stop Hypertension (DASH) Trial. *Am J Clin Nutr* 2001;74:80-89.

69. Appel LJ, Miller ER III, Ha Jee S, et al. Effect of dietary patterns on serum homocysteine. *Circulation* 2000;102:852-857.

70. Seamus P, Welton A, Chin MPH, et al. Effect of aerobic exercise on blood pressure: A meta-analysis of randomized, controlled trials. *Ann Intern* Med 2002;136:493-503.

71. Blair SN, Kohl HW, Paffenbarger RS, et al. Physical fitness and all-cause mortality: A prospective study of healthy and unhealthy men. *JAMA* 1995;273:1093-1098.

72. Myers J, Manish P, Froelicher V, et al. Exercise capacity and mortality among men referred for exercise testing. *N Engl J Med* 2002;346:793-801.

73. Manson JE, Greenland P, LaCroix AZ, et al. Walking compared with vigorous exercise for the prevention of cardiovascular events in women. *N Engl J Med* 2002;347:716-725.

74. Lee IM, Skerrett PJ. Physical activity and all-cause mortality: What is the dose-response relation? *Med Sci Sports Exerc* 2001;33(6 suppl):S459-S471.

75. Hambrecht R, Niebauer J, Marburger C, et al. Various intensities of leisure time physical activity in patients with coronary artery disease: Effects on cardiorespiratory fitness and progression of coronary atherosclerotic lesions. *J Am Coll Cardiol* 1993;22:468-477.

76. NIH Consensus Development Panel of Physical Activity and Cardiovascular Health. NIH Consensus Conference: Physical activity and cardiovascular health. *JAMA* 1996;276:241-246.

77. U.S. Department of Health and Human Services. *Physical Activity and Health: A Report of the Surgeon General.* Atlanta: U.S. Department of Health and Human Services, Centers for Disease Control and Prevention, National Center for Chronic Disease Prevention and Health Promotion, 1996.

78. The recommended quality and quantity of exercise for developing and maintaining cardiorespiratory and muscular fitness and flexibility in healthy adults. American College of Sports Medicine Position Stand. *Med Sci Sports Exerc* 1998;30:975-991.

79. Franklin BA (ed). *ACSM's Guidelines for Exercise Testing and Exercise Prescription.* Baltimore: Lippincott Williams & Wilkins, 2000.

80. Kraus WE, Houmard JA, Duscha BD, et al. Effects of the amount and intensity of exercise on plasma lipoproteins. *N Engl J Med* 2002;347:1483-1492.

81. Laughlin MH. Physical activity in prevention and treatment of coronary disease: The battle line is in exercise cell biology. *Med Sci Sports Exerc* 2004;36:352-362.

82. Maiorana A, O'Driscoll G, Taylor R, et al. Exercise and the nitric oxide vasodilator system. *Sports Med* 2003;33:1013-1035.

83. Hambrecht R, Fiehn E, Weigl C, et al. Regular physical exercise corrects endothelial dysfunction and improves exercise capacity in patients with chronic heart failure. *Circulation* 1998;98:2709-2715.

84. Manson JE, Hu FB, Rich-Edwards JW, et al. A prospective study of walking as compared with vigorous exercise in the prevention of coronary heart disease in women. *N Engl J Med* 1999;341:650-658.

85. Lee IM, Rexrode KM, Cook NR, et al. Physical activity and coronary heart disease in women: Is "no pain, no gain" passé? *JAMA* 2001;285:1447-1454.

86. Hakim A, Petrocitch H, Burchfield CM, et al. Effects of walking on mortality in nonsmoking, retired men. *N Engl J Med* 1998;338:94-99.

87. Dunn AL, Marcus BH, Kampert JB, et al. Comparison of lifestyle and structured interventions to increase physical activity and cardiorespiratory fitness. *JAMA* 1999;28:327-334.

88. Schulz R, Beach SR, Oves DG, et al. Association between depression and mortality in older adults: The Cardiovascular Health Study. *Arch Intern Med* 2000;160:1761-1768.

89. Angerer P, Siebert U, Kothny W, et al. Impact of social support, cynical hostility and anger expression on progression of coronary atherosclerosis. *J Am Coll Cardiol* 2000;36:1781-1789.

90. Frasure-Smith N, Lesperance F, Gravel G, et al. Social support, depression and mortality during the first year after myocardial infarction. *Circulation* 2000;101:1919-1924.

91. American Association of Cardiovascular and Pulmonary Rehabilitation. *Guidelines for Cardiac Rehabilitation and Secondary Prevention Programs*. Fourth Edition. Champaign, IL: Human Kinetics, 2004.

92. Blumenthal JA, Jinag MA, Babyak DA, et al. Stress management and exercise training in cardiac patients with myocardial ischemia: Effects on prognosis and evaluation of mechanisms. *Arch Intern Med* 1997;157:2213-2223.

93. Denolett J, Brutsaert DL. Reducing emotional distress improves prognosis in coronary heart disease: 9-year mortality in a clinical trial of rehabilitation. *Circulation* 2001;104:2018-2024.

94. Blumenthal JA, Babyak M, Wei J, et al. Usefulness of psychosocial treatment of mental stress-induced myocardial ischemia in men. *Am J Cardiol* 2002;89:164-168.

95. Williams RR. Genetics of atherosclerosis: Can early familial coronary heart disease be prevented? In: *Coronary Heart Disease Prevention*. Yanowitz FG (ed). New York: Marcel Dekker, 1992, pp. 45-70.

96. Stampfer MJ, Hu FB, Manson JE, et al. Primary prevention of coronary heart disease in women through diet and lifestyle. *N Engl J Med* 2000;343:16-22.

97. Stamler J, Stamler R, Neaton JD, et al. Low risk factor profile and long-term cardiovascular mortality and life expectancy: Findings for 5 large cohorts of young adult and middle-aged men and women. *JAMA* 1999;308:363-366.

98. Jomini V, Oppliger-Pasquali S, Wietlisbach V, et al. Contribution of major cardiovascular risk factors to familial premature coronary artery disease: The GENECARD project. *J Am Coll Cardiol* 2002;40:676-684.

99. Wood D. Established and emerging cardiovascular risk factors. *Am Heart J* 2001;141(2 suppl):S49-S57.

100. Mosca L, Grundy SM, Judelson D, et al. Guide to preventive cardiology for women. AHA/ACC Scientific Statement: Consensus Panel Statement. *Circulation* 1999;99:2480-2484.

101. Hulley S, Grady D, Bush T, et al. Randomized trial of estrogen plus progestin for secondary prevention of coronary heart disease in post-menopausal women: Heart and Estrogen/Progestin Replacement Study (HERS) Research Group. *JAMA* 1998;280:605-613.

102. Mosca L, Collins P, Herrington DM, et al. Hormone replacement therapy and cardiovascular disease. *Circulation* 2001;104:499-506.

103. Shlipak MG, Simon JA, Vittinghoff E, et al. Estrogen, progestin, lipoprotein (a), and the risk of recurrent coronary heart disease events after menopause. *JAMA* 2000;283:1845-1852.

104. Reddy KG, Noir RN, Sheehan HM, et al. Evidence that selective endothelial dysfunction may occur in the absence of angiographic or ultrasound atherosclerosis in patients with risk factors for atherosclerosis. *J Am Coll Cardiol* 1994;23:833-843.

105. Ludmer PL, Selwyn AP, Shook TL, et al. Paradoxical vasoconstriction induced by acetylcholine atherosclerotic coronary segments. *N Engl J Med* 1986;315:1046-1051.

106. Rozanski A, Qureshi E, Bauman M, et al. Peripheral arterial responses to treadmill exercise among healthy subjects and atherosclerosis patients. *Circulation* 2001;103:2084-2089.

107. Halcox JPJ, Schenke WH, Zalos G, et al. Prognostic value of coronary vascular endothelial dysfunction. *Circulation* 2002;106:653-658.

108. Al Suwaidi J, Homosaki S, Higano ST, et al. Long-term follow-up of patients with mild coronary artery disease and endothelial dysfunction. *Circulation* 2000;101:948-954.

109. Vita JA, Loscalzo J. Shouldering the risk factor burden: Infection, atherosclerosis, and the vascular endothelium. *Circulation* 2002;106:164-166.

110. Ross R. The pathogenesis of atherosclerosis: A perspective for the 1990s. *Nature* 1993;362:801.

111. McLenachan JM, Vita J, Fish DR, et al. Early evidence of endothelial vasodilator dysfunction at coronary branch points. *Circulation* 1990;82:1169-1173.

112. Targonski PV, Bonetti PO, Pumper GM, et al. Coronary endothelial dysfunction is associated with an increased risk of cerebrovascular events. *Circulation* 2003;107:2805-2809.

113. Schachinger V, Britten MB, Zeiher AM. Prognostic impact of coronary vasodilator dysfunction on adverse long-term outcomes of coronary heart disease. *Circulation* 2000;101:1899-1906.

114. Halcox JP, Schenke WH, Zalos G, et al. Prognostic value of coronary vascular endothelial dysfunction, *Circulation* 2002;106:653-658.

115. Chan SY, Mancini GB, Kuramotol L, et al. The prognostic importance of endothelial dysfunction and carotid atheroma burden in patients with coronary artery disease. *J Am Coll Cardiol* 2003;42:1037-1043.

116. Bugiardini R, Manfrini O, Pizzi C, et al. Endothelial function predicts future development of coronary artery disease. *Circulation* 2004;109:2518-2523.

117. von Mering GO, Arant CB, Wessel TR, et al. Abnormal coronary vasomotion as a prognostic indicator of cardiovascular events in women: Results from the National Heart, Lung, and Blood Institute-sponsored Women's Ischemia Syndrome Evaluation (WISE). *Circulation* 2004;109:722-725.

118. Gokce N, Keaney JF Jr, Hunter LM, et al. Predictive value of noninvasively determined endothelial dysfunction for long-term cardiovascular events in patients with peripheral vascular disease. *J Am Coll Cardiol* 2003;41:1769-1775.

119. Modena MG, Bonnetti L, Coppi F, et al. Prognostic role of reversible endothelial dysfunction in hypertensive postmenopausal women. *J Am Coll Cardiol* 2002;40:505-510.

120. Anderson TJ. Assessment and treatment of endothelial dysfunction. *J Am Coll Cardiol* 1999;34:631-638.

121. Hambrecht R, Fiehn E, Weigl C, et al. Regular physical exercise corrects endothelial dysfunction and improves exercise capacity in patients with chronic heart failure. *Circulation* 1998;98:2709-2715.

122. Hambrecht R, Wolf A, Gielen G. Effect of exercise on coronary endothelial function in patients with coronary artery disease. *N Engl J Med* 2000;342:454-460.

123. Higashi Y, Sasaki S, Kurisu S, et al. Regular aerobic exercise augments endothelium-dependent vascular relaxation in normotensive as well as hypertensive subjects. *Circulation* 1999;100:1194-1202.

124. Maiorana A, O'Driscoll G, Cheetham C, et al. The effect of combined aerobic and resistance exercise on vascular function in type 2 diabetes. *J Am Coll Cardiol* 2001;38:860-866.

125. Hornig B, Maier V, Drexler H, et al. Physical training improves endothelial function in patients with chronic heart failure. *Circulation* 1996;93:210-214.

126. Katz SD, Yuen J, Bijou R, et al. Training improves endothelium-dependent vasodilation in resistance vessels of patients with heart failure. *J Appl Physiol* 1997;82:1488-1492.

127. Walsh JH, Bilborough W, Maiorana A, et al. Exercise training improves conduit vessel function in patients with coronary artery disease. *J Appl Physiol* 2003;95:20-25.

128. Kobayashi N, Tsuruya Y, Iwasawa T, et al. Exercise training in patients with chronic heart failure improves endothelial function predominantly in the trained extremities. *Circ J* 2003;67:505-510.

129. Gokce N, Vita JA, Bader DS, et al. Effect of exercise on upper and lower extremity endothelial function in patients with coronary artery disease. *Am J Cardiol* 2002;90:124-127.

130. Goto C, Higashi Y, Kimura M, et al. Effect of different intensities of exercise on endothelium-dependent vasodilation in humans: Role of endothelium dependent nitric oxide and oxidative stress. *Circulation* 2003;108:530-535.

131. Hosokawa S, Hiasa Y, Takahashi T, Itoh S. Effects of regular exercise on coronary endothelial function in patients with a recent MI. *Circ J* 2003;67:221-224.

132. Maeda S, Miyauchi T, Kakiyama T, et al. Effects of exercise training of 8 weeks and detraining on plasma levels of endothelium-derived factors, endothelin-1, and nitric oxide in healthy young humans. *Life Sci* 2001;69:1005-1116.

133. DeSouza CA, Shapiro LF, Clevenger CM, et al. Regular aerobic exercise prevents and restores age-related declines in endothelium-dependent vasodilation in healthy men. *Circulation* 2000;102:1351-1357.

134. Ridker P, Buring JE, Shih J, et al. Prospective study of C-reactive protein and the risk of future cardiovascular events among apparently healthy women. *Circulation* 1998;98:731-733.

135. Folsom AR, Aleksic N, Catellier D, et al. C-reactive protein and incident coronary heart disease in the Atherosclerosis Risk in Communities (ARIC) study. *Am Heart J* 2002;144:233-238.

136. Ridker PM, Rifai N, Pfeffer M, et al. Inflammation, pravastatin, and the risk of coronary events after myocardial infarction in patients with average cholesterol levels. *Circulation* 1998;98:839-844.

137. Rossi E, Biascussi LM, Citterio F, et al. Risk of myocardial infarction and angina in patients with severe peripheral vascular disease: Predictive role of C-reactive protein. *Circulation* 2002;05:800-803.

138. Morrow DA, Ridker PM. C-reactive protein, inflammation, and coronary risk. *Med Clin North Am* 2000;84:149-161.

139. Ridker PM, Cushman M, Stampher MJ, et al. Comparison of C-reactive protein and low-density lipoprotein cholesterol levels in the prediction of first cardiovascular events. *N Engl J Med* 2002;347:1557-1565.

140. Pearson TA, Mensah GA, Alexander RW, et al. Markers of inflammation and cardiovascular disease: Application to clinical and public health practice. A statement for healthcare professionals from the Centers for Disease Control and Prevention and the American Heart Association. *Circulation* 2003;107:499-511.

141. Abramson JL, Vaccarino V. Relationship between physical activity and inflammation among apparently healthy middle-aged and older adults. *Arch Intern Med* 2002;161:1286-1292.

142. LaMonte MJ, Durstine JL, Yanowitz, FG, et al. Cardiorespiratory fitness and C-reactive protein among a tri-ethnic sample of women. *Circulation* 2002;106:403-406.

143. McCully KS. Vascular pathology of homocysteinemia: Implications for the pathogenesis of arteriosclerosis. *Am J Pathol* 1969;56:111-128.

144. Clarke R, Daly L, Robinson K, et al. Hyperhomocysteinemia: An independent risk factor for cardiovascular disease. *N Engl J Med* 1991;324:1149-1155.

145. Bostom AG, Silbershatz H, Rosenberg IH, et al. Nonfasting plasma total homocysteine levels and all-cause cardiovascular disease mortality in elderly Framingham men and women. *Arch Intern Med* 1999;159:1077-1080.

146. Mangoni A, Jackson SHD. Homocysteine and cardiovascular disease: Current evidence and future prospects. *Am J Med* 2002;112:556-565.

147. Schnyder G, Roffi M, Pin R, et al. Decreased rate of coronary restenosis after lowering of plasma homocysteine levels. *N Engl J Med* 2001;345:1593-1600.

148. Schnyder G, Roffi M, Flammer Y, et al. Effect of homocysteine-lowering therapy with folic acid, vitamin B_{12} and vitamin B_6 on clinical outcome after percutaneous coronary intervention: The Swiss Heart Study: A randomized controlled trial. *JAMA* 2002;288:973-979.

149. Willems FF, Wim R, Aengevaeren M, et al. Coronary endothelial function in hyperhomocysteinuria: Improvement after treatment with folic acid and cobalamin in patients with coronary artery disease. *J Am Coll Cardiol* 2002;40:766-772.

150. Vermeulen EGJ, Stehower CDA, Twisk JWR, et al. Effect of homocysteine-lowering treatment with folic acid plus B_6 on progression of subclinical atherosclerosis:

A randomized, placebo-controlled trial. *Lancet* 2000;355: 517-522.

151. Woo KS, Chook P, Lindy LT. Long-term improvement in homocysteine levels and arterial endothelial function after 1-year folic acid supplementation. *Am J Med* 2002;112:535-539.

152. Rosenberg IH. Is it time to standardize and to measure blood homocysteine levels in patients with heart disease? *Am J Med* 2002;112:582-583.

153. Chai AU, Abrams J. Homocysteine: A new cardiac risk factor. *Clin Cardiol* 2001;24:80-84.

154. de la Pena-Diaz A, Izaguirre-Avila R, Angles-Cano E. Lipoprotein Lp(a) and atherothrombotic disease. *Arch Med Res* 2000;31:353-359.

155. Danga G, Mehan R, Harpel PC, et al. Lipoprotein(a) and inflammation in human coronary atheroma: Association with the severity of clinical presentation. *J Am Coll Cardiol* 1998;32:2035-2042.

156. Armstrong VW, Cremer P, Eberle E, et al. The association between serum Lp(a) concentration and angiographically-assessed coronary atherosclerosis: Dependence on serum LDL levels. *Atherosclerosis* 1986;62:249-257.

157. Maher VM, Brown BG, Marcovina SM, et al. Effects of lowering elevated LDL-cholesterol on the cardiovascular risk of lipoprotein(a). *JAMA* 1995;274:1771-1774.

158. Cantin B, Gagnon F, Moorjani S, et al. Is lipoprotein(a) an independent risk factor for ischemic heart disease in men? The Quebec Cardiovascular Study. *J Am Coll Cardiol* 1998;31:519-525.

159. Seed M, Ayers KL, Humphries SE, Miller GJ. Lipoprotein(a) as a predictor of myocardial infarction in middle-aged men. *Am J Med* 2001;110:22-27.

160. Sharrett AR, Ballantyne CM, Coady SA, et al. Coronary heart disease prediction from lipoprotein cholesterol levels, triglycerides, lipoprotein(a), Apolipoproteins A-I and B, and HDL density subfractions: The Atherosclerosis Risk in Communities (ARIC) Study. *Circulation* 2001;104:1108-1113.

161. von Eckardstein A, Schulte H, Cullen P, Assman G. Lipoprotein(a) further increases the risk of coronary events in men with high global cardiovascular risk. *J Am Coll Cardiol* 2001;37:434-439.

162. Marcovina SM, Koschinsky ML. Lipoprotein(a) concentration and apolipoprotein(a) size: A synergistic role in advanced atherosclerosis. *Circulation* 1999;100: 1151-1153.

163. Hulley S, Grady D, Bush T, et al. Randomized trial of estrogen plus progestin for secondary prevention of coronary heart disease in postmenopausal women. *JAMA* 1998;280:605-613.

164. Gardner CD, Fortmann SP, Krauss RM. Small low density lipoprotein particles are associated with the incidence of coronary artery disease in men and women. *JAMA* 1996;276: 875-881.

165. Lemarche B, Tchemof A, Moorjani S, et al. Small, dense low-density lipoprotein particles as a predictor of the risk of ischemic heart disease in men. Prospective results from the Quebec cardiovascular study. *Circulation* 1997;96:69-75.

166. Dunn P, Meese R, Superko R, et al. Cardiovascular risk reduction is cost-effective in the real world. *Circulation* 1997;96(suppl):I-67.

167. Schrott H, Bittner V, Vittinghoff E, et al. Adherence to national cholesterol education program treatment goals in postmenopausal women with heart disease: The heart and estrogen/progestin replacement study (HERS). *JAMA* 1997;277:1281-1286.

168. McBride P, Schrott H, Plane M, et al. Primary care adherence to National Cholesterol Education Program guidelines for patients with coronary artery disease. *Arch Intern Med* 1998;158:1238-1244.

169. Sueta C, Chowdhury M, Boccusi S. Analysis of the degree of undertreatment of hyperlipidemia and congestive heart failure secondary to coronary artery disease. *Am J Cardiol* 1999;83:1303-1307.

170. Pearson T, Laurora I, Chu H, et al. The lipid treatment assessment project (L-TAP): A multicenter survey to evaluate the percentages of dyslipidemic patients receiving lipid-lowering therapy and achieving low-density lipoprotein cholesterol goals. *Arch Intern Med* 2000;160:459-467.

171. Qureshi AL, Suri FK, Guterman LR, et al. Ineffective secondary prevention in survivors of cardiovascular events in the US population. *Arch Intern Med* 2001;161: 1621-1628.

172. Fonarow GC, French WJ, Parsons LS, et al. Use of lipid-lowering medications at discharge in patients with myocardial infarction. *Circulation* 2001;87:38-44.

173. Fonarow GC, Gawlinski A, Moughrabi S, et al. Improved treatment of coronary heart disease by implementation of a Cardiac Hospitalization Atherosclerosis Management Program (CHAMP). *Am J Cardiol* 2001;87: 819-822.

174. Cao J, Savage P, Brochu M, et al. Prevalence of lipid-lowering therapy at cardiac rehabilitation entry: 2000 vs. 1996. *J Cardiopulm Rehabil* 2002;22:80-84.

175. Smith DA, Harnick D, Kilaru R. Comparison of physician-managed lipid-lowering care in patients with coronary heart disease in two time periods (1994 and 1999). *Am J Cardiol* 2001;88:1417-1419.

176. Phillips LS, Branch WT, Cook CB, et al. Clinical inertia. *Ann Intern Med* 2001;135:825-834.

177. Ades PA, Balady GJ, Berra K. Transforming exercise-based cardiac rehabilitation programs into secondary prevention centers: A national imperative. *J Cardiopulm Rehabil* 2001;21:263-272.

178. Ades PA. Cardiac rehabilitation and secondary prevention of coronary heart disease. *N Engl J Med* 2001;345: 892-902.

179. Roitman JL, LaFontaine T, Drimmer AM. A new model for risk stratification and delivery of cardiovascular rehabilitation services in the long-term clinical management of patients with coronary artery disease. *J Cardiopulm Rehabil* 1998;18:113-123.

180. Levknecht L, Schriefer J, Schriefer J, Maconis B. Combining case management, pathways, and report cards for secondary cardiac prevention. *Jt Comm J Qual Improv* 1997;23:162-174.

181. DeBusk RF, Houston-Miller N, Superko R, et al. A case-management system for coronary risk factor modification after acute myocardial infarction. *Ann Intern Med* 1994;120:721-729.

182. Gordon NF, Salmon RD, Mitchell BS, et al. Innovative approaches to comprehensive cardiovascular disease risk reduction in clinical and community-based settings. *Curr Atheroscler Rep* 2001;3:498-506.

183. Franklin BF, Bonzheim K, Warren J, et al. Effects of a contemporary, exercise-based rehabilitation and cardiovascular risk-reduction program on coronary patients with abnormal baseline risk factors. *Chest* 2002;122:338-343.

184. Gordon NF, English CD, Contractor AS, et al. Effectiveness of three models for comprehensive cardiovascular risk reduction. *Am J Cardiol* 2002;89:1263-1268.

185. Thomas RJ, Miller HN, Lamendola C, et al. National survey on gender differences in cardiac rehabilitation programs: patient characteristics and enrollment patterns. *J Cardiopulm Rehabil* 1996;16:402-412.

186. McAlister FA, Lawson FME, Teo KK, et al. Randomized trials of secondary prevention programs in coronary heart disease: systematic review. *Br Med J* 2001;323:957-962.

187. Sdringola S, Nakagawa K, Nakagawa Y, et al. Combined intense lifestyle and pharmacologic lipid treatment further reduce coronary events and myocardial perfusion abnormalities compared with usual-care cholesterol-lowering drugs in coronary artery disease. *J Am Coll Cardiol* 2003;41:263-272.

188. Williams MA, JL Fleg, PA Ades, BR Chaitman, et al. Secondary prevention of coronary heart disease in the elderly (with emphasis on patients ≥75 years of age). *Circulation* 2002;105:1735-1743.

Chapter 4

1. Barefoot J, Dahlstrom W, Williams R. Hostility, CHD, incidence, and total mortality: A 25-year follow-up of 255 physicians. *Psychosom Med* 1983;45:59-63.

2. Barefoot J, Helms M, Mark D, et al. Depression and long-term mortality risk in patients with coronary artery disease. *Am J Cardiol* 1996;78:613-617.

3. Frasure-Smith N, Lesperance F, Talajic M. Depression and 18-month prognosis after myocardial infarction. *Circulation* 1995;91:999-1005.

4. Frasure-Smith N, Lesperance F, Talajic M. Depression following myocardial infarction. *JAMA* 1993;270:1819-1825.

5. Iribarren C, Sidney S, Bild D, et al. Association of hostility with coronary artery calcification in young adults: The CARDIA study, Coronary Artery Risk Development in Young Adults. *JAMA* 2000;283:2546-2551.

6. Matthews K, Owens J, Kuller L, Sutton-Tyrell K, Jansen-McWilliams L. Are hostility and anxiety associated with carotid atherosclerosis in healthy postmenopausal women? *Psychosom Med* 1998;60:633-638.

7. Ornish D. *Dr. Dean Ornish's Program for Reversing Heart Disease.* New York: Random House, 1990.

8. Seigler IC, Costa PT, Brummett BH, et al. Patterns of change in hostility for college to midlife in the UNC alumni heart study predict high risk status. *Psychosom Med* 2003;65:738-745.

9. Allen R, Sheidt S. Empirical bases for cardiac psychology. In: *Heart and Mind.* Allen R, Sheidt S (eds). Washington, DC: American Psychological Association, 1996, pp. 63-123.

10. Lui M, Herridge ML. *Psychosocial Tools to Identify Hostility, Anger, and Depression: The Herridge Cardiopulmonary Questionnaire (HCQ) and Center for Epidemiologic Studies Depression Scale.* Syllabus for the American Association of Cardiovascular and Pulmonary Rehabilitation 17th Annual Meeting, 2002, pp. 407-413.

11. Clark NM, Becker MH. Theoretical models and strategies for improving adherence and disease management. In: *The Handbook of Health Behavior Change.* Second Edition. Shumaker SA (ed). New York: Springer, 1998, pp. 5-32.

12. King AC, Kiernan M. Physical activity promotion: antecedents. In: *ACSM's Resource Manual for Guidelines for Exercise Testing and Prescription.* Fourth Edition. Roitman J, Herridge M, Kelsey M, et al. (eds). Baltimore: Lippincott Williams & Wilkins, 2001, pp. 573-583.

13. Daly J, Sindone AP, Thompson DR, Hancock K, Chang E, Davidson P. Barriers to participation in and adherence to cardiac rehabilitation programs: A critical literature review. *Prog Cardiovasc Nurs* 2002;17:8-17.

14. Bandura A. Health promotion by social cognitive means. *Health Educ Behav* 2004;31:143-164.

15. Prochaska JO, DiClemente CC. Stages of change in the modification of problem behaviors. *Prog Behav Mod* 1992;28:184-214.

16. Donker FJ. Cardiac rehabilitation: A review of current developments. *Clin Psychol Rev* 2000;20:923-943.

17. Barefoot JC, Schroll M. Symptoms of depression, acute myocardial infarction, and total mortality in a community sample. *Circulation* 1996;93:1976-1980.

18. Carney RM, Freedland KE, Rich MW, Smith LJ, Jaffe AS. Ventricular disease and psychiatric depression in patients with coronary artery disease. *Am J Med* 1993;95:23-18.

19. Carney RM, Rich MW, Tevelde A. Major depressive disorder in coronary artery disease. *Am J Cardiol* 1987;60:1273-1275.

20. Lespérance F, Frasure-Smith N, Juneau M, Théroux P. Depression and 1-year prognosis following unstable angina. *Arch Intern Med* 2000;160:1354-1360.

21. Lespérance F, Frasure-Smith N. Depression in patients with cardiac disease: A practical review. *J Psychosom Res* 2000;48:379-391.

22. Musselman DL, Evans DL, Nemeroff CB. The relationship of depression to cardiovascular disease: Epidemiology, biology and treatment. *Arch Gen Psychiatry* 1998;5:580-592.

23. Herridge ML, Stimler CE, Southard DR, King ML. Depression screening in cardiac rehabilitation:

AACVPR Task Force Report. *J Cardiopulm Rehabil* 2005;25:14-21.

24. Lespérance F, Jaffe AS. Beyond the blues: Understanding the link between coronary artery disease and depression. Symposium presented at the 73rd Annual Scientific Sessions of the American Heart Association, New Orleans, LA, November 12-15, 2002.

25. Williams RB. Hostility (and other psychological risk factors): Effects on health and the potential for successful behavioral approaches to prevention and treatment. In: *Handbook of Health Psychology*. Baum A, Revenson TR, Singer JE (eds). Mahwah, NJ: Erlbaum, 2000, pp. 661-668.

26. O'Farrell P, Murray J, Hotz SB. Psychologic distress among spouses of patients undergoing cardiac rehabilitation. *Heart Lung* 2000;29:97-104.

27. Miller W, Rolnick S. *Motivational Interviewing: Preparing People to Change Addictive Behavior.* New York: Guilford, 1991.

28. Goldstein G, Depue J, Kazura A, Niauara R. Models for provider-patient interaction: Applications to health behavior change. In: *The Handbook of Health Behavior Change.* Second Edition. Shumaker SA (ed). New York: Springer, 1998, pp. 85-113.

29. Ware JE, Sherbourne CD. The MOS 36-item short-form health survey (SF-36): I. Conceptual framework and item selection. *Med Care* 1992;30:473-483.

30. Matthews KA, Jamison JW, Cottington EM. *Assessment of Type A, Anger, and Hostility: A Review of Scales Through 1982. Measuring Psychosocial Variables in Epidemiologic Studies of Cardiovascular Disease* (NIH Pub. No. 85-2270). Bethesda, MD: National Institutes of Health, 1985.

31. Radloff LS. The CES-D scale: A self-report depressive scale for research in the general population. *J Appl Psychol Measurement* 1977;1:385-401.

32. Beck AT, Steer RA, Brown GK. *Beck Depression Inventory—II Manual.* San Antonio, TX: Psychological Corporation, 1996.

33. Spielberger C, Gorsuch, R, Lusken R. *Manual for the State-Trait Anxiety Inventory.* Palo Alto, CA: Consulting Psychologists Press, 1970.

34. Beck AT, Steer RA. *Beck Anxiety Inventory Manual.* San Antonio, TX: The Psychological Corporation, 1990.

Chapter 5

1. Thompson PD, Buchner D, Piña IL, et al. AHA scientific statement. Exercise and physical activity in the prevention and treatment of atherosclerotic cardiovascular disease. *Circulation* 2003;107:3109-3116.

2. U.S. Department of Health and Human Services. *Physical Activity and Health: A Report of the Surgeon General.* Atlanta: U.S. Department of Health and Human Services, Centers for Disease Control and Prevention, National Center for Chronic Disease Prevention and Health Promotion, 1996.

3. Leon AS (ed). *Physical Activity and Cardiovascular Health: A National Consensus.* Champaign, IL: Human Kinetics, 1997.

4. Bouchard C, Dionne FT, Simoneau J, Boulay MR. Genetics of aerobic and anaerobic performances. *Exerc Sport Sci Rev* 1992;20:27-58.

5. Taylor HL, Klepetar E, Keys A, Parlin W, Blackburn H, Puchner T. Death rates among physically active and sedentary employees of the railroad industry. *Am J Pub Health* 1962;52:1697-1707.

6. Morris JN, Kagan A, Pattison DC, Gardner MJ, Raffle PAB. Incidence and prediction of ischemic heart disease in London busmen. *Lancet* 1966;2:553-559.

7. Paffenbarger RS, Hale WE. Work activity and coronary heart mortality. *N Engl J Med* 1975;292:545-550.

8. Paffenbarger RS, Hyde RT, Wing AL, Steinmetz CH. A natural history of athleticism and cardiovascular health. *JAMA* 1984;252:491-495.

9. Sesso HD, Paffenbarger RS, Lee IM. Physical activity and coronary heart disease in men: The Harvard Alumni Health Study. *Circulation* 2000;102:975-980.

10. Lee IM, Sesso HD, Paffenbarger RS. Physical activity and coronary heart disease risk in men: Does the duration of exercise episodes predict risk? *Circulation* 2000;102:981-986.

11. Morris JN, Everitt MG, Pollard R, Chave SPW, Semmence AM. Vigorous exercise in leisure time: Protection against coronary heart disease. *Lancet* 1980;2: 1207-1210.

12. Manson, JE, Hu FB, Rich-Edwards JW, et al. A prospective study of walking as compared with vigorous exercise in the prevention of coronary heart disease in women. *N Engl J Med* 1999;341:650-658.

13. Lee IM, Rexrode KM, Cook NR, Manson JE, Buring JE. Physical activity and coronary heart disease in women: Is "no pain, no gain" passé? *JAMA* 2001;285: 1447-1454.

14. Blair SN, Kohl HW III, Paffenbarger RS, Clark DG, Cooper KH, Gibbons LW. Physical fitness and all-cause mortality: A prospective study of healthy men and women. *JAMA* 1989;262:2395-2401.

15. Blair SN, Kohl HW III, Barlow CE, Paffenbarger RS, Gibbons LW, Macera CA. Changes in physical fitness and all-cause mortality: A prospective study of healthy and unhealthy men. *JAMA* 1995;273:1093-1098.

16. Sandvik L, Erikssen J, Thaulow E, Erikssen G, Mundal R, Rodahl K. Physical fitness as a predictor of mortality among healthy, middle-aged Norwegian men. *N Engl J Med* 1993;328:533-537.

17. Roger VL, Jacobsen SJ, Pellika PA, Miller TD, Bailey KR, Gersh BJ. Prognostic value of treadmill exercise testing: A population-based study in Olmsted county, Minnesota. *Circulation* 1998;98:2836-2841.

18. Goraya TY, Jacobsen SJ, Pellika PA, et al. Prognostic value of treadmill exercise testing in elderly persons. *Ann Intern Med* 2000;132:862-870.

19. Myers J, Prakash M, Froelicher V, Dat D, Partington S, Atwood JE. Exercise capacity and mortality among men

referred for exercise testing. *New Engl J Med* 2002;346: 793-801.

20. Kavanagh T, Mertens DJ, Hamm LF, et al. Prediction of long-term prognosis in 12,169 men referred for cardiac rehabilitation. *Circulation* 2002;106:666-671.

21. Kavanagh T, Mertens DJ, Hamm LF, et al. Peak oxygen intake and cardiac mortality in women referred for cardiac rehabilitation. *J Am Coll Cardiol* 2003;42:2139-2143.

22. Wannamethee SG, Shaper AG, Walker M. Physical activity and mortality in older men with diagnosed coronary heart disease. *Circulation* 2000;102:1358-1363.

23. Kallio V, Hamalainen H, Hakkila J, Luurila OJ. Reduction in sudden deaths by a multifactorial intervention programme after acute myocardial infarction. *Lancet* 1979;2:1091-1094.

24. Hamalainen H, Luurila OJ, Kallio V, Knuts LR, Arstila M, Hakkila J. Long-term reduction in sudden deaths after a multifactorial intervention programme in patients with myocardial infarction: 10-year results of a controlled investigation. *Eur Heart J* 1989;10:55-62.

25. O'Connor GT, Buring JE, Yusuf S, et al. An overview of randomized trials of rehabilitation with exercise after myocardial infarction. *Circulation* 1989;80:234-244.

26. Jolliffe JA, Rees K, Taylor RS, Oldridge N, Ebrahim S. Evidence-based rehabilitation for coronary heart disease. *The Cochrane Library* 2001;2:1-58.

27. Thompson PD, Moore GE. The cardiac risks of vigorous physical activity. In: *Physical Activity and Cardiovascular Health: A National Consensus*. Leon AS (ed). Champaign, IL: Human Kinetics, 1997, pp. 137-142.

28. Mittleman MA, Maclure M, Tolfer GH, Sherwood JB, Goldberg RJ, Muller JE. Triggering of acute myocardial infarction by heavy physical exertion: Protection against triggering by regular exertion. *N Engl J Med* 1993;329:1677-1683.

29. Siscovick DS, Weiss NS, Fletcher RH, Lasky T. The incidence of primary cardiac arrest during vigorous exercise. *N Engl J Med* 1984;311:874-877.

30. Maron BJ, Polliac LC, Roberts WO. Risk for sudden death associated with marathon running. *J Am Coll Cardiol* 1996;28:428-431.

31. Van Camp SP, Peterson RA. Cardiovascular complications of outpatient cardiac rehabilitation programs. *JAMA* 1986;256:1160-1163.

32. Burke AP, Farb A, Malcom GT, Liang YH, Smialek JE, Virmani R. Plaque rupture and sudden death related to exertion in men with coronary artery disease. *JAMA* 1999;281:921-926.

33. Hess OM, Buchi M, Kirkeeide R, et al. Potential role of coronary vasoconstriction in ischemic heart disease: Effect of exercise. *Eur Heart J* 1990;(II suppl B):58-64.

34. Curtis BM, O'Keefe JH. Autonomic tone as a cardiovascular risk factor: The dangers of chronic fight or flight. *Mayo Clin Proc* 2002;77:45-54.

35. Pellicia A, Spataro A, Granata J, Biffi A, Casselli G, Alabiso A. Coronary arteries in physiological hypertro-phy: Echocardiographic evidence of increased proximal size in elite athletes. *Int J Sports Med* 1990;11:120-126.

36. Haskell WL, Sims C, Myll J, Bortz WM, St. Goar FG, Alderman EL. Coronary artery size and dilating capacity in ultradistance runners. *Circulation* 1993;87:1076-1082.

37. Belardinelli R, Georgiou D, Ginzton L, Cianci G, Purcaro A. Effects of moderate exercise training on thallium uptake and contractile response to low-dose dobutamine in dysfunctional myocardium in patients with ischemic cardiomyopathy. *Circulation* 1998;97: 553-561.

38. Paffenbarger RS, Wing AL, Hyde RT, Jung DL. Physical activity and incidence of hypertension in college alumni. *Am J Epidemiol* 1983;117:245-257.

39. Seals DR, Hagberg JM. The effect of exercise training on human hypertension: A review. *Med Sci Sports Exerc* 1984;16:207-215.

40. Tran ZV, Weltman A. Differential effects of exercise on serum lipid and lipoprotein levels seen with changes in body weight: A meta-analysis. *JAMA* 1985;254:919-924.

41. Shah PK, Kaul S, Nilsson J, Cercek B. Exploiting the vascular protective effects of high-density lipoprotein and its apolipoproteins: An idea whose time for testing is coming, part I. *Circulation* 2001;104:2376-2683.

42. Mokdad AH, Bowman BA, Ford ES, Vinicor F, Marks JS, Koplan JP. The continuing epidemics of obesity and diabetes in the United States. *JAMA* 2001;286: 1195-1200.

43. Ross R, Rissanen J, Pedwell H, Clifford J, Shragge P. Influence of diet and exercise on skeletal muscle and visceral adipose tissue in men. *J Appl Physiol* 1996;81: 2445-2455.

44. Tchernof A, Nolan A, Sites CK, Ades PA, Poehlman ET. Weight loss reduces C-reactive protein levels in obese postmenopausal women. *Circulation* 2002;105: 564-569.

45. Ziccardi P, Nappo F, Giugliano G, et al. Reduction in inflammatory cytokine concentrations and improvement of endothelial functions in obese women after weight loss over one year. *Circulation* 2002;105:804-809.

46. McGuire MT, Wing RR, Hill JO. Behavioral strategies of individuals who have maintained long-term weight losses. *Obes Res* 1999;7:334-341.

47. Jakicic JM, Clark K, Coleman E, et al. American College of Sports Medicine position stand: Appropriate intervention strategies for weight loss and prevention of weight regain for adults. *Med Sci Sports Exerc* 2001;33: 2145-2156.

48. DiPietro L, Kohl HW III, Barlow CE, Blair SN. Improvements in cardiorespiratory fitness attenuate age-related weight gain in healthy men and women: The Aerobics Center Longitudinal Study. *Int J Obes* 1998;22:55-62.

49. Martinsen EW, Medhus A, Sandvik L. Effects of aerobic exercise on depression: A controlled study. *Br Med J (Clin Res Ed)* 1985;291:109.

50. Ades PA. Cardiac rehabilitation and secondary prevention of coronary heart disease. *N Engl J Med* 2001;345: 892-902.

51. Ford ES, Giles WH, Dietz WH. Prevalence of the metabolic syndrome among US adults: Findings from the third National Health and Nutrition Examination Survey. *JAMA* 2002;287:356-359.

52. Expert Panel on Detection, Evaluation, and Treatment of High Blood Cholesterol in Adults. Executive summary of the third report of the National Cholesterol Education Program (NCEP) expert panel on detection, evaluation, and treatment of high blood cholesterol in adults (Adult Treatment Panel III). *JAMA* 2001;285: 2486-2497.

53. Grundy SM, Hansen B, Smith SC, et al. AHA/NHLBI/ADA Conference Proceedings. Clinical management of metabolic syndrome. *Circulation* 2004;109:551-556.

54. Bjorntorp B, Fahlen M, Grimby G, et al. Carbohydrate and lipid metabolism in middle-aged, physically well-trained men. *Metabolism* 1972;21:1032-1044.

55. Knowler WC, Barrett-Connor E, Fowler SE, et al. Reduction in the incidence of type 2 diabetes with lifestyle intervention or metformin. *N Engl J Med* 2002;346:393-403.

56. Hu FB, Manson JE, Stampfer MJ, et al. Diet, lifestyle, and the risk of type 2 diabetes mellitus in women. *N Engl J Med* 2001;345:790-797.

57. Tuomilehto J, Lindstrom J, Eriksson JG, et al. Prevention of type 2 diabetes mellitus by changes in lifestyle among subjects with impaired glucose tolerance. *N Engl J Med* 2001;344:1343-1350.

58. Levy WC, Cerqueira MD, Harp GD, et al. Effect of endurance exercise training on heart rate variability at rest in healthy young and older men. *Am J Cardiol* 1998;82:1236-1241.

59. Tygesen H, Wettervik C, Wennerblom B. Intensive home-based exercise training in cardiac rehabilitation increases exercise capacity and heart rate variability. *Int J Card* 2001;79:175-182.

60. Squires RW. Coronary atherosclerosis. In: *American College of Sports Medicine. ACSM's Resource Manual for Guidelines for Exercise Testing and Prescription*. Fourth Edition. Philadelphia: Lippincott Williams & Wilkins, 2001, pp. 227-237.

61. Verma S, Anderson TJ. Fundamentals of endothelial function for the clinical cardiologist. *Circulation* 2002;105:546-549.

62. Hambrecht R, Wolf A, Gielen S, et al. Effect of exercise on coronary endothelial function in patients with coronary artery disease. *N Engl J Med* 2000;342:454-460.

63. Hambrecht R, Adams V, Erbs S, et al. Regular physical activity improves endothelial function in patients with coronary artery disease by increasing phosphorylation of endothelial nitric oxide synthase. *Circulation* 2003;107:3152-3158.

64. Dimmler S, Zeiher AM. Exercise and cardiovascular health. Get active to "AKTivate" your endothelial nitric oxide synthase. *Circulation* 2003;107:3118-3120.

65. Hambrecht R, Niebauer J, Marburger C, et al. Various intensities of leisure time physical activity in patients with coronary artery disease: Effects on cardiorespiratory fitness and progression of coronary atherosclerotic lesions. *J Am Coll Cardiol* 1993;22:468-477.

66. Koenig W, Ernst E. Exercise and thrombosis. *Coronary Artery Dis* 2000;11:123-127.

67. Ernst E. Regular exercise reduces fibrinogen levels: A review of longitudinal studies. *Br J Sports Med* 1993;27: 175-176.

68. Paramo JA, Olavide I, Barba J, et al. Long-term cardiac rehabilitation program favorably influences fibrinolysis and lipid concentrations in acute myocardial infarction. *Haematologica* 1998;83:519-524.

69. Lehman M, Keul J. Physical activity and coronary heart disease: Sympathetic drive and adrenaline-induced platelet aggregation. *Int J Sports Med* 1986;7(suppl 1): 34-37.

70. Ehsani AA, Martin WH, Heath GW, Coyle EF. Cardiac effects of prolonged and intense exercise training in patients with coronary artery disease. *Am J Cardiol* 1982;50:246-254.

71. Schuler G, Schlierf G, Wirth A, et al. Low-fat diet and regular, supervised physical exercise in patients with symptomatic coronary artery disease: Reduction of stress-induced myocardial ischemia. *Circulation* 1988;77:172-181.

72. Todd IC, Bradnam MS, Cooke MB, Ballantyne D. Effects of daily high-intensity exercise on myocardial perfusion in angina pectoris. *Am J Cardiol* 1991;68:1593-1599.

73. Laslett LJ, Paumer L, Amsterdam EA. Increase in myocardial oxygen consumption index by exercise training at the onset of ischemia in patients with coronary artery disease. *Circulation* 1985;71:958-962.

Chapter 6

1. Hung J, Goldwater D, Convertino VA, et al. Mechanisms for decreased exercise capacity after bed rest in normal middle-aged men. *Am J Cardiol* 1983;51:344-348.

2. Saltin B, Blomqvist G, Mitchell JH, et al. Response to exercise after bed rest and after training. *Circulation* 1968;38(suppl 7):1-78.

3. Myers J. Physiologic adaptations to exercise and immobility. In: *Cardiac Nursing*. Third Edition. Woods SL, Sivarijan-Froelicher ES, Halpenny CJ, Vanderhill Motzer S (eds). Philadelphia: Lippincott, 1995, pp. 147-162.

4. Ades PA. Cardiac rehabilitation and secondary prevention of coronary heart disease. *N Engl J Med* 2001;345: 892-902.

5. Agency for Health Care Policy and Research Clinical Practice Guidelines. *Cardiac Rehabilitation*. Washington, DC: U.S. Department of Health and Human Services, 1995.

6. Nelson RR, Gobel FL, Jorgensen CR, et al. Hemodynamic predictors of myocardial oxygen consumption

during static and dynamic exercise. *Circulation* 1974;50: 1179-1189.

7. Hammond HK, Froelicher VF. Normal and abnormal heart rate responses to exercise. *Prog Cardiovasc Dis* 1985;27:271-296.

8. Froelicher VF, Myers J. *Exercise and the Heart*. Fourth Edition. Philadelphia: Saunders, 2000.

9. Franciosa JA, Park M, Levine TH. Lack of correlation between exercise capacity and indexes of resting left ventricular performance in heart failure. *Am J Cardiol* 1981;47:33-39.

10. McKirnan MD, Sullivan M, Jensen D, et al. Treadmill performance and cardiac function in selected patients with coronary heart disease. *J Am Coll Cardiol* 1984;3: 253-261.

11. Myers J, Froelicher VF. Hemodynamic determinants of exercise capacity in chronic heart failure. *Ann Intern Med* 1991;115:377-386.

12. Sullivan MJ, Green HJ, Coff FR. Altered skeletal muscle metabolic response to exercise in chronic heart failure: Relation to skeletal muscle aerobic enzyme activity. *Circulation* 1991;84:1597-1607.

13. Hambrecht R, Niebauer J, Fiehn E, et al. Physical training in patients with stable chronic heart failure: Effects on cardiorespiratory fitness and ultrastructural abnormalities of leg muscles. *J Am Coll Cardiol* 1995;25: 1239-1249.

14. Myers J, Salleh A, Buchanan N, et al. Ventilatory mechanisms of exercise intolerance in chronic heart failure. *Am Heart J* 1992;124:710-719.

15. Wada O, Asanoi H, Miyagi K, et al. Importance of abnormal lung perfusion in excessive exercise ventilation in chronic heart failure. *Am Heart J* 1993;125:790-798.

16. Sullivan MJ, Higginbotham MB, Cobb FR. Increased exercise ventilation in patients with chronic heart failure: Intact ventilatory control despite hemodynamic and pulmonary abnormalities. *Circulation* 1988;73: 552-559.

17. Clark AL, Piepoli M, Coats AJS. Skeletal muscle and the control of ventilation on exercise: Evidence for metabolic receptors. *Eur J Clin Invest* 1995;25:299-305.

18. American Association of Cardiovascular and Pulmonary Rehabilitation. *Guidelines for Cardiac Rehabilitation Programs*. Fourth Edition Champaign, IL: Human Kinetics, 2004.

19. Blair SN, Cheng Y, Holder JS. Is physical activity or physical fitness more important in defining health benefits? *Med Sci Sports Exerc* 2001;33:S379-S399.

20. Myers J, Prakash M, Froelicher V, Do Dat, Partington S, Atwood E. Exercise capacity and mortality among men referred for exercise testing. *N Engl J Med* 2002;346: 793-801.

21. Dorn J, Naughton J, Imamura D, Trevisan M. Results of a multicenter randomized clinical trial of exercise and long-term survival in myocardial infarction patients: The National Exercise and Heart Disease Project. *Circulation* 1999;100:1764-1769.

22. Poliner LR, Dehmer GJ, Lewis SE, et al. Left ventricular performance in normal subjects. A comparison of the responses to exercise in the upright and supine position. *Circulation* 1980;62:528-536.

23. Levine BD, Lane LD, Buckey JC, et al. Left ventricular pressure-volume and Frank–Starling relations in endurance athletes: Implications for orthostatic tolerance and exercise performance. *Circulation* 1991;84:1016-1023.

24. Belardinelli R, Georgiou D, Cianci G, Berman N, Ginzton L, Purcaro A. Exercise training improves left ventricular diastolic filling in patients with dilated cardiomyopathy. *Circulation* 1995;91:2775-2784.

25. Brubaker PH. Clinical considerations and exercise responses of patients with primary left ventricular diastolic dysfunction. *Clin Exerc Physiol* 1999;1:5-12.

26. Kiowski W, Sutsch G, Schalcher C, Brunner HP, Oechslin E. Endothelial control of vascular tone in chronic heart failure. *J Cardiovasc Pharmacol* 1998;32:S67-S73.

27. Hambrecht R, Fiehn E, Weigl C, Gielen S, Hamann C, et al. Regular physical exercise corrects endothelial dysfunction and improves exercise capacity in patients with chronic heart failure. *Circulation* 1998;98: 2709-2715.

28. Linke A, Schoene N, Gielen S, et al. Endothelial dysfunction in patients with chronic heart failure: Systemic effects of lower-limb exercise training. *J Am Coll Cardiol* 2001;37:392-397.

29. Andersen P, Henriksson J. Capillary supply of the quadriceps femoris muscle of man: Adaptive response to exercise. *J Physiol (Lond)* 1977;270:677-691.

30. Saltin B, Gollnick PD. Skeletal muscle adaptability: Significance for metabolism and performance. In: *Handbook of Physiology. Skeletal Muscle*. Peachy LD, Adrian RH, Geiger SR (eds). Bethesda, MD: American Physiological Society, 1983, pp. 555-631.

31. Saltin B, Rowell LB. Functional adaptations to physical activity and inactivity. *Fed Proc* 1980;39:1506-1516.

32. Hudlick O. Growth of capillaries in skeletal and cardiac muscle. *Circ Res* 1982;50:451-456.

33. Ingjer F, Brodal P. Capillary supply of skeletal muscle fibers in untrained and endurance-trained women. *Eur J Appl Physiol* 1978;38:291-296.

34. Mancini DM, Henson D, LaManca J, Donchez L, Levine S. Benefit of selective respiratory muscle training on exercise capacity in patients with chronic congestive heart failure. *Circulation* 1995;91:320-329.

35. Mancini DM. Pulmonary factors limiting exercise capacity in patients with heart failure. *Prog Cardiovasc Dis* 1995;6:347-370.

36. Levine S, Weiser P, Gillen J. Evaluation of ventilatory muscle endurance training program in the rehabilitation of patents with chronic obstructive pulmonary disease. *Am Rev Respir Dis* 1986;133:400-406.

37. Parcy R, Reid W, Belman M. Respiratory muscle training. *Clin Chest Med* 1988;9:287-296.

38. Belman MJ. Ventilatory muscle training and unloading. In: *Principles and Practice of Pulmonary Rehabilitation*.

Casaburi R, Petty T (eds). Philadelphia: Saunders, 1993, pp. 225-240.

Chapter 7

1. American College of Sports Medicine. *ACSM's Guidelines for Exercise Testing and Prescription.* Sixth Edition. Franklin BA, Whaley, MH, Howley ET (eds). Baltimore: Lippincott, William & Wilkins, 2000.

2. Franklin BA. Revitalizing the conventional exercise stress test. *Am J Med Sports* 2002;4:190-194.

3. Convertino VA. Effect of orthostatic stress on exercise performance after bed rest: Relation to inhospital rehabilitation. *J Cardiac Rehabil* 1983;3:660-663.

4. Dunn AL, Marcus BH, Kampert JB, et al. Comparison of lifestyle and structured interventions to increase physical activity and cardiorespiratory fitness. *JAMA* 1999;281:327-334.

5. Andersen RE, Wadden TA, Bartlett SJ, et al. Effects of lifestyle activity vs structured aerobic exercise in obese women. *JAMA* 1999;281:335-340.

6. Franklin BA, Gordon S, Timmis GC. Amount of exercise necessary for the patient with coronary artery disease. *Am J Cardiol* 1992;69:1426-1432.

7. Porcari JP, McCarron R, Kline G, et al. Is fast walking an adequate training stimulus for 30 to 69 year-old men and women? *Phys Sportsmed* 1987;1:119-129.

8. Quell KJ, Porcari JP, Franklin BA, et al. Is brisk walking an adequate aerobic training stimulus for cardiac patients? *Chest* 2002;122:1852-1856.

9. Pollock ML, Miller HS, Janeway R, et al. Effects of walking on body composition and cardiovascular function of middle-aged men. *J Appl Physiol* 1971;30:126-130.

10. Evans BW, Cureton KJ, Purvis JW. Metabolic and circulatory responses to walking and jogging in water. *Res Q Exerc Sport* 1978;49:442-449.

11. Shoenfeld Y, Keren G, Shimoni T, et al. Walking: A method for rapid improvement of physical fitness. *JAMA* 1980;243:2062-2063.

12. Pollock ML, Gaesser GA, Butcher JD, et al. The recommended quantity and quality of exercise for developing and maintaining cardiorespiratory and muscular fitness, and flexibility in healthy adults. *Med Sci Sports Exerc* 1998;30:975-991.

13. Sady SP, Wortman M, Blanke D. Flexibility training: Ballistic, static or proprioceptive neuromuscular facilitation? *Arch Phys Med Rehabil* 1982;63:261-263.

14. American Association of Cardiovascular and Pulmonary Rehabilitation. *Guidelines for Cardiac Rehabilitation and Secondary Prevention Programs.* Third Edition. Champaign, IL: Human Kinetics, 1999.

15. Pollock ML, Franklin BA, Balady GJ, et al. Resistance exercise in individuals with and without cardiovascular disease: Benefits, rationale, safety, and prescription. *Circulation* 2000;101:828-833.

16. Pate RR, Pratt M, Blair SN, et al. Physical activity and public health: A recommendation from the Centers for Disease Control and Prevention and the American College of Sports Medicine. *JAMA* 1995;273:402-407.

17. Gordon NF, Kohl HW, Blair SN. Life style exercise: A new strategy to promote physical activity for adults. *J Cardiopulm Rehabil* 1993;13(3):161-163.

18. Swain DP, Franklin BA. $\dot{V}O_2$ reserve and the minimal intensity for improving cardiorespiratory fitness. *Med Sci Sports Exerc* 2002;34:152-157.

19. Swain DP, Franklin BA. Is there a threshold intensity for aerobic training in cardiac patients? *Med Sci Sports Exerc* 2002;34:1071-1075.

20. Casperson CJ, Powell KE, Christenson GM. Physical activity, exercise, and physical fitness. *Public Health Rep* 1985;100:125-131.

21. Leon AS, Norstrom J. Evidence of the role of physical activity and cardiorespiratory fitness in the prevention of coronary heart disease. *Quest* 1995;47:311-319.

22. Swain DP, Leutholtz BC. Heart rate reserve is equivalent to % $\dot{V}O_2$ Reserve, not to % $\dot{V}O_2$ max. *Med Sci Sports Exerc* 1997;29:410-414.

23. Swain DP, Leutholtz BC, King ME, et al. Relationship of % heart rate reserve and % $\dot{V}O_2$ reserve in treadmill exercise. *Med Sci Sports Exerc* 1998;30:318-321.

24. Swain DP. % $\dot{V}O_2$ reserve: A new method for exercise prescription. *ACSM's Health & Fitness Journal* 1999;3(5):10-14.

25. Karvonen M, Kentala K, Mustala O. The effects of training heart rate: A longitudinal study. *Ann Med Exp Biol* 1957;35:307-315.

26. Fox SM, Naughton JP, Gorman PA. Physical activity and cardiovascular health. III. The exercise prescription: Frequency and type of activity. *Mod Concepts Cardiovasc Dis* 1972;41:21-24.

27. Wilmore JH. Exercise prescription: Role of the physiatrist and allied health professional. *Arch Phys Med Rehabil* 1976;57:315-319.

28. Pandolf KB, Cafarelli E, Noble BJ, et al. Hyperthermia: Effect on exercise prescription. *Arch Phys Med Rehabil* 1975;56:524-526.

29. American Heart Association Committee on Exercise. *Exercise Testing and Training of Individuals With Heart Disease or at High Risk for Its Development: A Handbook for Physicians.* Dallas: American Heart Association, 1975.

30. Taylor HL, Haskell W, Fox SM III, et al. Exercise tests: A summary of procedures and concepts of stress testing for cardiovascular diagnosis and function evaluation. In: *Measurement in Exercise Electrocardiography (The Ernst Simonson Conference).* Blackburn H (ed). Springfield, IL: Charles C Thomas, 1969, p. 259.

31. Hossack KF, Bruce RA, Clark LJ. Influence of propranolol on exercise prescription of training heart rates. *Cardiology* 1980;65:47-58.

32. Chang K, Hossack KF. Effect of diltiazem on heart rate responses and respiratory variables during exercise:

Implications for exercise prescription and cardiac rehabilitation. *J Cardiac Rehabil* 1982;2:326-332.

33. Gibbons RJ, Balady GJ, Beasley JW, et al. ACC/AHA guidelines for exercise testing. A report of the American College of Cardiology/American Heart Association Task Force on Practice Guidelines (Committee on Exercise Testing). *J Am Coll Cardiol* 1997;30:260-311.

34. Gill TM, DiPietro L, Krumholz HM. Role of exercise stress testing and safety monitoring for older persons starting an exercise program. *JAMA* 2000;284:342-349.

35. Little WC, Constantinescu M, Applegate RJ, et al. Can coronary angiography predict the site of a subsequent myocardial infarction in patients with mild to moderate coronary artery disease? *Circulation* 1988;78:1157-1166.

36. Ambrose JA, Tannenbaum MA, Alexopoulos D, et al. Angiographic progression of coronary artery disease and the development of myocardial infarction. *J Am Coll Cardiol* 1988;12:56-62.

37. McConnell TR. Exercise prescription: When the guidelines do not work. *J Cardiopulm Rehabil* 1996;16:34-37.

38. Pollock ML, Gomes PS. Exercise prescription: With and without exercise testing. In: *Cardiac Rehabilitation: Guide to Procedures for the 21st Century*. Wenger NK, Smith E, Froelicher E, Comoss P (eds). New York: Marcel Dekker, 1999.

39. Joo KC, Brubaker PH, MacDougall A, et al. Exercise prescription using resting heart rate plus 20 or perceived exertion in cardiac rehabilitation. *J Cardiopulm Rehabil* 2004;24:178-184.

40. McConnell TR, Klinger TA, Gardner JK, et al. Cardiac rehabilitation without exercise tests for post-myocardial infarction and post-bypass surgery patients. *J Cardiopulm Rehabil* 1998;18:458-463.

41. Dressendorfer RH, Franklin BA, Cameron JL, et al. Exercise training frequency in early post-infarction cardiac rehabilitation: Influence on aerobic conditioning. *J Cardiopulm Rehabil* 1995;15:269-276.

42. Pollock ML, Gettman LR, Milesis CA, et al. Effects of frequency and duration of training on attrition and incidence of injury. *Med Sci Sports Exerc* 1977;9:31-36.

43. U.S. Department of Health and Human Services. *Physical Activity and Health: A Report of the Surgeon General*. Atlanta: U.S. Department of Health and Human Services, Centers for Disease Control and Prevention, National Center for Chronic Disease Prevention and Health Promotion, 1996.

44. Pollock ML. Quantification of endurance training programs. In: *Exercise and Sport Sciences Reviews*. Wilmore JH (ed). New York: Academic Press, 1973, p. 155.

45. Franklin BA. Exercise adds up like loose change. *ACSM's Health & Fitness Journal* 1999;3(4):38-39.

46. Fletcher GF, Balady GJ, Amsterdam EA, et al. Exercise standards for testing and training. A statement for healthcare professionals from the American Heart Association. *Circulation* 2001;104:1694-1740.

47. USDA/DHHS (U.S. Department of Agriculture/U.S. Department of Health and Human Services). *Nutrition and Your Health: Dietary Guidelines for Americans* (Home and Garden Bulletin No. 232). Sixth Edition.

Washington, DC: U.S. Department of Agriculture, U.S. Department of Health and Human Services, 2002.

48. Hambrecht R, Niebauer J, Marburger C, et al. Various intensities of leisure time physical activity in patients with coronary artery disease: Effects on cardiorespiratory fitness and progression of coronary atherosclerotic lesions. *J Am Coll Cardiol* 1993;22:468-477.

49. Clausen JP, Trap-Jensen J, Lassen NA. The effects of training on the heart rate during arm and leg exercise. *Scand J Clin Lab Invest* 1970;26:295-301.

50. Klausen K, Rasmussen B, Clausen JP, et al. Blood lactate from exercising extremities before and after arm or leg training. *Am J Physiol* 1974;227:67-72.

51. Rasmussen B, Klausen K, Clausen JP, et al. Pulmonary ventilation, blood gases and blood pH after training of the arms or the legs. *J Appl Physiol* 1975;38:250-256.

52. Henriksson J, Reitman JS. Time course of changes in human skeletal muscle succinate dehydrogenase and cytochrome oxidase activities and maximal oxygen uptake with physical activity and inactivity. *Acta Physiol Scand* 1977;99:91-97.

53. Franklin BA. Aerobic exercise training programs for the upper body. *Med Sci Sports Exerc* 1989;21:S141-S148.

54. Franklin BA, Vander L, Wrisley D, et al. Trainability of arms versus legs in men with previous myocardial infarction. *Chest* 1994;105:262-264.

55. Franklin BA. Exercise testing, training and arm ergometry. *Sports Med* 1985;2:100-119.

56. Frost G. The Playbuoy® exercise device. *Am Corr Ther J* 1977;31:156.

57. Grais SL, McClintock S, Franklin BA, et al. Myocardial and aerobic requirements for an upper body exerciser: Implications for cardiac rehabilitation. *Arch Phys Med Rehabil* 1991;72:563-566.

58. Amos K, Porcari JP, Bauer S, Wilson P. The safety and effectiveness of walking with ankle and wrist weights in cardiac rehabilitation patients. *J Cardiopulm Rehabil* 1992;12(4):254-260.

59. Oldridge NB, Connolly C. Oxygen uptake and heart rate during cross-country skiing and track walking after myocardial infarction. *Am Heart J* 1989;117:495-497.

60. Fardy PS, Webb D, Hellerstein HK. Benefits of arm exercise in cardiac rehabilitation. *Phys Sportsmed* 1977;5:30-41.

61. Goss FL, Robertson RJ, Auble TE, et al. Are treadmill-based exercise prescriptions generalizable to combined arm and leg exercise? *J Cardiopulm Rehabil* 1987;7:551-555.

62. Wetherbee S, Franklin BA, Hollingsworth V, et al. Relationship between arm and leg training work loads in men with heart disease: Implications for exercise prescription. *Chest* 1991;99:1271-1273.

63. Mc Cartney N, McKelvie RS, Martin J, et al. Weight-training-induced attenuation of the circulatory response of older males to weight lifting. *J Appl Physiol* 1993;74:1056-1060.

64. Hickson RC, Rosenkoetter MA, Brown MM. Strength training effects on aerobic power and short-term endurance. *Med Sci Sports Exerc* 1980;12:336-339.

65. Ades PA, Ballor DL, Ashikaga T, et al. Weight training improves walking endurance in healthy elderly persons. *Ann Intern Med* 1996;124:568-572.

66. Franklin BA, Bonzheim K, Gordon S, et al. Resistance training in cardiac rehabilitation. *J Cardiopulm Rehabil* 1991;11:99-107.

67. Feigenbaum MS, Pollock ML. Strength training: Rationale for current guidelines for adult fitness programs. *Phys Sportsmed* 1997;25:44-64.

Chapter 8

1. Kadish AH, Buxton AE, Kennedy HL, et al. ACC/AHA clinical competence statement on electrocardiography and ambulatory electrocardiography. A report of the ACC/AHA/ACP-ASIM Task Force on Clinical Competence (ACC/AHA Committee to Develop a Clinical Competence Statement on Electrocardiography and Ambulatory Electrocardiography). *Circulation* 2001;104:3169-3178.

2. Mirvis DM, Berson AS, Goldberger AL, et al. Instrumentation and practice standards for electrocardiographic monitoring in special care units. *Circulation* 1989;79:464-471.

3. Fletcher GF, Balady GJ, Amsterdam EA, et al. Exercise standards for testing and training: A statement for healthcare professionals from the American Heart Association. *Circulation* 2001;104:1694-1740.

4. Wanderman KL, Loutaty G, Ovsyshcher I, Cantor A, Gussarsky Y, Gueron M. Choice of electrocardiographic leads for recording the earliest QRS onset in noninvasive measurements. *Circulation* 1981;63:933-937.

5. Selvester RH, Velasquez DW, Elko PP, Cady LD. Intraventricular conduction defect (IVCD), real or fancied, QRS duration in 1,254 normal adult white males by a multilead automated algorithm. *J Electrocardiol* 1990;23(suppl):118-22.

6. MacFarlane PW, Lawrie TDV. *Comprehensive Electrocardiology: Theory and Practice in Health and Disease*. New York: Pergamon, 1989.

7. Drew BJ, Ide, B. Importance of accurate lead placement. *Progr Cardiovasc Nurs* 1994;Spring:44.

8. Wagner GS. *Marriott's Practical Electrocardiography*. 10th Edition. Baltimore: Williams & Wilkins, 2001.

9. Maurer MS, Shefrin EA, Fleg JL. Prevalence and prognostic significance of exercise-induced supraventricular tachycardia in apparently healthy volunteers. *Am J Cardiol* 1995;75:788-792.

10. Josephson M. *Clinical Cardiac Electrophysiology: Techniques and Interpretations*. Third Edition. Philadelphia: Lippincott Williams & Wilkins, 2002.

11. Gibbons RJ, Balady GJ, Bricker JT, et al. ACC/AHA 2002 guideline update for exercise testing: Summary article: A report of the American College of Cardiology/American Heart Association Task Force on Practice Guidelines (Committee to Update the 1997 Exercise Testing Guidelines). *Circulation* 2002;106:1883-1892.

12. Yeh SJ, Lin FC, Wu DL. The mechanisms of exercise provocation of supraventricular tachycardia. *Am Heart J* 1989;117:1041-1049.

13. Gooch AS. Exercise testing for detecting changes in cardiac rhythm and conduction. *Am J Cardiol* 1972;30:741-746.

14. Vedin JA, Wilhelmsson CE, Wilhelmsen L, Bjure J, Ekstrom-Jodal B. Relation of resting and exercise-induced ectopic beats to other ischemic manifestations and to coronary risk factors. Men born in 1913. *Am J Cardiol* 1972;30:25-31.

15. Olgin JE, Zipes DP. Specific arrhythmias: Diagnosis and treatment. In: *Heart Disease: A Textbook of Cardiovascular Medicine*. Sixth Edition. Braunwald E, Zipes DP, Libby P (eds). Philadelphia: Saunders, 2001, pp. 815-889.

16. Ortiz J, Nozaki A, Shimizu A, Khrestian C, Rudy Y, Waldo AL. Mechanism of interruption of atrial flutter by moricizine. Electrophysiological and multiplexing studies in the canine sterile pericarditis model of atrial flutter. *Circulation* 1994;89:2860-2869.

17. Cosio FG, Lopez Gil M, Arribas F, Palacios J, Goicolea A, Nunez A. Mechanisms of entrainment of human common flutter studied with multiple endocardial recordings. *Circulation* 1994;89:2117-2125.

18. Nagai N, Nagai K, Chun SJ, et al. Roles of the suprachiasmatic nucleus and vasoactive intestinal peptide in the response of plasma arginine vasopressin to osmotic challenge. *Endocrinology* 1996;137:504-507.

19. Evans T. *ECG Interpretation Cribsheets*. San Francisco: Ring Mountain Press, 1996.

20. Frolkis JP, Pothier CE, Blackstone EH, Lauer MS. Frequent ventricular ectopy after exercise as a predictor of death. *N Engl J Med* 2003;348:781-790.

21. Drew BJ, Scheinman MM. ECG criteria to distinguish between aberrantly conducted supraventricular tachycardia and ventricular tachycardia: Practical aspects for the immediate care setting. *Pacing Clin Electrophysiol* 1995;18:2194-2208.

22. Yuzuki Y, Horie M, Makita T, Watanuki M, Takahashi A, Sasayama S. Exercise-induced second-degree atrioventricular block. *Jpn Circ J* 1997;61:268-271.

23. Barold SS, Jais P, Shah DC, Takahashi A, Haissaguerre M, Clementy J. Exercise-induced second-degree AV block: Is it type I or type II? *J Cardiovasc Electrophysiol* 1997;8:1084-1086.

24. Sumiyoshi M, Nakata Y, Yasuda M, et al. Clinical and electrophysiologic features of exercise-induced atrioventricular block. *Am Heart J* 1996;132:1277-1281.

25. Byrne JM, Marais HJ, Cheek GA. Exercise-induced complete heart block in a patient with chronic bifascicular block. *J Electrocardiol* 1994;27:339-342.

26. Behar S, Zissman E, Zion M, et al. Prognostic significance of second-degree atrioventricular block in inferior wall acute myocardial infarction. SPRINT Study Group. *Am J Cardiol* 1993;72:831-834.

27. Sandberg L. Studies on electrocardiographic changes during exercise tests. *Acta Med Scand* 1961;169(suppl 365):1-117.

28. Boran KJ, Oliveros RA, Boucher CA, Beckmann CH, Seaworth JF. Ischemia-associated intraventricular conduction disturbances during exercise testing as a predictor of proximal left anterior descending coronary artery disease. *Am J Cardiol* 1983;51:1098-1102.

29. Grady TA, Chiu AC, Snader CE, et al. Prognostic significance of exercise-induced left bundle-branch block. *JAMA* 1998;279:153-156.

30. Kligfield P, Hochreiter C, Okin PM, Borer JS. Transient loss of complete bundle branch block patterns during exercise. *Am J Cardiol* 1995;75:523-525.

31. Haisty WK, Pahlm O, Wagner NB, et al. Performance of the automated complete Selvester QRS scoring system in normal subjects and patients with single and multiple myocardial infarction. *J Am Coll Cardiol* 1992;19: 341-346.

32. Mirvis DM, Goldberger AL. Electrocardiography. In: *Heart Disease*. Sixth Edition. Braunwald EZD, Libby P (eds). Philadelphia: Saunders, 2001, pp. 82-128.

33. Braat SH, Brugada P, den Dulk K, van Ommen V, Wellens HJ. Value of lead V4R for recognition of the infarct coronary artery in acute inferior myocardial infarction. *Am J Cardiol* 1984;53:1538-1541.

34. Wung SF, Drew BJ. New electrocardiographic criteria for posterior wall acute myocardial ischemia validated by a percutaneous transluminal coronary angioplasty model of acute myocardial infarction. *Am J Cardiol* 2001;87:970-974,A4.

35. Mark DB, Hlatky MA, Lee KL, Harrell FE Jr, Califf RM, Pryor DB. Localizing coronary artery obstructions with the exercise treadmill test. *Ann Intern Med* 1987;106: 53-55.

36. Goldschlager N, Selzer A, Cohn K. Treadmill stress tests as indicators of presence and severity of coronary artery disease. *Ann Intern Med* 1976;85:277-286.

37. Martin CM, McConahay DR. Maximal treadmill exercise electrocardiography. Correlations with coronary arteriography and cardiac hemodynamics. *Circulation* 1972;46:956-962.

38. Michaelides AP, Psomadaki ZD, Dilaveris PE, et al. Improved detection of coronary artery disease by exercise electrocardiography with the use of right precordial leads. *N Engl J Med* 1999;340:340-345.

39. Chouhan L, Krone RJ, Keller A, Eisenkramer G. Utility of lead V4R in exercise testing for detection of coronary artery disease. *Am J Cardiol* 1989;64:938-939.

40. Braat SH, Kingma JH, Brugada P, Wellens HJ. Value of lead V4R in exercise testing to predict proximal stenosis of the right coronary artery. *J Am Coll Cardiol* 1985;5: 1308-1311.

41. Shry EA, Eckart RE, Furgerson JL, Stajduhar KC, Krasuski RA. Addition of right-sided and posterior precordial leads during stress testing. *Am Heart J* 2003;146: 1090-1094.

42. Sabapathy R, Bloom HL, Lewis WR, Amsterdam EA. Right precordial and posterior chest leads do not increase detection of positive response in electrocardiogram during exercise treadmill testing. *Am J Cardiol* 2003;91:75-77.

Chapter 9

1. American Heart Association. *2004 Heart and Stroke Statistical Update.* Dallas: American Heart Association, 2004.

2. Mosca L, Ferris A, Fabunmi R, Robertson RM. Tracking women's awareness of heart disease. An American Heart Association national survey. Circulation 2004;109: 573-579.

3. Tofler GH, Stone PH, Muller JE. Effects of gender and race on prognosis after myocardial infarction: Adverse prognosis for women, particularly black women. *J Am Coll Cardiol* 1987;9:473-482.

4. Fibrinolytic Therapy Trialists (FTT) Collaborative Group. Indications for fibrinolytic therapy in suspected acute myocardial infarction: Collaborative overview of early mortality and major morbidity results from all randomized trials of more than 1000 patients. *Lancet* 1994;343:311-322.

5. Chandra NC, Zeigelstein RC, Rogers WJ, et al. Observations of the treatment of women in the United States with myocardial infarction. *Arch Intern Med* 1998;158: 981-988.

6. Mosca L, Manson JE, Sutherland SE, Langer RD, Manolio T, Barrett-Connor E. Cardiovascular disease in women. A statement for healthcare professionals from the American Heart Association. *Circulation* 1997;96: 2468-2482.

7. Cummings SR, Black DM, Rubin SM. Lifetime risks of hip, Colles' or vertebral fracture and coronary artery disease among white postmenopausal women. *Arch Intern Med* 1989;149:2445-2448.

8. Eaker ED, Kronmal R, Kennedy JW, Davis K. Comparison of the long-term, post-surgical survival of women and men in the Coronary Artery Surgery Study (CASS). *Am Heart J* 1989;117:71-80.

9. Cannistra LB, Balady GJ, O'Mallley CJ, Weiner DA, Ryan TJ. Comparison of the clinical profile and outcome of women and men in cardiac rehabilitation. *Am J Cardiol* 1992;69:1274-1279.

10. Maynard C, Althouse R, Cerqueira M, Olsufka M, Kennedy JW. Underutilization of thrombolytic therapy in eligible women with acute myocardial infarction. *Am J Cardiol* 1990;68:529-530.

11. McLaughlin TJ, Soumerai SB, Willison DJ, et al. Adherence to national guidelines for drug treatment of suspected acute myocardial infarction: Evidence for undertreatment in women and elderly. *Arch Intern Med* 1996;156:799-805.

12. Scirica BM, Moliterno DJ, Every NR, et al. Differences between men and women in the management of unstable angina pectoris (the GUARANTEE registry). *Am J Cardiol* 1999;84:1145-1150.

13. Miller M, Byington R, Hunninghake D, et al. for the Prospective Randomized Evaluation of the Vascular Effects of Norvasc Trial (PREVENT) investigators. Sex bias and underutilization of lipid-lowering therapy in patients with coronary artery disease at academic

medical centers in the United States and Canada. *Arch Intern Med* 2000;160:343-347.

14. Wenger N. Coronary heart disease: Diagnostic decision making. In: *Cardiovascular Health and Disease in Women.* Douglas PS (ed). Philadelphia: Saunders, 1993, pp. 28-36.

15. Antiplatelet Trialists' Collaboration. Collaborative overview of randomized trials of antiplatelet therapy—I: prevention of death, myocardial infarction, and stroke by prolonged antiplatelet therapy in various categories of patients. *BMJ* 1994;308:81-106.

16. Pedersen TR, for the Scandinavian Simvastatin Survival Study Group. Randomised trial of cholesterol lowering in 4444 patients with coronary heart disease: The Scandinavian Simvastatin Survival Study (4S). *Lancet* 1994;344:1383-1389.

17. Downs JR, Clearfield M, Weis S, et al. Primary prevention of acute coronary events with lovastatin in men and women with average cholesterol levels. Results of AFCAPS/TexCAPS. *JAMA* 1998;339:1349-1357.

18. Tobin JN, Wassertheil-Smoller S, Wexler JP, et al. Sex bias in considering coronary bypass surgery. *Ann Intern Med* 1987;107:19-25.

19. Weitzman S, Cooper L, Chambless L, et al. Gender, racial, and geographic differences in the performance of cardiac diagnostic and therapeutic procedures for hospitalized acute myocardial infarction in four states. *Am J Cardiol* 1997;79:722-726.

20. Lavie CJ, Milani RV. Effects of cardiac rehabilitation and exercise training on exercise capacity, coronary risk factors, behavioral characteristics, and quality of life in women. *Am J Cardiol* 1995;75:340-343.

21. Thomas RJ, Miller NH, Lamendola C, et al. National survey on gender differences in cardiac rehabilitation programs: Patient characteristics and enrollment patterns. *J Cardiopulm Rehabil* 1996;16:402-412.

22. Mosca L, Appel LJ, Benjamin EJ, et al. Evidence-based guidelines for the prevention of cardiovascular disease in women. *Circulation* 2004;109:672-693.

23. Kannel WB, Feinleib M. Natural history of angina pectoris in the Framingham study. *Am J Cardiol* 1972;29:154-163.

24. Chaitman BR, Bourassa MG, Davis K, et al. Angiographic prevalence of high-risk coronary artery disease in patient subsets (CASS). *Circulation* 1981;64:360-367.

25a. Robertson RM. Women and cardiovascular disease. The risks of misperception and the need for action. *Circulation* 2001;103:2318-2320.

25b. Lansky AJ, Hochman JS, Ward PA, et al. *Circulation* 2005;111(7):940-953.

26. Kudenchek P, Maynard C, Martin J, Wirkus M, Weaver WD. Comparison of presentation, treatment, and outcome of acute myocardial infarction in men versus women (the Myocardial Infarction Triage and Intervention Registry). *Am J Cardiol* 1996;78:9-14.

27. Merz CB, Kelsey SF, Pepine CJ, et al. The Women's Ischemia Syndrome Evaluation (WISE) study: Protocol design, methodology, and feasibility report. *J Am Coll Cardiol* 1999;33:1453-1461.

28. Pepine CJ, Balaban RS, Bonow RO, et al. Women's Ischemia Syndrome Evaluation: Current status and future research directions. Section 1. Diagnosis of stable ischemia and ischemic heart disease. *Circulation* 2004;109:e44-e46.

29. Johnson BD, Kelsey SF, Bairey Merz CN. Clinical risk assessment in women: Chest discomfort. Report from the WISE study. In: *Coronary Disease in Women: Evidence-Based Diagnosis and Treatment.* Shaw LJ, Redberg RF (eds). Totowa, NJ: Humana Press, 2003, pp. 129-141.

30. Douglas PS, Ginsberg GS. The evaluation of chest pain in women. *N Engl J Med* 1996:334:1311-1315.

31. Waters DD, Halphen C, Theroux P, et al. Coronary artery disease in young women: Clinical and angiographic features and correlation with risk factors. *Am J Cardiol* 1978;42:41-47.

32. Bullemer F, Graham KJ, Pankow J, Meszaros T, Flygenring BP. Gender-related differences in risk factors of young patients with symptomatic coronary artery disease. Abstract. *J Am Co*

33. Mosca L, Grundy SM, Judelson D, et al. Guide to preventive cardiology for women: AHA/ACC Scientific Statement Consensus panel statement. *Circulation* 1999;99:2480-2484.

34. Mosca L, Appel LJ, Benjamin EJ, et al. Evidence-based guidelines for cardiovascular disease prevention in women. *J Am Coll Cardiol* 2004;43:900-921.

35. Willet WC, Green A, Stampfer W, et al. Relative and absolute excess risks of coronary heart disease among women who smoke cigarettes. *N Engl J Med* 1987;317: 1303-1309.

36. Hansen EF, Andersen LT, Von Eyben FE. Cigarette smoking and age at first acute myocardial infarction, and influence of gender and extent of smoking. *Am J Cardiol* 1993;71:1439-1442.

37. Manolio TA, Pearson TA, Wenger NK, Barrett-Connor E, Payne GH, Harlan WR. Cholesterol and heart disease in older persons and women: Review of an NHLBI workshop. *Ann Epidemiol* 1992;2:161-176.

38. Bass KM, Newschaffer CJ, Klag MJ, Bush TL. Plasma lipoprotein levels as predictors of cardiovascular death in women. *Arch Intern Med* 1993;153:2209-2216.

39. *Executive Summary of the Third Report of the National Cholesterol Education Program (NCEP) Expert Panel on Detection, Evaluation, and Treatment of High Blood Cholesterol in Adults (Adult Treatment Panel III).* Bethesda, MD: U.S. Department of Health and Human Services, Public Health Service, National Institutes of Health. *JAMA* 2001;285:2486-2497.

40. Kannel WB, Wilson PW. Risk factors that attenuate the female coronary disease advantage. *Arch Intern Med* 1995;155:57-61.

41. Manson JE, Spelsberg A. Risk modification in the diabetic patient. In: *Prevention of Myocardial Infarction.* Manson JE, Ridker PM, Gaziano JM, Hennekens CH (eds). New York: Oxford University Press, 1996, pp. 241-273.

42. Palmer J, Rosenberg L, Shapiro S. Reproductive factors and the risk of myocardial infarction. *Am J Epidemiol* 1992;136:408-416.

43. Tsang T, Barnes ME, Gersh BJ, Hayes SN. Risks of coronary heart disease in women: Current understanding and evolving concepts. *Mayo Clin Proc* 2000;75:1289-1303.

44. Stampfer M, Colditz G. Estrogen replacement therapy and coronary heart disease: A quantitative assessment of the epidemiologic evidence. *Prev Med* 1991;20:47-63.

45. Grady D, Rubin SM, Petitti DB, et al. Hormone therapy to prevent disease and prolong life in post-menopausal women. *Ann Intern Med* 1992;117:1016-1037.

46. Sullivan JM, Vander Zwaag R, Hughes JP, et al. Estrogen replacement and coronary artery disease. *Arch Intern Med* 1990;150:2557-2562.

47. Writing Group for the Women's Health Initiative Investigators. Risks and benefits of estrogen plus progestin in healthy postmenopausal women. *JAMA* 2002;288:321-333.

48. Matthews KA, Kuller LH, Wing RR, Meilahn EN, Plantinga P. Prior to use of estrogen replacement therapy, are users healthier than nonusers? *Am J Epidemiol* 1996;143:971-978.

49. Hulley S, Grady D, Bush T, et al. Heart and Estrogen/Progestin Replacement Study (HERS) Research Group. Randomized trial of estrogen plus progestin for secondary prevention of coronary heart disease in postmenopausal women. *JAMA* 1998;280:605-613.

50. Alexander KP, Newby LK, Hellkamp MS, et al. Initiation of hormone replacement therapy after acute myocardial infarction is associated with more cardiac events during follow-up. *J Am Coll Cardiol* 2001;38:1-7.

51. Grodstein F, Manson JE, Stampfer MJ. Postmenopausal hormone use and secondary prevention of coronary events in the Nurses' Health Study. A prospective, observational study. *Ann Intern Med* 2001;135:1-8.

52. Herrington DM, Reboussin DM, Brosnihan, et al. Effects of estrogen replacement on the progression of coronary-artery atherosclerosis. *N Engl J Med* 2000;343:522-529.

53. Mosca L, Collins P, Herrington DM, et al. Hormone replacement therapy and cardiovascular disease. A statement for healthcare professionals from the American Heart Association. *Circulation* 2001;104:499-503.

54. Delmas PD. Treatment of postmenopausal osteoporosis. *Lancet* 2002;359:2018-2026.

55. Hlatky MA, Pryor DB, Harrell FE, Califf RM, Mark DB, Rosati RA. Factors affecting sensitivity and specificity of exercise electrocardiography: Multivariable analysis. *Am J Med* 1984;77:64-71.

56. Barolsky SM, Gilbert CA, Farugui A, et al. Differences in electrocardiographic response to exercise of women and men: A non-Bayesian factor. *Circulation* 1979;60:1021-1027.

57. Morise AP, Diamond GA. A comparison of the accuracy of exercise electrocardiography in men and women using biased and unbiased populations. *Am Heart J* 1995;130:741-747.

58. Taillefer R, DePuey G, Udelson J, Beller GA, Latour Y, Reeves F. Comparative diagnostic accuracy of TI-201 and Tc-99m Sestamibi SPECT imaging (perfusion and ECG-gated SPECT) in detecting coronary artery disease in women. *J Am Coll Cardiol* 1997;29:69-77.

59. Hachamovitch R, Berman DS, Kiat H, et al. Effective risk stratification using exercise myocardial perfusion SPECT in women: Gender-related differences in prognostic nuclear testing. *J Am Coll Cardiol* 1996;28:34-44.

60. Mieres, JH, Shaw LJ, Arai A, et al. AHA scientific statement. Role of noninvasive testing in the clinical evaluation of women with suspected coronary artery disease. *Circulation* 2005;111:682-696.

61. Sawada SG, Ryan T, Fineberg NS, Armstrong WF, McHenry PL, Feigenbaum H. Exercise echocardiographic detection of coronary artery disease in women. *J Am Coll Cardiol* 1989;14:1440-1447.

62. Heupler S, Metha R, Lobo A, Leung D, Marwick TH. Prognostic implications of exercise echocardiography in women with known or suspected coronary artery disease. *J Am Coll Cardiol* 1997;30:414-420.

63. Paffenbarger RS, Hyde RT, Wing A, Hsieh C. Physical activity, all-cause mortality, and longevity of college alumni. *N Eng J Med* 1986;314:605-613.

64. Manson JE, Stampfew MJ, Colditz GA, Willett WC, Speizer FE, Hennekens CH. A prospective study of exercise and incidence of myocardial infarction in women. *Circulation* 1993;88:I-220.

65. Leon A, Connett J, Jacobs DR, Raurama R. Leisure time physical activity levels and risk of coronary heart disease and death. The Multiple Risk Factor Intervention Trial. *JAMA* 1987;258:2388-2395.

66. Kushi LH, Fee RM, Folsom AR, Mink PJ, Anderson KE, Sellers TA. Physical activity and mortality in postmenopausal women. *JAMA* 1997;277:1287-1292.

67. O'Connor GT, Buring JE, Yusuf S, et al. An overview of randomized trial of rehabilitation with exercise after myocardial infarction. *Circulation* 1989;80:234-244.

68. Lemaitre RN, Heckbert SR, Psaty BM, Siscovick DS. Leisure-time physical activity and the risk of nonfatal myocardial infarction in postmenopausal women. *Arch Intern Med* 1995;155:2302-2308.

69. Ades PA, Waldmann ML, Polk DM, Coflesky JT. Referral patterns and exercise response in the rehabilitation of female coronary patients aged ≥ 62 years. *Am J Cardiol* 1992; 69:1422-1425.

70. Lavie CJ, Milani RV. Effects of cardiac rehabilitation and exercise training on exercise capacity, coronary risk factors, behavioral characteristics, and quality of life in women. *Am J Cardiol* 1995;75:340-343.

71. Kavanagh T, Hamm LF, Shephard RJ, et al. Can women benefit from exercise cardiac rehabilitation? In: *Advances in Cardiopulmonary Rehabilitation*. Jobin J, Maltais F, LeBlanc P, Simard C (eds). Champaign, IL: Human Kinetics, 2000, pp. 78-88.

72. Balady GJ, Jette D, Scheer J, Downing J. Changes in exercise capacity following cardiac rehabilitation in patients stratified according to age and gender. Results of the Massachusetts Association of Cardiovascular and Pulmonary Rehabilitation Multicenter Database. *J Cardiopulmonary Rehabil* 1996;16:38-46.

73. Owens JF, Matthews KA, Wing RR, Kuller LH. Can physical activity mitigate effects of aging in middle-aged women? *Circulation* 1992;85:1265-1270.

74. Wood PD, Stefanick ML, Williams PT, Haskell WL. The effects on plasma lipoproteins of a prudent weight-reducing diet, with or without exercise in overweight men and women. *N Engl J Med* 1991;325:461-466.

75. Wing R, Matthews K, Kuller L, Meilahn E, Plantinga P. Waist to hip ratio in middle-aged women. *Arterioscler Thromb* 1991;11:1250-1257.

76. Wasserman DH, Zinman B. Fuel homeostasis. In: *The Health Professional's Guide to Diabetes and Exercise.* Ruderman N, Devlin JT (eds). Alexandria, VA: American Diabetes Association, 1995, pp. 29-47.

77. Wei M, Gibbons LW, Mitchell TL, Kasmpert JB, Lee CD, Blair SN. The association between cardiorespiratory fitness and impaired fasting glucose and type 2 diabetes in men. *Ann Intern Med* 1999;130:80-96.

78. Hu FB, Sigal RJ, Rich-Edwards JW, et al. Walking compared with vigorous physical activity and risk of type 2 diabetes in women. *JAMA* 1999;282:1433-1439.

79. Reaven PD, Barrett-Connor EL, Edelestein S. Relation between leisure-time physical activity and blood pressure in older women. *Circulation* 1991;83:559-565.

80. Ishikawa K, Ohta T, Zhang J, Hashimoto S, Tanaka H. Influence of age and gender on exercise training-induced blood pressure reduction in systemic hypertension. *Am J Cardiol* 1999;84:192-196.

81. Blumenthal JA, Sherwood A, Gullette EC, et al. Exercise and weight loss reduce blood pressure in men and women with mild hypertension. *Arch Intern Med* 2000;160:1947-1958.

82. Durstine JL, Haskell WL. Effects of exercise training on plasma lipids and lipoproteins. *Exerc Sport Sci Rev* 1994;22:477-521.

83. Williams PT. High-density lipoprotein cholesterol and other risk factors for coronary heart disease in female runners. *N Engl J Med* 1996;334:1298-1303.

84. Stefanick M, Mackey S, Sheehan M, Ellsworth N, Haskell W, Wood P. Effects of diet and exercise in men and postmenopausal women with low levels of HDL cholesterol and high levels of LDL cholesterol. *N Engl J Med* 1998;339:12-20.

85. Warner JG, Brubaker PH, Zhu Y, et al. Long-term (5 year) changes in HDL cholesterol in cardiac rehabilitation patients. Do sex differences exist? *Circulation* 1995;92:773-777.

86. Loose MS, Fernhall B. Differences in quality of life among male and female cardiac rehabilitation participants. *J Cardiopulm Rehabil* 1995;15:225-231.

87. Hamm LF, Leon AS. Exercise training for the coronary patient. In: *Rehabilitation of the Coronary Patient.* Wenger NK (ed). New York: Churchill Livingstone, 1993, pp. 367-402.

88. Moore SM, Kramer FM. Women's and men's preferences for cardiac rehabilitation program features. *J Cardiopulmonary Rehabil* 1996;16:163-168.

89. Johnson PA, Manson JE. Cardiology patient page. How to make sure the beat goes on. Protecting a woman's heart. *Circulation* 2005;111:e28-e33.

Chapter 10

1. Mittelmark MB, Psaty BM, Rautaharju PM, et al. Prevalence of cardiovascular diseases among older adults: The Cardiovascular Health Study. *Am J Epidemiol* 1993;137:311-317.

2. National Center for Health Statistics. *Current Estimates from the National Health Interview Survey, 1995* (DHS Publication PHS 98-1527). Hyattsville, MD: U.S. Department of Health and Human Services, CDC, 1998.

3. Bild DE, Fitzpatrick A, Fried LP, et al. Age-related trends in cardiovascular morbidity and physical functioning in the elderly: The Cardiovascular Health Study. *J Am Geriatr Soc* 1993;41:1047-1056.

4. Wenger NK (ed). *Cardiovascular Disease in the Octogenarian and Beyond.* London: Martin Dunitz, 1999.

5. Sollott SJ, Lakatta EG. Normal aging changes in the cardiovascular system. *Cardiol Elderly* 1993;1:349-358.

6. Fleg JL, Lakatta EG. Role of muscle loss in the age-associated reduction in VO_2 max. *J Appl Physiol* 1988;65:1147-1151.

7. Lernfelt B, Wikstrand J, Svanborg A, et al. Aging and left ventricular function in elderly healthy people. *Am J Cardiol* 1991;68:547-549.

8. Rutan GH, Hermanson B, Bild DE, et al. Orthostatic hypotension in older adults. The Cardiovascular Health Study. *Hypertension* 1992;19(Part 1):508-519.

9. Bharati S, Lev M. Pathologic changes of the conduction system with aging. *Cardiol Elderly* 1994;2:152-160.

10. Lindroos M, Kupari M, Heikkilä J, et al. Prevalence of aortic valve abnormalities in the elderly: An echocardiographic study of a random population sample. *J Am Coll Cardiol* 1993;21:1220-1225.

11. Wenger NK, Furberg CD, Pitt E. *Coronary Heart Disease in the Elderly* (Working Conference on the Recognition and Management of Coronary Heart Disease in the Elderly, National Institutes of Health, Bethesda, MD, 1985). New York: Elsevier Science, 1986.

12. Graves EJ. *Summary, 1989 National Hospital Discharge Survey: Advance Data From Vital and Health Statistics No. 199.* Hyattsville, MD: National Center for Health Statistics, 1991, pp. 1-12.

13. Pepine CJ, Abrams J, Marks RG, et al. for the TIDES Investigators. Characteristics of a contemporary

population with angina pectoris. *Am J Cardiol* 1994;74: 226-231.

14. Paul SD, O'Gara PT, Mahjoub ZA, et al. Geriatric patients with acute myocardial infarction: Cardiac risk factor profiles, presentation, thrombolysis, coronary interventions, and prognosis. *Am Heart J* 1996;131: 710-715.

15. Marcus FI, Friday K, McCans J, et al. Age-related prognosis after acute myocardial infarction (the Multicenter Diltiazem Postinfarction trial). *Am J Cardiol* 1990;65:559-566.

16. Vaccarino V, Berkman LF, Mendes de Leon CF, et al. Functional disability before myocardial infarction in the elderly as a determinant of infarction severity and postinfarction mortality. *Arch Intern Med* 1997;157:2196-2204.

17. Nadelmann J, Frishman WH, Ooi WL, et al. Prevalence, incidence and prognosis of recognized and unrecognized myocardial infarction in persons aged 75 years or older: The Bronx Aging Study. *Am J Cardiol* 1990;66: 533-537.

18. Solomon CG, Lee TH, Cook EF, et al, for the Chest Pain Study Group. Comparison of clinical presentation of acute myocardial infarction in patients older than 65 years of age to younger patients: The Multicenter Chest Pain Study experience. *Am J Cardiol* 1989;63:772-776.

19. Gurwitz JH, McLaughlin TJ, Willison DJ, et al. Delayed hospital presentation in patients who have had acute myocardial infarction. *Ann Intern Med* 1997;126:593-599.

20. Fibrinolytic Therapy Trialists' (FTT) Collaborative Group. Indications for fibrinolytic therapy in suspected acute myocardial infarction: Collaborative overview of early mortality and major morbidity results from all randomised trials of more than 1000 patients. *Lancet* 1994;343:311-322.

21. Thiemann DR, Coresh J, Schulman SP, et al. Lack of benefit for intravenous thrombolysis in patients with myocardial infarction who are older than 75 years. *Circulation* 2000;101:2239-2246.

22. Berger AK, Schulman KA, Gersh GS, et al. Primary coronary angioplasty vs thrombolysis for the management of acute myocardial infarction in elderly patients. *JAMA* 1999;282:341-348.

23. Krumholtz HM, Radford MJ, Wang Y, et al. Early β-blocker therapy for acute myocardial infarction in elderly patients. *Ann Intern Med* 1999;131:648-654.

24. Krumholtz HM, Radford MJ, Wang Y, et al. National use and effectiveness of β-blockers for treatment of elderly patients after acute myocardial infarction. National Cooperative Cardiovascular Project. *JAMA* 1998;280:623-629.

25. McClellan M, McNeil BJ, Newhouse JP. Does more intensive treatment of acute myocardial infarction in the elderly reduce mortality? Analysis using instrumental variables. *JAMA* 1994;272:859-866.

26. Pashos CL, Newhouse JP, McNeil BJ. Temporal changes in the care and outcomes of elderly patients with acute

myocardial infarction, 1987 through 1990. *JAMA* 1993;270:1832-1836.

27. Gottlieb S, Goldbourt U, Boyko V, et al, for the SPRINT and Thrombolytic Survey Groups. Improved outcome of elderly patients (≥75 years of age) with acute myocardial infarction from 1981-1983 to 1992-1994 in Israel. *Circulation* 1997;95:342-350.

28. Smith SC, Blair SN, Bonow RO, et al. AHA/ACC guidelines for preventing heart attack and death in patients with atherosclerotic cardiovascular disease: 2001 update. *Circulation* 2001;104:1577-1579.

29. Ciaroni S, Delonca J, Righetti A. Early exercise testing after acute myocardial infarction in the elderly: Clinical evaluation and prognostic significance. *Am Heart J* 1993;126:304-311.

30. Wenger NK. Populations with special needs for exercise rehabilitation. Elderly coronary patients. In: *Rehabilitation of the Coronary Patient*. Third Edition. Wenger NK, Hellerstein HK (eds). New York: Churchill Livingstone, 1992, pp. 415-420.

31. Lavie CJ, Milani RV. Effects of cardiac rehabilitation programs on exercise capacity, coronary risk factors, behavioral characteristics, and quality of life in a large elderly cohort. *Am J Cardiol* 1995;76:177-179.

32. Wenger NK, Froelicher ES, Smith LK, et al. *Cardiac Rehabilitation* (Clinical Practice Guideline No. 17, AHCPR Publication No. 96-0672). Bethesda, MD: U.S. Department of Health and Human Services, Public Health Service, Agency for Health Care Policy and Research, National Heart, Lung, and Blood Institute, 1995.

33. Ades PA, Waldmann ML, Poehlman ET, et al. Exercise conditioning in older coronary patients: Submaximal lactate response and endurance capacity. *Circulation* 1993;88:572-577.

34. Lavie CJ, Milani RV. Benefits of cardiac rehabilitation and exercise training in elderly women. *Am J Cardiol* 1997;79:664-666.

35. Pollock ML, Carroll JF, Graves JE, et al. Injuries and adherence to walk/jog and resistance training programs in the elderly. *Med Sci Sports Exerc* 1991;23: 1194-1200.

36. Berkman LF, Leo-Summers L, Horwitz RI. Emotional support and survival after myocardial infarction: A prospective, population-based study of the elderly. *Ann Intern Med* 1992;117:1003-1009.

37. Gersh BJ, Kronmal RA, Schaff HV, et al. Long-term (5-year) results of coronary bypass surgery in patients 65 years or older: A report from the Coronary Artery Surgery Study. *Circulation* 1983;68(suppl II):II-190–II-199.

38. Edwards FH, Carey JS, Grover FL, et al. Impact of gender on coronary bypass operative mortality. *Ann Thorac Surg* 1998;66:125-131.

39. Peterson ED, Cowper PA, Jollis JG, et al. Outcomes of coronary artery bypass graft surgery in 24 461 patients aged 80 years or older. *Circulation* 1995;92(suppl II): 85-91.

40. Weintraub WS, Clements SD, Ware J, et al. Coronary artery surgery in octogenarians. *Am J Cardiol* 1991;68: 1530-1534.

41. Barzilay JI, Kronmal RA, Bittner V, et al. Coronary artery disease and coronary artery bypass grafting in diabetic patients aged ≥65 years (reports from the Coronary Artery Surgery Study [CASS] Registry). *Am J Cardiol* 1994;74:334-339.

42. Kelsey SF, Miller DP, Holubkov R, et al. Results of percutaneous transluminal coronary angioplasty in patients ≥65 years of age (from the 1985 to 1986 National Heart, Lung, and Blood Institute's Coronary Angioplasty Registry). *Am J Cardiol* 1990;66:1033-1038.

43. Bedotto JB, Rutherford BD, McConahay DR, et al. Results of multivessel percutaneous transluminal coronary angioplasty in persons aged 65 years and older. *Am J Cardiol* 1991;67:1051-1055.

44. Jackman JD, Navetta FI, Smith JE, et al. Percutaneous transluminal coronary angioplasty in octogenarians as an effective therapy for angina pectoris. *Am J Cardiol* 1991;68:116-119.

45. Taddei CFG, Weintraub WS, Douglas JS Jr, et al. Influence of age on outcome after percutaneous transluminal coronary angioplasty. *Am J Cardiol* 1999;84:245-251.

46. Popma JJ, Satler LF, Mintz GS, et al. Coronary angioplasty and new device therapy. *Cardiol Elderly* 1993;1: 62-70.

47. National High Blood Pressure Education Program Working Group. National High Blood Pressure Education Program Working Group Report on Hypertension in the Elderly. *Hypertension* 1994;23:275-285.

48. Staessen J, Amery A, Fagard R. Editorial review. Isolated systolic hypertension in the elderly. *J Hypertens* 1990;8:393-405.

49. Applegate WB. Hypertension in elderly patients. *Ann Intern Med* 1989;110:901-915.

50. Amery A, Birkenhäger W, Brixko R, et al. Efficacy of antihypertensive drug treatment according to age, sex, blood pressure, and previous cardiovascular disease in patients over the age of 60. *Lancet* 1986;2:589-592.

51. Glynn RJ, Chae CU, Guralnik JM, et al. Pulse pressure and mortality in old people. *Arch Intern Med* 2000;160: 2765-2772.

52. SHEP Cooperative Research Group. Prevention of stroke by antihypertensive drug treatment in older persons with isolated systolic hypertension: Final results of the Systolic Hypertension in the Elderly Program (SHEP). *JAMA* 1991;265:3255-3264.

53. Staessen JA, Fagard R, Thijs I, et al. Randomized double-blind comparison of placebo and active treatment for older patients with isolated systolic hypertension. *Lancet* 1997;350:757-764.

54. Gueyffier F, Bulpit C, Boissel J-P, et al. Antihypertensive drugs in very old people: A sub-group meta analysis of randomized controlled trials. *Lancet* 1999;353:793-796.

55. Joint National Committee on Prevention, Detection, Evaluation, and Treatment of High Blood Pressure. The seventh report of the Joint National Committee on Prevention, Detection, Evaluation, and Treatment of High Blood Pressure. *Hypertension* 2003;42:1206-1252.

56. Whelton PK, Appel LJ, Espeland MA, et al., for the TONE Collaborative Research Group. Sodium reduction and weight loss in the treatment of hypertension in older persons: A randomized controlled Trial of Nonpharmacologic Interventions in the Elderly (TONE). *JAMA* 1998;279:839-846.

57. Mulrow CD, Cornell JA, Herrera CR, et al. Hypertension in the elderly: Implications and generalizability of randomized trials. *JAMA* 1994;272:1932-1938.

58. Elliott WJ, Weir DR, Black HR. Cost-effectiveness of the lower treatment goal (of JNC VI) for diabetic hypertensive patients. *Arch Intern Med* 2000;160:1277-1283.

59. Smith WM. Epidemiology of congestive heart failure. *Am J Cardiol* 1985;55:3A-8A.

60. Konstam MA, Dracup K, Baker D, et al. *Heart Failure: Evaluation and Care of Patients with Left-Ventricular Systolic Dysfunction* (Clinical Practice Guideline No. 11. AHCPR Publication No. 94-0612). Rockville, MD: Agency for Health Care Policy and Research, Public Health Service, U.S. Department of Health and Human Services, June 1994.

61. Vasan RS, Benjamin EJ, Levy D. Prevalence, clinical features and prognosis of diastolic heart failure: An epidemiologic perspective. *J Am Coll Cardiol* 1995;26: 1565-1574.

62. The CONSENSUS Trial Study Group. Effects of enalapril on mortality in severe congestive heart failure: Results of the Cooperative North Scandinavian Enalapril Survival Study (CONSENSUS). *N Engl J Med* 1987;316:1429-1435.

63. The SOLVD Investigators. Effect of enalapril on survival in patients with reduced left ventricular ejection fractions and congestive heart failure. *N Engl J Med* 1991;325:293-302.

64. Cohn JN, Johnson G, Ziesche S, et al. A comparison of enalapril with hydralazine-isosorbide dinitrate in the treatment of chronic congestive heart failure. *N Engl J Med* 1991;325:303-310.

65. Chapman D, Wang T, Gheorghiade M. Therapeutic approaches to heart failure in elderly patients. *Cardiol Elderly* 1994;2:89-97.

66. De Bock V, Mets T, Romagnoli M, et al. Captopril treatment of chronic heart failure in the very old. *J Gerontol* 1994;49:M148-M152.

67. Packer M, Bristow MR, Cohn JN, et al. The effect of carvedilol on morbidity and mortality in patients with chronic heart failure. *N Engl J Med* 1996;334:1349-1355.

68. CIBIS-II Investigators and Committees. The Cardiac Insufficiency Bisoprolol Study II (CIBIS II): A randomized trial. *Lancet* 1999;353:9-13.

69. MERIT-HF Study Group. Effect of metoprolol CR/XL in chronic heart failure: Metoprolol CR/XL Randomised Intervention Trial in Congestive Heart Failure (MERIT-HF). *Lancet* 1999;353:2001-2007.

70. Pitt B, Zannad F, Remme WJ, et al. The effect of spironolactone on morbidity and mortality in patients with severe heart failure. Randomized Aldactone Evaluation Study Investigators. *N Engl J Med* 1999;341:709-717.

71. Rich MW, Beckham V, Wittenberg C, et al. A multidisciplinary intervention to prevent the readmission of elderly patients with congestive heart failure. *N Engl J Med* 1995;333:1190-1195.

72. Rich MW, Gray DB, Beckham V, et al. Effect of a multidisciplinary intervention on medication compliance in elderly patients with congestive heart failure. *Am J Med* 1996;101:270-276.

73. Martin A, Benbow LJ, Butrous GS. Five-year follow-up of 101 elderly subjects by means of long-term ambulatory cardiac monitoring. *Eur Heart J* 1984;5:592-596.

74. Fleg JL, Kennedy HL. Cardiac arrhythmias in a healthy elderly population: Detection by 24-hour ambulatory electrocardiography. *Chest* 1982;81:302-307.

75. Kantelip JP, Sage E, Duchene-Marullaz P. Findings on ambulatory electrocardiographic monitoring in subjects older than 80 years. *Am J Cardiol* 1986;57:398-401.

76. Ryder KM, Benjamin EJ. Epidemiology and significance of atrial fibrillation. *Am J Cardiol* 1999;84:131R-138R.

77. Wolf PA, Abbott RD, Kannel WB. Atrial fibrillation: A major contributor to stroke in the elderly. *Arch Intern Med* 1987;147:1561-1564.

78. Stroke Prevention in Atrial Fibrillation Investigators. Stroke prevention in atrial fibrillation study: Final results. *Circulation* 1991;84:527-539.

79. Frishman WH, Heiman M, Karpenos A, et al. Twenty-four-hour ambulatory electrocardiography in elderly subjects: Prevalence of various arrhythmias and prognostic implications (report from the Bronx Longitudinal Aging Study). *Am Heart J* 1996;132:297-302.

80. Shen W-K, Hayes DL. Pacing the octogenarians and nonagenarians: Should age be a consideration for pacing and outcome analysis of pacing in the very elderly? *Cardiol Elderly* 1994;2:161-170.

81. Culliford AT, Galloway AC, Colvin SB, et al. Aortic valve replacement for aortic stenosis in persons aged 80 years and over. *Am J Cardiol* 1991;67:1256-1260.

82. Lund O, Nielsen TT, Magnussen K, et al. Valve replacement for calcified aortic stenosis in septuagenarians infers normal life-length. *Scand J Thorac Cardiovasc Surg* 1991;25:37-44.

83. Turina J, Hess O, Sepulcri F, et al. Spontaneous course of aortic valve disease. *Eur Heart J* 1987;8:471-483.

84. Zaidi AM, Fitzpatrick AP, Keenan DJM, et al. Good outcomes from cardiac surgery in the over 70s. *Heart* 1999;82:134-137.

85. World Health Organization Study Group. *Epidemiology and Prevention of Cardiovascular Diseases in Elderly People* (WHO Technical Report Series 853). Geneva: World Health Organization, 1995.

86. Tervahauta M, Pekkanen J, Nissinen A. Risk factors of coronary heart disease and total mortality among elderly men with and without preexisting coronary heart disease: The Finnish Cohorts of the Seven Countries Study. *J Am Coll Cardiol* 1995;26:1623-1629.

87. Kannel WB, Doyle JT, Shephard RJ, et al. 18th Bethesda Conference. Cardiovascular Disease in the Elderly. Prevention of cardiovascular disease in the elderly. *J Am Coll Cardiol* 1987;10(suppl A):25A-28A.

88. *Third Report of the National Cholesterol Education Program (NCEP) Expert Panel on Detection, Evaluation, and Treatment of High Blood Cholesterol in Adults (Adult Treatment Panel) Executive Summary* (NIH Publication No. 01-3670). Bethesda, MD: U.S. Department of Health and Human Services, Public Health Service, National Institutes of Health, National Heart, Lung, and Blood Institutes, 2001.

89. Denke MA, Grundy SM. Hypercholesterolemia in elderly persons: Resolving the treatment dilemma. *Ann Intern Med* 1990;112:780-792.

90. Sacks FM, Tonkin AM, Shepherd J, et al. Effect of pravastatin on coronary disease events in a subgroups defined by coronary risk factors: The Prospective Pravastatin Pooling Project. *Circulation* 2000;102:1893-1900.

91. Ganz DA, Kuntz KM, Jacobson GA, et al. Cost-effectiveness of 3-hydroxy-3-methylglutaryl coenzyme A reductase inhibitor therapy in older patients with myocardial infarction. *Ann Intern Med* 2000;132:780-787.

92. Carlson LA, Rosenhamer G. Reduction of mortality in the Stockholm Ischaemic Heart Disease Secondary Prevention Study by combined treatment with clofibrate and nicotinic acid. *Acta Med Scand* 1988;223:405-418.

93. British Heart Protection Study. Available at: www.hpsinfo.org. Accessed March 2002.

94. LaCroix AZ, Lang J, Scherr P, et al. Smoking and mortality among older men and women in three communities. *N Engl J Med* 1991;324:1619-1625.

95. Hermanson B, Omenn GS, Kronmal RA, et al., Beneficial six-year outcome of smoking cessation in older men and women with coronary artery disease. Results from the CASS registry. *N Engl J Med* 1988;319:1365-1369.

96. Williams MA, Fleg JL, Ades PA, et al. Secondary prevention of coronary heart disease in the elderly (with emphasis on patients ≥75 years of age). An American Heart Association Scientific Statement from the Council on Clinical Cardiology Subcommittee on Exercise, Cardiac Rehabilitation, and Prevention. *Circulation* 2002;105:1735-1743.

97. Fiore MC, Bailey WC, Cohen SJ, et al. *Treating Tobacco Use and Dependence*. Rockville, MD: Clinical Practice Guideline. U.S. Department of Health and Human Services, Public Health Service, 2000.

98. Ades PA, Ballor DL, Ashikaga T, et al. Weight training improves walking endurance in healthy elderly persons. *Ann Intern Med* 1996;124:568-572.

99. Paffenbarger RS Jr, Hyde RT, Wing AL, et al. Physical activity, all-cause mortality, and longevity of college alumni. *N Engl J Med* 1986;314:605-613.

100. Braith RW, Pollock ML, Lowenthal DT, et al. Moderate- and high-intensity exercise lowers blood pressure in normotensive subjects 60 to79 years of age. *Am J Cardiol* 1994;73:1124-1128.

101. Reaven PD, Barrett-Connor E, Edelstein S. Relation between leisure-time physical activity and blood pressure in older women. *Circulation* 1991;83:559-565.

102. Hakim AA, Petrovitch H, Burchfiel CM, et al. Effects of walking on mortality among nonsmoking retired men. *N Engl J Med* 1998;338:94-99.

103. Kushi LH, Fee RM, Folsom AR, et al. Physical activity and mortality in postmenopausal women. *JAMA* 1997;277:1287-1292.

104. Fried LP, Kronmal RA, Newman AB, et al. Risk factors for 5-year mortality in older adults. *JAMA* 1998;279:585-592.

105. MacMahon S, Rodger A. The effects of blood pressure reduction in older patients: An overview of five randomized controlled trials in elderly hypertensives. *J Clin Exp Hypertens* 1993;15:967-978.

106. Vokonas PS, Kannel WB. Epidemiology of coronary heart disease in the elderly. In: *Cardiovascular Disease in the Elderly Patient*. Tresch DD, Aronow WS (eds). New York: Dekker, 1994, pp. 91-123.

107. Turcato E, Bosello O, Francesco VD, et al. Waist circumference and abdominal sagittal diameter as surrogates of body fat distribution in the elderly: Their relation with cardiovascular risk factors. *Int J Obes Relat Metab Disord* 2000;24:1005-1010.

108. Mertens DJ, Kavanagh T, Campbell RB, et al. Exercise without dietary restriction as a means to long-term fat loss in the obese cardiac patient. *J Sports Med Phys Fitness* 1998;38:310-316.

109. Vokonas PS, Kannel WB. Diabetes mellitus and coronary heart disease in the elderly. *Clin Geriatr Med* 1996;2:69-78.

110. Kirwan JP, Kohrt WM, Wojta DM, et al. Endurance exercise training reduces glucose-stimulated insulin levels in 60- to 70-year-old men and women. *J Gerontol* 1993;48:M84-M90.

111. Hertog MGL, Feskens EJM, Hollman PCH, et al. Dietary antioxidant flavonoids and risk of coronary heart disease: The Zutphen Elderly Study. *Lancet* 1993;342:1007-1011.

112. Schauffler HH, D'Agostino RB, Kannel WB. Risk for cardiovascular disease in the elderly and associated Medicare costs: The Framingham Study. *Am J Prev Med* 1993;9:146-154.

113. Williams MA, Maresh CM, Esterbrooks DJ, et al. Early exercise training in patients older than age 65 years compared with that in younger patients after acute myocardial infarction or coronary artery bypass grafting. *Am J Cardiol* 1985;55:263-266.

114. Ades PA, Hanson JS, Gunther JGS, Tonino RP. Exercise conditioning in the elderly coronary patient. *J Am Geriatr Soc* 1987;35:121-124.

115. Lanie CJ, Milani RV. Disparate effects of improving aerobic exercise capacity and quality of life after cardiac rehabilitation in young and elderly coronary patients. *J Cardiopulm Rehabil* 2000;20:235-240.

116. Ståhle A, Mattson E, Rydén L, Unden A-L, Nordlander R. Improved physical fitness and quality of life following training of elderly patients after acute coronary events. A 1 year follow-up randomized controlled study. *Eur Heart J* 1999;20:1475-1484.

117. Hung C, Daub B, Black B, et al. Exercise training improves overall physical fitness and quality of life in older women with coronary artery disease. *Chest* 2004;126:1026-1031.

118. Hakim AA, Petrovitch H, Burchfiel CM, et al. Effects of walking on mortality among nonsmoking retired men. *New Engl J Med* 1998;338:94-99.

119. Wenger NK. Physical inactivity and coronary heart disease in elderly patients. *Clin Geriatr Med* 1996;12:79-88.

120. Pollock ML, Franklin BA, Balady GJ, et al. Resistance exercise in individuals with and without cardiovascular disease: Benefits, rationale, safety, and prescription. *Circulation* 2000;101:823-828.

121. Fiatarone MA, O'Neill EF, Ryan ND, et al. Exercise training and nutritional supplementation for physical frailty in very elderly people. *N Engl J Med* 1994;330:1769-1775.

122. Wannamethee SG, Shaper AG, Walker M. Physical activity and mortality in older men with diagnosed heart disease. *Circulation* 2000;102:1358-1363.

123. Lavie CJ, Milani RV, Littman AB. Benefits of cardiac rehabilitation and exercise training in secondary coronary prevention in the elderly. *J Am Coll Cardiol* 1993;22:678-683.

124. Ades PA, Waldmann ML, Polk D, Coflesky JT. Referral patterns and exercise response in the rehabilitation of female coronary patients aged ≥62 years. *Am J Cardiol* 1992;69:1422-1425.

Chapter 11

1. American Diabetes Association. Report of the Expert Committee on the Diagnosis and Classification of Diabetes Mellitus. *Diabetes Care* 2002;25(suppl 1):S5-S20.

2. National Diabetes Information Clearinghouse. *Diabetes Statistics* (NIH publication 99-3926). Bethesda, MD: National Institute of Diabetes and Digestive and Kidney Diseases, 1999.

3. American Diabetes Association. *Therapy for Diabetes Mellitus and Related Disorders*. Lebovitz HE (ed). Alexandria, VA: American Diabetes Association, 1998.

4. American Diabetes Association. Screening for diabetes. *Diabetes Care* 2002;25(suppl 1):S21-S24.

5. American Diabetes Association. Standards of medical care for patients with diabetes mellitus. *Diabetes Care* 2002;25(suppl 1):S33-S49.

6. Grundy SM, Benjamin IJ, Burke GL, et al. Diabetes and cardiovascular disease: A statement for healthcare professionals from the American Heart Association. *Circulation* 1999;100:1134-1146.

7. American Diabetes Association. Evidence-based nutrition principles and recommendations for the treatment

and prevention of diabetes and related complications. *Diabetes Care* 2002;25(suppl 1):S50-S60.

8. American Diabetes Association. Diabetes mellitus and exercise (position statement). *Diabetes Care* 2000;23(suppl 1):S50-S54.

9. American College of Sports Medicine. *ACSM's Guidelines for Exercise Testing and Prescription.* Sixth Edition. Franklin BA, Whaley MH, Howley ET, et al. (eds). Philadelphia: Lippincott Williams & Wilkins, 2000.

10. American Diabetes Association. Exercise and NIDDM (technical review). *Diabetes Care* 1993;16(suppl 2): 64–68.

11. Gordon NF. The exercise prescription. In: *American Diabetes Association: Handbook of Exercise in Diabetes.* Ruderman N, Devlin JT, Schneider SH, Kriska A (eds). Alexandria, VA: American Diabetes Association, 2002, pp. 269-288.

12. Fletcher GF, Balady G, Blair SN, et al. Benefits and recommendations for physical activity programs for all Americans (statement on exercise). *Circulation* 1986;94: 857-862.

13. Thompson PD, Funk EJ, Carleton RA, Sturner WQ. Incidence of death during jogging in Rhode Island from 1975 through 1980. *JAMA* 1982;247:2535-2538.

14. Siscovick DS, Weiss NS, Fletcher RH, Lasky T. The incidence of primary cardiac arrest during vigorous exercise. *N Engl J Med* 1984;311:874-877.

15. Kohl HW, Gordon NF, Powell KE, et al. Physical activity, physical fitness and sudden cardiac death. *Epidemiol Rev* 1992;14:37-58.

16. Thompson PD, Klocke FJ, Levine BD, Van Camp SP. Task force 5: Coronary artery disease. *Med Sci Sports Exercise* 1994;26:S271-S275.

17. Gordon NF. *Diabetes. Your Complete Exercise Guide.* Champaign, IL: Human Kinetics, 1993.

18. *American Diabetes Association. Handbook of Exercise in Diabetes.* Ruderman N, Devlin JT, Schneider SH, Kriska A (eds). Alexandria, VA: American Diabetes Association, 2002.

19. Marrero DG. Initiation and maintenance of exercise in patients with diabetes. In: *American Diabetes Association. Handbook of Exercise in Diabetes.* Ruderman N, Devlin JT, Schneider SH, Kriska A (eds). Alexandria, VA: American Diabetes Association, 2002, pp. 289-309.

20. Wasserman DH, Davis SN, Zinman B. Fuel metabolism during exercise in health and disease. In: *American Diabetes Association: Handbook of Exercise in Diabetes.* Ruderman N, Devlin JT, Schneider SH, Kriska A (eds). Alexandria, VA: American Diabetes Association, 2002, pp. 63-99.

21. Berger M. Adjustment of insulin and oral agent therapy. In: *American Diabetes Association: Handbook of Exercise in Diabetes.* Ruderman N, Devlin JT, Schneider SH, Kriska A (eds). Alexandria, VA: American Diabetes Association, 2002, pp. 365-376.

22. Fletcher GF, Balady G, Froelicher VF, et al. A statement for health professionals from the American Heart Association. Exercise standards. *Circulation* 1995;91: 580-612.

23. Miller WJ, Sherman WM, Ivy JL. Effect of strength training on glucose tolerance and post-glucose insulin response. *Med Sci Sports Exerc* 1984;16:539-543.

24. Durak EP, Jovanovic-Peterson L, Peterson CM. Randomized cross-over study of effect of resistance training on glycemic control, muscular strength, and cholesterol in type I diabetic men. *Diabetes Care* 1990;13: 1039-1043.

25. Hornsby WG, Chatlin RD. Resistance training. In: *American Diabetes Association: Handbook of Exercise in Diabetes.* Ruderman N, Devlin JT, Schneider SH, Kriska A (eds). Alexandria, VA: American Diabetes Association, 2002, pp. 311-319.

26. Vranic M, Wasserman D. Exercise, fitness, and diabetes. In: *Exercise, Fitness, and Health.* Bouchard C, Shephard RJ, Stephens T, et al. (eds). Champaign, IL: Human Kinetics, 1990, pp. 467-490.

27. De Busk RF, Stenestrand U, Sheehan M, Haskell WL. Training effects of long versus short bouts of exercise in healthy subjects. *Am J Cardiol* 1990;65:1010-1013.

28. De Busk RF, Haskell WL. Do multiple short bouts of exercise really produce the same benefits as single long bouts? *Am J Cardiol* 1991;67:326.

29. American College of Sports Medicine: The recommended quantity and quality of exercise for developing and maintaining cardiorespiratory and muscular fitness and flexibility in healthy adults (position stand). *Med Sci Sports Exerc* 1998;30:975-991.

Chapters 12 and 13

1. American Heart Association. *Heart Disease and Stroke Statistics—2004 Update.* Dallas: American Heart Association, 2004.

2. Eriksson H. Heart failure: A growing public health problem. *J Intern Med* 1995;237:135-141.

3. Vasan RS, Benjamin EL, Levy D. Prevalence, clinical features and prognosis of diastolic heart failure: An epidemiologic perspective. *J Am Coll Cardiol* 1995;26: 1565-1574.

4. Senni M, Tribouilloy CM, Rodenheffer RJ, et al. Congestive heart failure in the community: A study of all incident cases in Olmsted County, Minnesota, in 1991. *Circulation* 1998;98:2282-2289.

5. Pina IL, Apstein CS, Balady GJ, et al. Exercise and heart failure. A statement from the American Heart Association Committee on Exercise, Rehabilitation, and Prevention. *Circulation* 2003;107:1210-1225.

6. Jugdutt BI, Michorowski BL, Kappadoga CT. Exercise training after anterior Q wave myocardial infarction: Importance of regional left ventricular function and topography. *J Am Coll Cardiol* 1988;12:362-372.

7. Giannuzzi P, Tavazzi L, Temporelli PL, et al. Long-term physical training and left ventricular remodeling after

anterior myocardial infarction: Results of the Exercise in Anterior Myocardial Infarction (EAMI) trial: EAMI Study Group. *J Am Coll Cardiol* 1993;22:1821-1829.

8. Giannuzzi P, Temporelli PL, Corra U, et al. Attenuation of unfavourable remodeling by exercise training in postinfarction patients with left ventricular dysfunction. Results of the Exercise in Left Ventricular Dysfunction (ELVD) trial. *Circulation* 1997;96:1790-1797.

9. Dubach P, Myers J, Dziekan G, et al. Effect of exercise training on left ventricular volumes and contractility in chronic heart failure: Application of MRI. *Eur Heart J* 1995;16:8.

10. Dubach P, Myers J, Dziekan G, et al. Effect of exercise training on myocardial remodeling in patients with reduced left ventricular function after myocardial infarction. Application of magnetic resonance imaging. *Circulation* 1997;985:2060-2067.

11. Dubach P, Myers J, Dziekan G, et al. Effect of high intensity exercise training on central hemodynamic responses to exercise in men with reduced left ventricular function. *J Am Coll Cardiol* 1997;29:1591-1598.

12. Sullivan MJ, Higginbotham MB, Cobb FR. Exercise training in patients with severe left ventricular dysfunction. Hemodynamic and metabolic effects. *Circulation* 1988;78:506-515.

13. Sullivan MJ, Higginbotham MB, Cobb FR. Exercise training in patients with chronic heart failure delays ventilatory anaerobic threshold and improves submaximal exercise performance. *Circulation* 1989;79: 324-329.

14. Coats AJS, Adamopoulos S, Meyer TE, et al. Effects of physical training in chronic heart failure. *Lancet* 1990;335:63-66.

15. Wilson JR, Martin JL, Ferraro N. Impaired skeletal muscle nutritive flow during exercise in patients with congestive heart failure: Role of cardiac pump dysfunction as determined by the effect of dobutamine. *Am J Cardiol* 1984;53:1308-1315.

16. Kavanagh T, Yacoub MH, Mertens DJ, et al. Cardiorespiratory responses to exercise training after orthotopic cardiac transplantation. *Circulation* 1988;77: 162-171.

17. Franciosa JA, Park M, Levine TB. Lack of correlation between exercise capacity and indexes of resting left ventricular performance in heart failure. *Am J Cardiol* 1981;47:33-39.

18. Belardinelli R, Georgiou D, Ginzton L, et al. Effects of moderate exercise training on thallium uptake and contractile response to low-dose dobutamine of dysfunctional myocardium in patients with ischemic cardiomyopathy. *Circulation* 1998;97:553-561.

19. Belardinelli R, Georgiou D, Cianci G, Berman N, Ginzton L, Purcaro A. Exercise training improves left ventricular diastolic filling in patients with dilated cardiomyopathy. Clinical and prognostic implications. *Circulation* 1995;91:2775-2784.

20. Wilson JR, Fink L, Maris J, et al. Evaluation of energy metabolism in skeletal muscle of patients with heart failure with gated phosphorous-31 nuclear magnetic resonance. *Circulation* 1985;71:57-62.

21. Anker SD, Ponikowski PP, Clark AL, et al. Cytokines and neurohormones relating to body composition alterations in the wasting syndrome of chronic heart failure. *Eur Heart J* 1999;20:683-693.

22. Arcaro G, Cretti A, Balzano S, et al. Insulin causes endothelial dysfunction in humans. Sites and mechanisms. *Circulation* 2002;105:576-582.

23. Levine B, Kalmine J, Mayer L, Fillit H, Packer M. Elevated circulating levels of tumour necrosis factor in severe chronic heart failure. *N Engl J Med* 1990;323: 236-241.

24. Anker SD, Volterrani M, Swan JW, et al. Hormonal changes in cardiac cachexia. *Eur Heart J* 1995;16(suppl): 359.

25. Belardinelli R, Georgiou D, Scocco V, Barstow TJ, Purcaro A. Low intensity exercise training in patients with chronic heart failure. *J Am Coll Cardiol* 1995;26: 975-982.

26. Stratton JR, Dunn JF, Adamopoulos S, et al. Training partially reverses muscle metabolic abnormalities during exercise in heart failure. *J Appl Physiol* 1994;76: 1575-1582.

27. Hambrecht R, Fiehn E, Yu J, et al. Effects of endurance training on mitochondrial infrastructure and fiber type distribution in skeletal muscle of patients with stable chronic heart failure. *J Am Coll Cardiol* 1997;29:1067-1073.

28. Fink L, Wilson J, Ferraro N. Exercise ventilation and pulmonary artery wedge pressure in chronic stable congestive heart failure. *Am J Cardiol* 1986;249-253.

29. Clark AL, Coats AJS. Usefulness of arterial blood gas estimations during exercise in patients with chronic heart failure. *Br Heart J* 1994;71:528-530.

30. Lipkin DP, Canepa-Anson R, Stephens MR, Poole-Wilson PA. Factors determining symptoms in heart failure: Comparison of fast and slow exercise tests. *Br Heart J* 1986;55:439-445.

31. Mancini DM, Henson D, LaManca J, et al. Respiratory muscle function and dyspnea in patients with chronic congestive heart failure. *Circulation* 1992;86: 909-919.

32. Mancini DM, Henson D, LaManca J, Donchez L, Levine S. Benefit of selective respiratory muscle training on exercise capacity in patients with chronic congestive heart failure. *Circulation* 1995;91:320-329.

33. Beniaminovitz A, Lang CC, LaManca J, Mancini DM. Selective low-level leg muscle training alleviates dyspnea in patients with heart failure. *J Am Coll Cardiol* 2002;40:1602-1608.

34. Wilson JR, Mancini DM, Ferraro N, Egler J. Effect on dichloroacetate on the exercise performance of patients with heart failure. *J Am Coll Cardiol* 1988;12: 1464-1469.

35. Piepoli M, Clark AL, Coats AJS. Muscle metaboreceptors in haemodynamic, autonomic and ventilatory

responses to exercise in man. *Am J Physiol* 1995;269(*Heart Circ Physiol* 38)H1428-H1436.

36. Piepoli M, Clark AL, Volterrani M, Adamopoulos S, Sleight P, Coats AJS. Contribution of muscle afferents to the haemodynamic, autonomic and ventilatory responses to exercise in patients with chronic heart failure. Effects of physical training. *Circulation* 1996;93:940-952.

37. Grassi G, Seravalle G, Cattaneo BM, et al. Sympathetic activation and loss of reflex sympathetic control in mild congestive heart failure. *Circulation* 1995;92:3206.

38. Francis GS, Goldsmith SR, Levine TB, et al. The neurohormonal axis in congestive heart failure. *Ann Intern Med* 1984;101:370-377.

39. Cohen JN, Levine TB, Olivari MT, et al. Plasma norepinephrine as a guide to prognosis in patients with chronic congestive heart failure. *N Engl J Med* 1984;311:819.

40. Hartley LH, Mason JW, Hogan RP, et al. Multiple hormonal responses to graded exercise in relation to physical training. *J Appl Physiol* 1972;33:602-606.

41. McCrimmon DR, Cunningham DA, Rechnitzer PA, et al. Effect of training on plasma catecholamines in post myocardial infarction patients. *Med Sci Sports* 1976;8:152-156.

42. Coats AJ, Adamopoulos S, Radaelli A, et al. Controlled trial of physical training in chronic heart failure. Exercise performance, hemodynamics, ventilation, and autonomic function. *Circulation* 1992;85:2119-2131.

43. Shemesh J, Grossman E, Peleg E, et al. Norepinephrine and atrial natriuretic peptide responses to exercise testing in rehabilitated and nonrehabilitated men with ischemic cardiomyopathy after healing of anterior wall myocardial infarction. *Am J Cardiol* 1995;75:1072-1074.

44. Braith RW, Welsch MA, Feigenbaum MS, Kleuss HA, Pepine CJ. Neurohormone activation in heart failure is modified by endurance exercise. *J Am Coll Cardiol* 1999;34:1170-1175.

45. Larsen AI, Aukrust P, Aarsland T, Dickstein K. Effect of aerobic exercise training on plasma levels of tumor necrosis factor alpha in patients with heart failure. *Am J Cardiol* 2001;88:805-808.

46. Hornig B, Maier V, Drexler H. Physical training improves endothelial function in patients with chronic heart failure. *Circulation* 1996;93:210-214.

47. Hambrecht R, Fiehn E, Weigl C, et al. Regular physical exercise corrects endothelial dysfunction and improves exercise capacity in patients with chronic heart failure. *Circulation* 1998;98:2709-2715.

48. Linke A, Schoene N, Gielen S, et al. Endothelial dysfunction in patients with chronic heart failure: Systemic effects of lower-limb exercise training. *J Am Coll Cardiol* 2001;37:392-397.

49. Hambrecht R, Wolf A, Gielen S, et al. Effect of exercise on coronary endothelial function in patients with coronary artery disease. *N Engl J Med* 2000;342:454-460.

50. Belardinelli R, Georgiou D, Cianci G, Purcaro A. Randomized, controlled trial of long-term moderate exercise training in chronic heart failure. Effects on functional capacity, quality of life, and clinical outcome. *Circulation* 1999;99:1173-1182.

51. Weber KT, Janicki JS. Cardiopulmonary exercise testing for evaluation of chronic cardiac failure. *Am J Cardiol* 1985;55:22A-31A.

52. Cohn JN, Johnson GR, Shabetai R, et al. Ejection fraction, peak exercise oxygen consumption, cardiothoracic ratio, ventricular arrhythmias, and plasma norepinephrine, as determinants of prognosis in heart failure. *Circulation* 1993;87(suppl VI):5-16.

53. Chua TP, Ponikowski P, Harrington D, et al. Clinical correlates and prognostic significance of the ventilatory response to exercise in chronic heart failure. *J Am Coll Cardiol* 1997;29:1585-1590.

54. Kleber FX, Vietzke G, Wernecke KD, et al. Impairment of ventilatory efficiency in heart failure: Prognostic impact. *Circulation* 2000;101:2803-2809.

55. Ponikowski P, Francis DP, Piepoli MF, et al. Enhanced ventilatory response to exercise in patients with chronic heart failure and preserved exercise tolerance: Marker of abnormal cardiorespiratory reflex control and predictor of poor prognosis. *Circulation* 2001;103:967-972.

56. Mancini DM, Eisen H, Kussmaul W, Mull R, Edmunds LH. Value of peak oxygen consumption for optimal timing of cardiac transplantation in ambulatory patients with heart failure. *Circulation* 1991;84:778-786.

57. U.S. Department of Health and Human Services. Agency for Health Care Policy and Research. *Clinical Practice Guideline No. 17: Cardiac Rehabilitation* (ACHR Publication No. 96-0672). Washington, DC: Agency for Health Care Policy and Research, October 1995.

58. Working Group on Cardiac Rehabilitation and Exercise Physiology and Working Group on Heart Failure of the European Society of Cardiology. Recommendations for exercise training in chronic heart failure patients. *Eur Heart J* 2001;22:125-135.

59. Meyer K, Samek L, Schwaibold M, et al. Interval training in patients with severe chronic heart failure: Analysis and recommendations for exercise procedures. *Med Sci Sports Exerc* 1997;29:306-312.

60. McKelvie RS, Teo KK, Roberts R, et al. Effects of exercise training in patients with heart failure: The Exercise Rehabilitation Trial (EXERT). *Am Heart J* 2002;144:23-30.

61. Kavanagh T, Myers MG, Baigrie RS, Mertens DJ, Sawyer P, Shephard RJ. Quality of life and cardiorespiratory function in chronic heart failure: Effects of 12 months' aerobic training. *Heart* 1996;76:42-49.

62. McKelvie RS, McCartney N, Tomlinson CW, et al. Comparison of hemodynamic responses to cycling and resistance exercise in congestive heart failure secondary to ischemic cardiomyopathy. *Am J Cardiol* 1995;76:977-979.

63. Meyer K, Hajric R, Westbrook S, et al. Hemodynamic responses during leg press exercise in patients with chronic congestive heart failure. *Am J Cardiol* 1999;83:1537-1543.

64. Wilson JR, Groves J, Rayos G. Circulatory status and response to cardiac rehabilitation in patients with heart failure. *Circulation* 1996;94:1567-1572.

65. Hertz MI, Taylor DO, Trulock EP, et al. The registry of the international society for heart and lung transplantation: Nineteenth official report-2002. *J Heart Lung Transplant* 2002;21:950-970.

66. Tischler MD, Lee RT, Plappert T, Mudge GH, St. John Sutton M, Parker JD. Serial assessment of left ventricular function and mass after orthotopic heart transplantation: A 4-year longitudinal study. *J Am Coll Cardiol* 1992;19:60-66.

67. Kao AC, Van Tright III P, Shaeffer-McCall GS, et al. Central and peripheral limitations to upright exercise in untrained cardiac transplant recipients. *Circulation* 1994;89:2605-2615.

68. Borow KM, Neumann A, Arensman FW, Yacoub MH. Left ventricular contractility and contractive reserve in humans after cardiac transplantation. *Circulation* 1985;71:866-872.

69. Kao AC, Van Tright P III, Shaeffer-McCall GS, et al. Allograft diastolic dysfunction and chronotropic incompetence limit cardiac output response to exercise two to six years after heart transplantation. *J Heart Lung Transplant* 1995;14:11-22.

70. Hausdorf G, Banner NR, Mitchell A, Khaghani A, Martin M, Yacoub M. Diastolic function after cardiac and heart-lung transplantation. *Br Heart J* 1989;62:123-132.

71. Paulus WJ, Bronzwaer JGF, Felice H, Kishan N, Wellens F. Deficient acceleration of left ventricular relaxation during exercise after heart transplantation. *Circulation* 1992;86:1175-1185.

72. Beck W, Barnard CN, Schrire V. Heart rate after cardiac transplantation. *Am J Physiol* 1969;218:475-484.

73. Carleton RA, Heller SJ, Najaf H, Clark JG. Hemodynamic performance of a transplanted human heart. *Circulation* 1969;40:447-452.

74. Campeau L, Pospisil L, Grondin P, Dydra I, LePage G. Cardiac catheterization findings at rest and after exercise in patients following cardiac transplantation. *Am J Cardiol* 1970;25:523-528.

75. Pope SE, Stinson EB, Daughters GT, Schroeder JS, Ingels NB, Alderman EL. Exercise response of the denervated heart in long-term cardiac transplant recipients. *Am J Cardiol* 1978;46:213-218.

76. Yusuf SA, Mitchell A, Yacoub MH. Interrelation between donor and recipient heart rates during exercise after heterotopic cardiac transplantation. *Br Heart J* 1985;54:173-178.

77. de Marneffe M, Jacobs P, Haaradt R, Englert E. Variations of normal sinus node function in relation to age: Role of autonomic influence. *Eur Heart J* 1986;7:662-672.

78. Jose A, Collison D. The normal range and determinants of the intrinsic heart rate in man. *Cardiovasc Res* 1970;4:160-167.

79. Bernardi L, Keller R, Sanders M, et al. Respiratory sinus arrhythmia in the denervated human heart. *J Appl Physiol* 1989;67:1447-1455.

80. Alexopoulos D, Yusuf S, Johnston JA, Bostock J, Sleight P, Yacoub MH. The 24 hour heart rate behavior in long-term survivors of cardiac transplantation. *Am J Cardiol* 1988;61:880-884.

81. Pflugfelder PW, Purves PD, McKenzie FN, Kostuk WJ. Cardiac dynamics during supine exercise in cyclosporine treated orthotopic heart transplant recipients: Assessments by radionuclide angiography. *J Am Coll Cardiol* 1987;10:336-341.

82. Dempsey PJ, Cooper T. Supersensitivity of the chronically denervated feline heart. *Am J Physiol* 1968;215:1245-1249.

83. Yusuf S, Theodoropoulos S, Mathias CJ, et al. Increased sensitivity of the denervated transplanted human heart to isoprenaline both before and after beta-adrenergic blockade. *Circulation* 1987;75:696-704.

84. Bantle JP, Nath KA, Sutherland DER, Najaran JES, Ferris TF. Effects of cyclosporine on the renin-angiotensin-aldosterone system and potassium excretion in transplant recipients. *Arch Intern Med* 1985;145:505-508.

85. Thompson ME, Shapiro AP, Johnsen AM, et al. New onset of hypertension following cardiac transplantation: A preliminary report and analysis. *Transplant Proc* 1983;15:2573-2577.

86. Jarowenko MV, Flechner SM, Van Buren CT, Lorber MI, Kahan BD. Influence of cyclosporine on post-transplant blood pressure response. *Am J Kidney Dis* 1987;10:98-103.

87. Loughran TP Jr, Deeg HJ, Dahlberg S, Kennedy MS, Storb R, Thomas ED. Incidence of hypertension after marrow transplantation among 112 patients randomized to either cyclosporine or methotrexate as graft-versus-host disease prophylaxis. *Br J Hematol* 1985;59:547-553.

88. Braith RW, Plunkett MB, Mills RM. Cardiac output responses during exercise in volume-expanded heart transplantation recipients. *Am J Cardiol* 1998;81:1-5.

89. Perini R, Orizio C, Gamba A, Veicsteinas A. Kinetics of heart rate and catecholamines during exercise in humans. *Eur J Appl Physiol* 1993;66:500-506.

90. Schuler S, Thomas D, Thebken M, et al. Endocrine response to exercise in cardiac transplant patients. *Transplant Proc* 1987;19:2506-2509.

91. Braith RW, Clapp L, Brown T, et al. Rate-responsive pacing improves exercise tolerance in heart transplant recipients. *J Cardiopulmonary Rehabil* 2000;20:377-382.

92. Braith RW, Limacher MC, Mills RM, Leggett SH, Pollock ML, Staples ED. Exercise-induced hypoxemia in heart transplant recipients. *J Am Coll Cardiol* 1993;22:767-776.

93. Casan P, Sanchis J, Cladellas M, Amengual MJ, Caralps JM. Diffusing lung capacity and cyclosporine in patients with heart transplants. *Heart Transplant* 1987;6:54-56.

94. Kraemer MD, Kubo SH, Rector TS, Brunsvold N, Denk AJ. Pulmonary and peripheral vascular factors are important determinants of peak exercise oxygen uptake in patients with heart failure. *J Am Coll Cardiol* 1993;21:641-648.

95. Ville N, Mercier J, Varray A, Albat B, Messner-Pellene P, Prefaut C. Exercise tolerance in heart transplant patients with altered pulmonary diffusion capacity. *Med Sci Sports Exerc* 1998;30:339-344.

96. Braith RW, Limacher MC, Leggett SH, Pollock ML. Skeletal muscle strength in heart transplant patients. *J Heart Lung Transplant* 1993;12:1018-1023.

97. Bussieres LM, Pflugfelder PW, Taylor AW, Noble EG, Kostuk WK. Changes in skeletal muscle morphology and biochemistry after cardiac transplantation. *Am J Cardiol* 1997;79:630-634.

98. Stark RP, McGinn AL, Wilson RF. Chest pain in cardiac-transplant recipients. *N Engl J Med* 1991;324:1791-1794.

99. Fallen EL, Kamath MV, Ghista DN, Fitchett D. Spectral analysis of heart rate variability following human heart transplantation: Evidence for functional reinnervation. *J Auton Nerv Syst* 1988;23:199-206.

100. Rudas L, Pflugfelder PW, Menkis AAH, Novick RJ, McKenzie FN, Kostuk WJ. Evolution of heart rate responsiveness after orthotopic cardiac transplantation. *Am J Cardiol* 1991;68:232-236.

101. Folino AF, Buja G, Miorelli M, et al. Heart rate variability in patients with orthotopic heart transplantation: Long-term follow-up. *Clin Cardiol* 1993;16:539-542.

102. Schwaiger M, Hutchins GD, Rosenspire K, et al. Evidence for regional catecholamine uptake and storage sites in the transplanted human heart by positron emission tomography. *J Clin Invest* 1991;87:1681-1690.

103. Kaye DM, Esler M, Kingwell B, McPherson G, Esmore D, Jennings G. Functional and neurochemical evidence for partial cardiac sympathetic reinnervation after cardiac transplantation in humans. *Circulation* 1993;88:1110-1118.

104. Wilson RF, Christensen BV, Olivari MT, Simon A, White CW, Laxson DD. Evidence for structural sympathetic reinnervation after orthotopic cardiac transplantation in humans. *Circulation* 1991;83:1210-1220.

105. Wilson RF, Laxson DD, Christensen BV, McGinn AL, Kubo SH. Regional differences in sympathetic reinnervation after human orthotopic cardiac transplantation. *Circulation* 1993;88:165-171.

106. Wharton J, Polak JM, Gordon L, et al. Immunohistochemical demonstration of human cardiac innervation before and after transplantation. *Circ Res* 1990;66:900-912.

107. Lord SW, Brady S, Holt NND, Mitchell L, Dark JH, McComb JM. Exercise response after cardiac transplantation: Correlation with sympathetic reinnervation. *Heart* 1996;75:40-43.

108. Kobashigawa JA, Leaf DA, Lee N, et al. A controlled trial of exercise rehabilitation after heart transplantation. *N Engl J Med* 1999;340:272-277.

109. McGregor CGA. Cardiac transplantation: Surgical considerations and early postoperative management. *Mayo Clin Proc* 1992;67:577-585.

110. Naughton P, Haider R. Methods of exercise testing. In: *Exercise Testing and Exercise Training in Coronary Heart Disease.* Naughton JP, Hellerstein HK (eds). New York: Academic Press, 1973, pp. 79-91.

111. Lerman J, Bruce RA, Sivarajan E, Pettet GEM, Trimble S. Low-level dynamic exercises for earlier cardiac rehabilitation: Aerobic and hemodynamic responses. *Arch Phys Med Rehabil* 1976;57:355-360.

112. Savin WM, Haskell WL, Schroeder JS, Stinson EB. Cardiorespiratory responses of cardiac transplant patients to graded, symptom-limited exercise. *Circulation* 1980;62:55-60.

113. Lipkin DP. The role of exercise training in chronic heart failure. *Br Heart J* 1987;58:559-566.

114. Brubaker PH, Berry MJ, Brozena SC, et al. Relationship of lactate and ventilatory thresholds in cardiac transplant patients. *Med Sci Sports Exerc* 1993;25:191-196.

115. Gaer J. Physiological consequences of complete cardiac denervation. *Br J Hosp Med* 1992;48:220-224.

116. Ehrman JK, Keteyian SJ, Levine AB, et al. Exercise stress tests after cardiac transplantation. *Am J Cardiol* 1993;71:1372-1373.

117. Braith RW, Mills RM, Welsch MA, Keller JW, Pollock ML. Resistance exercise training restores bone mineral density in heart transplant recipients. *J Am Coll Cardiol* 1996;28:1471-1477.

118. Braith RW, Welsch MA, Mills RM, et al. Resistance exercise prevents glucocorticoid-induced myopathy in heart transplant recipients. *Med Sci Sports Exerc* 1998;30:483-489.

119. Braith RW, Edwards DG. Role of cardiac rehabilitation in heart failure and cardiac transplantation. In: *Clinical Exercise Testing.* Weisman EM, Zeballos RJ (eds). Basel, Switzerland: Karger, 2002, pp. 120-138.

120. Winder W, Hagberg J, Hickson R, Ehsani A, McLane J. Time course of sympathoadrenal adaptation to endurance exercise testing in man. *J Appl Physiol* 1978;45:370-374.

121. Duncan JJ, Farr JE, Upton SJ, Hagan RD, Oglesby ME, Blair SN. The effects of aerobic exercise on plasma catecholamines and blood pressure in patients with mild hypertension. *JAMA* 1985;254:2609-2613.

122. American College of Sports Medicine. *ACSM's Guidelines for Exercise Testing and Prescription.* Fifth Edition. Philadelphia: Williams & Wilkins, 1995, pp. 206-210.

123. Squires RW, Arthur PR, Gau GT, Muri A, Lambert WB. Exercise after cardiac transplantation: A report of two cases. *J Cardiac Rehabil* 1983;3:570-574.

124. Savin WM, Gordon E, Green S, et al. Comparison of exercise training effects in cardiac denervated and innervated humans. Abstract. *J Am Coll Cardiol* 1983;1:722.

125. Sieurat P, Roquebrune JP, Frinneiser D, et al. Monitoring and rehabilitation of heterotopic transplantation patients during the period of convertescence [in French]. *Arch Mal Coeur* 1986;2:210-216.

126. Degré S, Niset G, Desmet JM, et al. Effects de l'entraînement physique sur le coeur humain dénervé après transplantation cardiaque orthotopique. *Ann Cardiol Angeiol* 1986;35:147-149.

127. Niset G, Cousty-Degré C, Degré S. Psychosocial and physical rehabilitation after heart transplantation: 1-year follow-up. *Cardiology* 1988;75:311-317.

128. Keteyian S, Ehrman J, Fedel F, Rhoads K. Heart rate-perceived exertion relationship during exercise in orthotopic heart transplant patients. *J Cardiopulmon Rehabil* 1990;10:287-293.

129. Keteyian S, Shepard R, Ehrman J, et al. Cardiovascular responses of heart transplant patients to exercise training. *J Appl Physiol* 1991;70:2627-2631.

130. Ehrman J, Keteyian S, Fedel F, Rhoads K, Levine B, Shepard R. Ventilatory threshold after exercise training in orthotopic heart transplant patients. *J Cardiopulmon Rehabil* 1992;12:126-130.

131. Daida H, Squires RW, Allison TG, Johnson BD, Gau GT. Sequential assessment of exercise tolerance in heart transplantation compared with coronary artery bypass surgery after phase II cardiac rehabilitation. *Am J Cardiol* 1996;696-700.

132. Geny B, Saini J, Mettauer B, et al. Effect of short-term endurance training on exercise capacity, haemodynamics and atrial natriuretic peptide secretion in heart transplant recipients. *Eur J Appl Physiol* 1996;73:259-266.

133. Lampert E, Oyono-Enguéllé S, Mettauer B, Freund H, Lonsdorfer J. Short endurance training improves lactate removal ability in patients with heart transplants. *Med Sci Sports Exerc* 1996;28:801-807.

134. Niset G, Poortmans JR, Leclercq R, et al. Metabolic implications during a 20-km run after heart transplantation. *Int J Sports Med* 1985;6:340-343.

135. Kavanagh T, Yacoub M, Campbell R, Mertens D. Marathon running after cardiac transplantation. *J Cardiopulm Rehabil* 1986;6:16-20.

136. Kavanagh T, Mertens DJ, Shephard RJ, et al. Long-term cardiorespiratory results of exercise training following cardiac transplantation. *Am J Cardiol* 2003;91:190-194.

137. Kavanagh T, Mertens DJ, Hamm LF. Prediction of long-term prognosis in 12 169 men referred for cardiac rehabilitation. *Circulation* 2002;106:666-671.

138. ExTraMATCH Collaborative. Exercise training meta-analysis of trials in patients with chronic heart failure (ExTraMATCH). *Br Med J* 2004;328:189-196.

Appendix A

1. Dorland W. *Dorland's Illustrated Medical Dictionary*. Philadelphia: Saunders, 2000.

2. Yusuf S, Hawken S, Ounpuu S, et al. Effect of potentially modifiable risk factors associated with myocardial infarction in 52 countries (the INTERHEART study): case-control study. *Lancet* 2004;364:937-952.

3. Smith SC Jr, Greenland P, Grundy SM. AHA conference proceedings. Prevention conference V: Beyond secondary prevention: Identifying the high-risk patient for primary prevention: Executive summary. American Heart Association. *Circulation* 2000;101:111-116.

4. Wilson PW, D'Agostino RB, Levy D, Belanger AM, Silbershatz H, Kannel WB. Prediction of coronary heart disease using risk factor categories. *Circulation* 1998;97:1837-1847.

5. Lipid Research Clinics Program. The Lipid Research Clinics coronary primary prevention trial results. I. Reduction in incidence of coronary heart disease. II. The relationship of reduction in incidence of coronary heart disease to cholesterol lowering. *JAMA* 1984;251:351-364.

6. Scandinavian Simvastatin Survival Study Group. Randomised trial of cholesterol lowering in 4444 patients with coronary heart disease: The Scandinavian Simvastatin Survival Study (4S). *Lancet* 1994;344:1383-1389.

7. Shepherd J, Cobbe SM, Ford I, et al. Prevention of coronary heart disease with pravastatin in men with hypercholesterolemia. *N Engl J Med* 1995;333:1301-1313.

8. Sacks FM, Pfeffer MA, Moye LA, et al. The effect of pravastatin on coronary events after myocardial infarction in patients with average cholesterol levels. *N Engl J Med* 1996;335:1001-1009.

9. Downs JR, Clearfield M, Weis S, et al. Primary prevention of acute coronary events with lovastatin in men and women with average cholesterol levels: Results of AFCAPS/TexCAPS. *JAMA* 1998;279:1615-1622.

10. Heart Protection Study. Available at: www.hpsinfo.org. Accessed April 20, 2002.

11. Castelli WP. Lipids, risk factors and ischaemic heart disease. *Atherosclerosis* 1996;124(suppl):S1-S9.

12. Forsen T, Eriksson J, Qiao Q, Tervahauta M, Nissinen A, Tuomilehto J. Short stature and coronary heart disease: A 35-year follow-up of the Finnish cohorts of the Seven Countries Study. *J Intern Med* 2000;248:326-332.

13. Daniels SR, Morrison JA, Sprecher DL, Khoury P, Kimball TR. Association of body fat distribution and cardiovascular risk factors in children and adolescents. *Circulation* 1999;99:541-545.

14. Hopkins PN, Williams RR. A survey of 246 suggested coronary risk factors. *Atherosclerosis* 1981;40:1-52.

15. Libby P, Ridker PM, Maseri A. Inflammation and atherosclerosis. *Circulation* 2002;105:1135-1143.

16. Ridker PM, Rifai N, Stampfer MJ, et al. Plasma concentration of interleukin-6 and the risk of future myocardial infarction among apparently healthy men. *Circulation* 2000;101:1767-1772.

17. Ridker PM, Rifai N, Pfeffer M, et al. Elevation of tumor necrosis factor-[alpha] and increased risk of recurrent coronary events after myocardial infarction. *Circulation* 2000;101:2149-2153.

18. Hwang SJ, Ballantyne CM, Sharrett AR, et al. Circulating adhesion molecules VCAM-1, ICAM-1, and E-selectin in carotid atherosclerosis and incident coronary heart disease cases. The Atherosclerosis Risk in Communities (ARIC) study. *Circulation* 1997;96:4219-4225.

19. Ridker PM, Stampfer MJ, Rifai N. Novel risk factors for systemic atherosclerosis: A comparison of C-reactive protein, fibrinogen, homocysteine, lipoprotein(a)

and standard cholesterol screening as predictors of peripheral arterial disease. *JAMA* 2001;285:2481-2485.

20. Ridker PM, Glynn RJ, Hennekens CH. R-reactive protein adds to the predictive value of total and HDL cholesterol in determining risk of first myocardial infarction. *Circulation* 1998;97:2007-2011.

21. Ridker PM, Hennekens CH, Buring JE, Rifai N. C-reactive protein and other markers of inflammation in the prediction of cardiovascular disease in women. *N Engl J Med* 2000;342:836-843.

22. Ridker PM, Rifai N, Pfeffer MA, Sacks F, Braunwald E. Long-term effects of pravastatin on plasma concentration of C-reactive protein. *Circulation* 1999;100:230-235.

23. Ridker PM, Hennekens CH, Rifai N, Buring JE, Manson JE. Hormone replacement therapy and increased plasma concentration of C-reactive protein. *Circulation* 1999;100:713-716.

24. Cushman M, Legault C, Barrett-Connor E, et al. Effect of postmenopausal hormones on inflammation-sensitive proteins: The Postmenopausal Estrogen/Progestin Interventions (PEPI) Study. *Circulation* 1999;100:717-722.

25. Geffken D, Cushman M, Burke G, Polak J, Sakkinen P, Tracy R. Association between physical activity and markers of inflammation in a healthy elderly population. *Am J Epidemiol* 2001;153:242-260.

26. Pearson TA, Mensah G, Alexander RW, et al. Markers of inflammation and cardiovascular disease: Application to clinical and public health practice: A statement for healthcare professionals from the Centers for Disease Control and Prevention and the American Heart Association. *Circulation* 2003;107:499-511.

27. Seymour RA, Steele JG. Is there a link between periodontal disease and coronary heart disease? *Br Dent J* 1998;184:33-38.

28. Danesh J, Collins R, Peto R. Chronic infections and coronary heart disease: Is there a link? *Lancet* 1997;350:430-436.

29. Gupta S, Leathem EW, Carrington D, Mendall MA, Kaski JC, Camm AJ. Elevated *Chlamydia pneumoniae* antibodies, cardiovascular events, and azithromycin in male survivors of myocardial infarction. *Circulation* 1997;96:404-407.

30. Gurfinkel E, Bozovich G, Livellara S, Testa E, Beck E, Mautner B. Antibiotic effects on unstable angina: The final report of the ROXIS trial. *Eur Heart J* 1999;20:121-127.

31. Sinasalo J, Mattila K, Valtonen V. Effect of 3 months of antimicrobial treatment with clarithromycin in acute non-Q-wave coronary syndrome. *Circulation* 2002;105:1555-1560.

32. Libby P, Egan D, Skarlatos S. Role of infectious agents in atherosclerosis and restenosis. *Circulation* 1997;96:4095-4103.

33. Folsom AR. Antibiotics for prevention of myocardial infarction? Not yet! *JAMA* 1999;281:461-462.

34. Grayston JT, Kronmal RA, Jackson LA, et al. Azithromycin for secondary prevention of coronary events. *New Engl J Med* 2005;352:1637-1645.

35. Cannon CP, Braunwald E, McCabe CH, et al. Antibiotic treatment of chlamydia pneumoniae after acute coronary syndrome. *New Eng J Med* 2005;352:1646-1654.

36. Hansson GK. Inflammation, atherosclerosis, and coronary artery disease. *New Engl J Med* 2005;352:1685-1695.

Index

Note: The italicized *f* and *t* following page numbers refer to figures and tables, respectively.

About the AACVPR

History and Purpose

Founded in 1985, the American Association of Cardiovascular and Pulmonary Rehabilitation (AACVPR) is dedicated to the professional development of its members through networking and educational opportunities. Central to the mission is improving the quality of life for patients and their families.

Mission Statement

To reduce morbidity, mortality, and disability from cardiovascular and pulmonary diseases through education, prevention, rehabilitation, research, and aggressive disease management.

Fast Facts

- Founded in 1985
- 2002 membership: 2,600 (and growing)
- Oversees the well-respected Program Certification for Cardiac and Pulmonary Rehabilitation programs
- Members are behavioral scientists, cardiovascular physicians, nutritionists/dieticians, cardiovascular nurses, cardiopulmonary physical therapists, exercise physiologists, pulmonary nurses, exercise rehabilitation specialists, pulmonary physicians, and respiratory therapists
- Headquarters: 401 N. Michigan Ave., Suite 2200, Chicago, IL 60611; 312-321-5146.
- Promotes advocacy for reimbursement issues in Washington, DC

Membership Benefits

Be part of a national network of professionals dedicated to the advancement of cardiovascular and pulmonary rehabilitation. Members receive the following:

Timely Information

- The bimonthly *Journal of Cardiopulmonary Rehabilitation*, a well-respected publication that features the most current research as well as clinical and practical information about the science of rehabilitation
- *Monthly News and Views*, AACVPR's e-mailed newsletter that provides the latest updates from the association and its affiliate societies, as well as practical information for daily practice
- Access to the members-only section of the AACVPR Web site
- E-mail updates of timely information regarding federal and state guidelines, reimbursement, and other issues of concern to professionals in the field

Influence

- Opportunities to join colleagues to promote the quality of patient care through efforts in Washington, DC, and to increase reimbursement for cardiac and pulmonary rehab services

Quality Education

- Members' discount to attend the AACVPR annual meeting
- Members' discount for new proposed distance-learning formats
- Members' discount on a wide variety of AACVPR publications and programs

Benchmarking and Standards of Care

- Members' discount for program certification and recertification applications
- Participation in a new AACVPR Mentorship program

Networking

- A complimentary copy of the membership directory, published annually
- Access to the members-only section of the Web site
- Opportunity to participate in the national network of professionals dedicated to the advancement of cardiac and pulmonary care

Professional Growth

- Access to the AACVPR career link—an on-line listing of nationwide job opportunities
- Invitation to submit articles to the *Journal of Cardiopulmonary Rehabilitation* and *News and Views* and to present your research at the annual meeting
- Opportunity to apply for AACVPR grants and scholarships
- Volunteer to serve on national committees with nationally recognized experts in the field

Publications

- *Journal of Cardiopulmonary Rehabilitation* (published bimonthly)
- *News and Views of AACVPR* (published quarterly)
- *Guidelines for Cardiac Rehabilitation and Secondary Prevention Programs,* third edition
- *Guidelines for Pulmonary Rehabilitation Programs,* second edition
- *How to Inform Payers and Influence Payment for Cardiac and Pulmonary Rehabilitation Services*

- Bibliography: *Outcomes of Pulmonary Rehabilitation*
- Bibliography: *Outcomes of Cardiac Rehabilitation*
- Annual membership and programs directory
- Outcomes tool resource guide
- Educational resource guide
- Annual meeting syllabus
- Agency for Health Care Policy and Research, *Clinical Practice Guideline for Cardiac Rehabilitation*
- Agency for Health Care Policy and Research, *Patient Guide: Recovering from Heart Problems Through Cardiac Rehabilitation*
- Fitness Products Council, *How to Buy Exercise Equipment for the Home*
- Agency for Health Care Policy and Research, *Cardiac Rehabilitation as Secondary Prevention: Quick Reference for Clinician*

It's Easy to Apply

To apply for membership, select one of these fast and easy methods:

- By mail: Complete the enclosed form and mail it to AACVPR headquarters.
- Online: Go to www.aacvpr.org and complete the online form or print out the form and mail it to AACVPR headquarters (address on application).

With either method of application, please include credit card information or a check for the dues amount in U.S. funds. If you wish to receive additional applications, or if you have any questions, please call headquarters at 312-321-5146, or send an e-mail to aacvpr@sba.com.

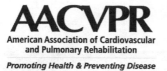

American Association of Cardiovascular and Pulmonary Rehabilitation
Membership Application

Name_____

Professional Degree _____
(Please list no more than two)

Job Title _____

Place of Employment_____

Mailing Address_____

City _____

State/Province_____

Zip Code/Postal Code _____

Country _____

This address is: ❏ Home   ❏ Business

(The above address will be used for mailings and will be listed in the Membership Directory.)

Email:_____

(Be sure to include your email address for frequent Regulatory Updates and the monthly News and Views. The AACVPR does not distribute email addresses to other groups).

Daytime Phone: (   )_____

Fax: (   ) _____

Are you a current member of your state/regional society?

❏ Yes   ❏ No

General Information

Where did you hear about the AACVPR?

❏ From an AACVPR Member

❏ Was a Previous Member—Year(s)

❏ Journal of Cardiopulmonary Rehabilitation

❏ Professional Colleague

❏ State/Regional Society

❏ University/School

❏ Other

What made you decide to join the AACVPR? _____

_____

Membership Categories

❏ Member
Membership Fee $150
Shall be any interested person of majority age who is a nurse, physician, medical scientist, allied health-care practitioner or educator, and who in his or her professional endeavors, is regularly involved in some aspect of cardiovascular and/or pulmonary rehabilitation. Members have AACVPR voting privileges.

Which of these categories best represents you?
Check only one:
❏ Behavioral Scientist
❏ Cardiopulmonary Physical Therapist
❏ Exercise Rehabilitation Specialist
❏ Cardiovascular Physician
❏ Exercise Physiologist
❏ Pulmonary Physician
❏ Nutritionist/Dietician
❏ Pulmonary Nurse
❏ Respiratory Therapist
❏ Cardiovascular Nurse
❏ Other _____

Are you certified by a professional association?
❏ Yes   ❏ No

Association Name _____

Certification _____

Does your current employer support individual AACVPR membership?
❏ Yes   ❏ No

❏ Student Member
Membership Fee $75

A Student Member shall be any interested undergraduate or graduate college student currently carrying the equivalent of at least one half of a full-time academic load for one year, as defined by the university or college of attendance. The area of study must be in a medical or allied health curriculum. Student Membership also applies to physicians-in-training, including residents and interns.

To qualify as a Student Member, one must submit a copy of his or her current student identification card along with this completed application.

Educational Institution _____

Major _____

Year Degree Expected_____

❏ Associate Member
Membership Fee $150

Shall be any person with an interest in cardiovascular and /or pulmonary rehabilitation, but not currently eligible for classification as a Member or Student Member. Dues are established by the Board of Directors and may be changed at its discretion. Associate Member privileges include a subscription to the AACVPR newsletter and placement on the Association mailing list.

Primary Occupation_____

Place of Employment_____

Current Program Involvement

In what area(s) do you spend the majority of your practice?

Check one:

❏ In-patient Cardiovascular/Pulmonary/Vascular

❏ Out-patient Cardiovascular/Pulmonary/Vascular

❏ In-patient & Out-patient Cardiovascular/Pulmonary/Vascular

Who is your employer?

❏ Hospital   ❏ Educational Institution

❏ Physician/Group practice   ❏ Other: _____

How many new out-patients would you estimate are seen in your program annually?

❏ Less than 100   ❏ 101-200 patients

❏ 201-300 patients   ❏ Over 300 patients

How many new in-patients would you estimate are seen in your program annually?

❏ Less than 100   ❏ 101-500 patients

❏ 501-1000 patients   ❏ Over 1000 patients

❏ Does not apply

Which of the following best describes the emphasis of your work environment?

❏ 100% rehabilitation

❏ 75% rehabilitation/25% prevention

❏ 50% rehabilitation/50% prevention

❏ 25% rehabilitation/75% prevention

Membership Agreement

I certify that the above information is correct and I agree to abide by the Code of Ethical and Professional conduct of the American Association of Cardiovascular and Pulmonary Rehabilitation. Visit the AACVPR Web site for the code of ethics.

Signature _____ Date _____

Payment

Purchase orders are not accepted.
Payment must accompany application.

❏ Check (Payable to AACVPR; US Funds Only)

❏ MC/Visa/American Express—Exp. Date _____

Cardholder's Name _____

Card Number _____

Cardholder's City/State _____

Cardholder's Signature _____

Heart and Lung Foundation Contribution Opportunities

The Heart and Lung Foundation strives to assist the AACVPR in becoming the recognized leader in professional and public education for the field of cardiopulmonary rehabilitation through:

- **Education**
- **Service/Outreach**
- **Research**

All donations are tax deductible.

Yes, I want to do my part to advance my profession by pledging the following:

❏ $25.. Foundation Supporter

❏ $50.. Foundation Member

❏ $100.. Foundation Partner

❏ $250.. Foundation Sponsor

❏ $500.. Foundation Patron

❏ $1,000....................................... Foundation Benefactor

Foundation benefactors will be acknowledged on the AACVPR Web site.

AACVPR membership is effective July through June 30. Membership is not pro-rated; however, members joining after march 1 will be deferred until July 1. Membership dues are non-refundable, nor deductible as a charitable contribution. Membership dues may be deductible as an ordinary and necessary business expense. Consult your tax advisor for information.

Please send completed application to:

AACVPR National Office

401 N Michigan Avenue, Suite 2200

Chicago, IL 60611

Telephone: 312-321-5146

Email: aacvpr@sba.com

Web site: www.aacvpr.org

Credit Card Users may fax application to:

312-245-1085